Women at Risk

Issues in the Primary Prevention of AIDS

AIDS Prevention and Mental Health

Series Editors:

David G. Ostrow, M.D., Ph.D., and Jeffrey A. Kelly, Ph.D.
Medical College of Wisconsin
Milwaukee, Wisconsin

Methodological Issues in AIDS Behavioral Research
Edited by David G. Ostrow, M.D., Ph.D., and Ronald C. Kessler, Ph.D.

Preventing AIDS: Theories and Methods of Behavioral Interventions
Edited by Ralph J. DiClemente, Ph.D., and John L. Peterson, Ph.D.

Women at Risk: Issues in the Primary Prevention of AIDS
Edited by Ann O'Leary, Ph.D., and Loretta Sweet Jemmott, R.N., Ph.D.

Women at Risk

Issues in the Primary Prevention of AIDS

Edited by

Ann O'Leary, Ph.D.

Rutgers University, Busch Campus
New Brunswick, New Jersey

and

Loretta Sweet Jemmott, R.N., Ph.D

University of Pennsylvania
Philadelphia, Pennsylvania

Plenum Press • New York and London

Library of Congress Cataloging-in-Publication Data

O'Leary, Ann.
Women at risk: issues in the primary prevention of AIDS / edited by Ann O'Leary and Loretta Sweet Jemmott.
p. cm. -- (AIDS prevention and mental health)
Includes bibliographical references and index.
ISBN 0-306-45041-0
1. AIDS (Disease)--United States--Prevention. 2. Women--Diseases--United States--Prevention. 3. Women--Health and hygiene--United States.. 4. AIDS (Disease)--Social aspects. I. O'Leary, Ann. II. Jemmott, Loretta Sweet. III. Series.
RA644.A25O38 1995
616.97'92'0082--dc20 95-20474
CIP

ISBN 0-306-45041-0

A Division of Plenum Publishing Corporation
233 Spring Street, New York, N. Y. 10013

10 9 8 7 6 5 4 3 2 1

Printed in the United States of America

Contributors

Priscilla Alexander • National Task Force on Prostitution, New York, NY 10025

Joyce Anastasia • Columbia University School of Nursing, New York, NY 10032

Sevgi O. Aral • Department of Health and Human Services, U.S. Public Health Service, Centers for Disease Control and Prevention, Atlanta, GA 30333

Vivian Brown • PROTOTYPES, Culver City, CA 90230

Veronica Catan • Columbia University School of Social Work, New York, NY 10032

Judith Blackfield Cohen • Project AWARE, Oakland, CA 94612

M. Isabel Fernandez • Department of Psychiatry, University of Miami, Miami, FL 33136

Mindy Thompson Fullilove • The Community Research Group, New York State Psychiatric Institute, New York, NY 10032

Erica L. Gollub • AIDS Activities Coordinating Office, Department of Public Health, Philadelphia, PA 19146

John B. Jemmott III • Department of Psychology, Princeton University, Princeton, NJ 08554

Loretta Sweet Jemmott • University of Pennsylvania School of Nursing, Philadelphia, PA 19104

Gail Kennedy • The Community Research Group, New York State Psychiatric Institute, New York, NY 10032

Kathleen M. Morrow • Department of Psychology, Western Michigan University, Kalamazoo, MI 49008

Adeline Nyamathi • UCLA School of Nursing, Los Angeles, CA 90024

Ann O'Leary • Department of Psychology, Rutgers University, New Brunswick, NJ 08903

Beatriz Perez • The Community Research Group, New York State Psychiatric Institute, New York, NY 10032

Jennifer Pranke • Department of Psychology, Rutgers University, New Brunswick, NJ 08903

Marcela Raffaelli • Department of Psychology, University of Nebraska, Lincoln, NE 68588-0308

Mary Jane Rotheram-Borus • Division of Social and Community Psychiatry, Department of Psychiatry, University of California, Los Angeles, Los Angeles, CA 90024

Judith N. Wasserheit • Department of Health and Human Services, U.S. Public Health Service, Centers for Disease Control and Prevention, Atlanta, GA 30333

Gloria Weissman • Health Resources and Services Administration, Rockville, MD 20857

Foreword

AIDS is the fourth leading cause of death among women of childbearing age and is increasing by about 8% a year in this group.* And yet, our understanding of the impact of HIV and AIDS on women's lives remains fragmented and incomplete. After a decade of struggling with mounting surveys of risk behavior, clinical trials, and behavioral interventions that were based primarily on experience with gay communities in large cities and, subsequently, on the needs of injection drug users, we have not given programs for women the attention they require if they are to be meaningful, effective, and gender appropriate. This book will introduce the reader to the range of complex issues of HIV and AIDS in women's lives.

Ann O'Leary and Loretta Sweet Jemmott have assembled an impressive list of authors who have contributed chapters from different disciplinary viewpoints. The reader will find information on prevention programs that have been effective for adolescent girls, on culturally specific strategies for African American and Latina women, and on the multiple issues of substance use and HIV that need to be faced by any outreach and intervention programs for drug-using women.

The issue of culture becomes even more paramount in programs for women in the developing world. The inclusion of a chapter giving an international perspective on women provides the relevant sociocultural background for viewing the impact of HIV and AIDS on women's lives by highlighting the importance of gender inequities between women and men, women's inferior status in society, and the context of women's sexual behavior.

Women at Risk: Issues in the Primary Prevention of AIDS is a very timely book and unique as a resource for anyone who wants information on the critical issues of the HIV epidemic as it affects women and on gender-specific prevention programs that have proven effective or that should be mounted and evaluated. Overall, this book provides us with a

*"AIDS Program Suspended," *New York Times,* May 12, 1995, p. 18.

composite of the multiple needs of different groups of women and, thus, an overall statement about the impact of HIV and AIDS on all of our lives.

Anke A. Ehrhardt, Ph.D.
New York State Psychiatric Institute, and
Columbia University College of Physicians and Surgeons
New York, New York

Preface

The acquired immunodeficiency syndrome (AIDS) epidemic is devastating the lives of millions of women, while many millions more are at risk for infection at this time. Women who engage in heterosexual intercourse are the group most rapidly becoming infected with human immunodeficiency virus (HIV) in the United States. Globally, heterosexual transmission accounts for the vast majority of new infections, with women representing at least half these cases. Further, many women infected with HIV transmit the virus to their unborn offspring or leave their children orphaned, thus magnifying the tragedy that AIDS brings to families.

Unlike other health-related behaviors, maintaining safety with respect to sexually transmitted disease requires the cooperation of another person, namely, the individual's sex partner. For this reason, social and other contextual factors are of great importance in controlling this epidemic. Gender roles, cultural expectations regarding sexual attitudes and behavior, and issues of economic inequality and dependence, violence, and empowerment are critically relevant to women's abilities to protect themselves from HIV infection.

Many of the subpopulations of women most affected by this disease have been inadequately studied in research generally and within the context of the AIDS epidemic specifically. These groups include drug-using women, African American women, Latina women (particularly Puerto Ricans), women living in nonindustrialized countries, sex workers, and women experiencing physical and sexual abuse in the past or the present. Another group, lesbian women, is almost completely unstudied but may become a high-risk group in the near future.

Our introductory Chapter 1 reviews the very small number of published controlled risk-reduction intervention studies and discusses general barriers to AIDS prevention efforts for women. Chapters 2 and 3 review two general issues in primary prevention for women: the link between HIV and other epidemic sexually transmitted diseases and the current status of, and need for, women-controlled prevention technologies. Chapters 4 through 11 focus on the special needs of several subpopulations of women affected by this epidemic. Our closing remarks in Chapter 12 emphasize the need for controlled intervention research in this area and point to several unanswered questions and unmet needs.

This book is the first to address issues of primary prevention of AIDS for women. Our forthcoming book in this series, *Women and AIDS: Coping and Care,* will discuss topics relevant to the lives of women already affected by this epidemic.

We wish to acknowledge the contributions of Mariclaire Cloutier at Plenum Publishing, who encouraged us to undertake this work initially and who provided decisive guidance at a critical juncture; and Jeff Kelly, who helped us to overcome some hurdles along the way. The contributors to this work should also be thanked for their patience and scholarly efforts. We also thank Cornelia Nicholson and Jennifer Pranke for their untiring assistance with many details involved in completing the book. We are also grateful to the agencies that have funded our own research: the National Institute of Mental Health, the National Institute of Nursing Research, the National Institute for Child Health and Human Development, and the American Foundation for AIDS Research. Finally, we wish to thank Sonia O'Leary and John B. Jemmott III, for their patience, love, and support during our work on this project.

Ann O'Leary
Loretta Sweet Jemmott

Contents

Chapter 3. Women-Centered Prevention Techniques and Technologies

Erica L. Gollub

Chapter 4. Childhood Sexual Abuse and AIDS: Issues and Interventions

Beatriz Perez, Gail Kennedy, and Mindy Thompson Fullilove

Chapter 5. Preventing AIDS in Female Adolescents

Mary Jane Rotheram-Borus, Loretta Sweet Jemmott, and John B. Jemmott III

Chapter 6. African American Women and HIV-Risk-Reduction Issues

Loretta Sweet Jemmott, Veronica Catan, Adeline Nyamathi, and Joyce Anastasia

Chapter 10. Women and AIDS in Developing Countries

Marcela Raffaelli and Jennifer Pranke

Chapter 11. Lesbian Women and HIV/AIDS: An Appeal for Inclusion

Kathleen M. Morrow

Chapter 12. Future Directions

Ann O'Leary and Loretta Sweet Jemmott

1

General Issues in the Prevention of AIDS in Women

ANN O'LEARY and LORETTA SWEET JEMMOTT

INTRODUCTION

As many authors in this volume indicate, women are increasingly represented among AIDS cases in the United States and are the demographic group most rapidly becoming infected. Further, most HIV transmission that takes place now, both in the United States and globally, occurs during heterosexual intercourse. Worldwide, it is estimated that 71% of HIV transmission has occurred through heterosexual contact (Ehrhardt, 1992).

While many issues relevant to womens' lives have arisen during the course of this epidemic (Ickovics & Rodin, 1992; O'Leary, Jemmott, Suarez-Al-Adam, AlRoy, & Fernandez, 1993b), primary prevention is at present among the most important objectives for those concerned about limiting the tragedy that HIV disease and its consequences bring to women, children, and men alike. Until very recently, the male latex condom was the only device available in the United States for the prevention of HIV transmission during vaginal intercourse, and it remains the primary strategy recommended in AIDS prevention efforts. Since the female condom is easily detected by the partner, it fails to eliminate many possible negative partner reactions. Thus, women can protect themselves only by avoiding intercourse altogether, relying on antibody testing (and thus on their partners' fidelity and honesty), or obtaining the cooperation of their partners in the use of condoms. Unfortunately, obtaining such cooperation can be a formidable task, even in loving and egalitarian relationships. Condom requests are

---

ANN O'LEARY • Department of Psychology, Rutgers University, New Brunswick, NJ 08903. *LORETTA SWEET JEMMOTT* • University of Pennsylvania School of Nursing, Philadelphia, PA 19104.

Women at Risk: Issues in the Primary Prevention of AIDS, edited by Ann O'Leary and Loretta Sweet Jemmott. Plenum Press, New York, 1995.

often perceived as possible indicants of infidelity or distrust or of sexually transmitted disease (STD) or HIV infection. Some men fear loss of sexual pleasure with the use of condoms and may reject them for that reason; others may wish to impregnate their partners. Chapter 3 discusses the importance of the development of female-centered prevention technologies, such as topical virucides, for the future. At present, however, the only known effective devices to prevent HIV transmission are problematic for many women.

In this chapter we attempt two tasks, recognizing a certain tension that exists between them. First, we wish to highlight the many difficulties and barriers to HIV protection experienced by women, particularly the low-income women at highest risk for HIV infection. We will describe individual, social, and structural problems, the solutions to which must ultimately come from individuals, communities, and society at large. Second, we will nevertheless describe experience among women in high-risk communities with some programs for HIV risk reduction that have been rigorously evaluated, some of which were found to be successful, indicating that many women do possess the resources and strength to protect themselves despite these barriers. Finally, we will suggest some important areas for future work in this area.

WOMEN AND HIV RISK: EFFECTS OF POVERTY

At present, AIDS in the United States affects predominantly the inner-city poor, with African American and Hispanic women being very disproportionately affected (see Chapters 6 and 7). About 73% of mothers with HIV-infected children receive public assistance (Shayne & Kaplan, 1991). Poverty potentiates HIV risk in many ways. Injected-drug use is much more common in low-income communities, contributing to initial infection rates early in the epidemic. Other STDs that potentiate HIV risk cluster in poor communities, as discussed in Chapter 2. Further, many of the poverty-related factors for HIV risk internationally, discussed in Chapter 10, apply to America's inner-city poor as well. For example, many women in the United States exchange sex for money, housing, gifts, or other favors, as in other countries, and exchange of sex for addictive drugs such as crack is common in the United States (e.g., Schilling *et al.*, 1994).

It has also been suggested that the stresses and difficulties encountered by the poor may contribute to HIV risk by displacing HIV infection among the list of concerns on peoples' minds (Amaro, 1988; Marin & Marin, 1991; Nyamathi & Vasquez, 1989). Indeed, female respondents in one study listed AIDS below several other life problems in seriousness (Kalichman, Hunter, & Kelly, 1992). In a study of injection-drug users (IDUs), residential instability was found to predict sexual risk for HIV transmission (Brown & Weissman, 1993).

RELATIONSHIP FACTORS AND HIV RISK

As indicated above, perhaps the most critical feature of many behavior changes that might prevent the sexual transmission of HIV is that they require the cooperation of another person, namely, the woman's sex partner. Some women also fear that they will lose desired partners if they insist on condom use or other safer sex behaviors, since condoms may suggest infidelity, and nonpenetrative sexual techniques such as mutual masturbation may be unacceptable to partners or to the women themselves. Of particular concern is the prevalence in low-income communities of domestic violence and coerced sex, which may render the recommendation of condom use useless or even dangerous. That domestic violence is prevalent in the communities most at risk for HIV is apparent to anyone who has worked closely with women in these communities, as is the gross inadequacy of present mechanisms for protecting women. Unfortunately, remarkably little research has even begun to address issues even of population prevalence or the degree of association of domestic violence with the stress of poverty. (The paucity of data is even more pronounced for emotional abuse, which could also be damaging in terms of HIV risk.) Pioneering research conducted in the 1970s (Strauss, Gelles, & Steinmetz, 1980) indicated that the unemployed, the less educated, and those with fewer financial resources were more likely to be in abusive relationships. However, few data exist to inform AIDS prevention efforts today on the populations (defined culturally, behaviorally, and/or geographically) most affected both by HIV and by domestic abuse.

There are some more recent data to indicate the relevance of domestic violence for HIV risk. In a focus group study, while participants failed to reveal abuse in their own lives, they commented that other women experience it, as illustrated by one respondent's statement, "It probably happens . . . in 90% of marriages and relationships where women live alone" (Fullilove, Fullilove, Haynes, & Gross, 1990). In one study, 31% of drug-using, incarcerated women in New York reported being physically abused by a spouse (El-Bassel *et al.*, 1994). In another recent study, 48 Latina participants in an HIV risk reduction program were interviewed, after their participation, regarding physical, emotional, and sexual abuse (Suarez-Al-

Adam, 1995). It was found that more than half the respondents had suffered some form of physical abuse at the hands of their partners during the study period (about 5 months); on average, women reported that their partners had committed 2.3 physically abusive acts. In addition, 23% of the women reported that their partners had forced them to engage in unwanted sexual activity. In a large study of female IDUs and partners of IDUs, 28% reported adult physical abuse and 20%, adult sexual abuse (reported in Weissman & Brown, 1995); in another similar study, physical abuse was reported by 45% of respondents, and 31% reported forced sex by a main partner (Weissman & Brown, 1995). Unfortunately, while AIDS prevention experts report anecdotal evidence for adverse consequences of condom recommendations for women in violent relationships, and while consideration of this possibility has been published (Cohen, 1991; Worth, 1989), systematic research on this topic is lacking. However, some studies have shown that women who expect their partners to react negatively (but not necessarily violently) to condom requests engage in riskier behavior (Harlow, Quina, Morokoff, Rose, & Grimley, 1993; O'Leary *et al.*, 1993a).

What psychosocial factors might be important in enabling women to protect themselves from HIV? That female "empowerment" is the ultimate requirement for success in HIV risk reduction is widely recognized (e.g., Levine *et al.*, 1993). Ultimately, changes in gender roles may require longer-term processes, possibly ones similar to the "consciousness raising" practiced by middle-class women in the 1970s. In the shorter term, however, women may be able to gain skills in the specific domain of condom negotiation with partners and thus be able to protect themselves from HIV. In the research literature on AIDS prevention, the self-efficacy construct of Bandura (1986) comes the closest to that of empowerment within specific realms such as condom negotiation.

SELF-EFFICACY AND SAFER SEX

Given the difficulties that women may experience in protecting themselves with male partners, they need good negotiation skills and strong confidence, or self-efficacy, in their ability to persuade partners to use condoms. Self-efficacy beliefs have been shown to be associated with successfully achieving safer sex in several studies. Self-efficacy operates by affecting people's behavior choices, the amount of effort they will exert in performing the behavior, and the degree of persistence they will display in the face of difficulty. Self-efficacy enhancement takes place through systematic skill-building through modeling (demonstrating the behavior) and practice of increasingly difficult skills (Bandura, 1986). Self-efficacy beliefs regarding safer sex ability are relevant in three domains (O'Leary, 1992): technical use of condoms and nonpenetrative sexual techniques; negotiation with partners; and self-control as related to use of alcohol, other drugs, and sexual arousal. Negotiation self-efficacy has been associated with higher rates of condom use by commercial sex workers (Corby & Wolitski, 1992), other disadvantaged women (LoConte, O'Leary, & Labouvie, 1993; O'Leary *et al.*, 1993a), and adolescents (Catania *et al.*, 1989; Harlow *et al.*, 1993; J. B. Jemmott, L. S. Jemmott, Spears, Hewitt, & Cruz-Collins, 1992). A recent study of black female adolescents demonstrated that increases in self-efficacy were associated with increased behavioral intention to practice safer sex (L. S. Jemmott & J. B. Jemmott, 1992).

Given that safer-sex negotiation skills are more critical for women, it is not surprising that self-efficacy perceptions were found in one recent study to be more closely linked to behavior safety for women than for men (LoConte *et al.*, 1993). Further, results from a recent evaluation of an HIV risk reduction program for college students suggest that low-intensity interventions that do not provide extensive individualized skill-building may be ineffective for women and even erode their efficacy beliefs by causing them to experience failure in negotiation efforts (O'Leary, Jemmott, Goodhart, Gebelt, & Boccher-Lattimore, 1994).

EVALUATED AIDS PREVENTION PROGRAMS FOR WOMEN

A small number of published studies have evaluated high-intensity prevention programs for women. A large-scale intervention study for IDU women and female sex partners of IDUs is described in Chapter 8. Several other intervention studies are at present under way (described in Moore, Harrison, & Doll, 1994). Such programs typically combine risk education with individualized skill-building for condom use and negotiation. One study with a pretest–posttest design demonstrated increases in condom use intentions among adolescent black women following a single-session intervention (L. S. Jemmott & J. B. Jemmott, 1992); a similar study produced significant increases in self-efficacy and intentions to use condoms in a 105-minute social cognitive skills-building intervention relative to an attention control and a no-intervention control (J. B. Jemmott *et al.*, 1992). Another study with a pretest–posttest design increased intended behavior change among low-income adult women attending Women, Infants, and Children clinics (Flaskerud & Nyamathi, 1990).

A few published studies have used randomized experimental designs to demonstrate the effects of intervention on actual behavior. A large study of black male and female adolescents demonstrated a significant effect of a 5-hour intervention that was significant at 6 months (but not at 3 months) postintervention, after removal of outliers. While control group participants reported an average of 0.57 day of unprotected intercourse in the previous 3 months, intervention group participants reported an average of 0.16 day. While results were not reported by gender, no indication of intervention moderation by gender was obtained, indicating that the females were able to achieve risk reduction of a magnitude comparable to that of the males.

A recent study designed for Latina women compared a one-session informational intervention with a 2-hour skills-building one (Nyamathi, Flaskerud, Bennett, Leake, & Lewis, 1994). No differences between groups in risk reduction were observed 2 weeks later, although both groups reported less activity with multiple partners. These results are difficult to interpret, as it is possible that all subjects were responding to demand.

Another study that also examined self-efficacy mediation was reported recently (Maibach & Flora, 1993). At-risk women were randomized to view one of three risk-reduction videotapes. One tape presented information only; another, information plus modeling of risk-reduction behaviors (i.e., negotiation sequences were presented); and the third had the aforenamed two components plus requests for cognitive rehearsal of the modeled behaviors by the participant (i.e., the women mentally practices negotiating safer sex with her partner). All three tapes contained a recommendation for condom use. Participants were assessed for changes in self-efficacy and a variety of behaviors 1 month later. As predicted by the investigators, self-efficacy rose the least in the information-only condition and the most in the information plus modeling plus rehearsal condition. In terms of actual behavior change, the rehearsal group reported buying more condoms and talking more to friends about HIV than the information-only group; however, no differences emerged for actual reduction of risk, i.e., using condoms, number of partners, number of partners using condoms, or even reporting any behavioral changes in response to the interventions.

Other randomized studies have used more intensive skill-building interventions. For example, Schilling, El-Bassel, Schinke, Gordon, and Nichols (1991) randomized women on methadone maintenance to receive a five-session skill-building intervention or to a control condition. The intervention included skill training in condom use and negotiation with partners. Significant increases in condom use, measured on a 4-point Likert scale, and in perceptions of control over AIDS were obtained, although number of sex partners did not change and number of risk encounters was not assessed. Further, condom use remained significantly more frequent among intervention participants at a 15-month follow-up (El-Bassel & Schilling, 1992).

Another study in which a similar five-session intervention was delivered to inner-city women attending a primary care clinic produced significant reductions in risk behavior at a 3-month follow-up relative to members of a health promotion control group (Kelly *et al.*, 1994). Condom use and negotiation as well as identifying and managing antecedents of risk acts were practiced in the groups. Percentage of condom use among those who were having sex rose from 26% to 56% among women in the HIV risk reduction group, but increased only from 26% to 32% in the control group, while the mean number of unprotected intercourse acts in the previous 3 months decreased from 14 to 12 in the experimental group, but increased from 13 to 15 in the control group. While not large, this latter effect was statistically significant.

Another recent study tested a four-session intervention against a health promotion control and a no-intervention control among inner-city pregnant single women (Hobfall, Jackson, Lavin, Britton, & Shepherd, 1994). The intervention included, in addition to modeling and practice for negotiation skill-building, cognitive imagining of negative and positive outcomes to build motivation. Again, some statistically significant effects were obtained, although it should be noted that analyses were conducted only for participants who completed at least three of four intervention sessions. Frequency of condom and spermicide use, assessed with a 4-point scale, changed significantly among treated women postintervention. Although both control groups increased in condom use, an ANCOVA in which baseline level was used as the covariate produced a nonsignificant treatment-group-by-time (postintervention to follow-up) interaction, suggesting maintenance of change. Number of intercourse events did not change significantly, and number of unprotected encounters was not reported. Redemption of condom coupons increased significantly in both the AIDS prevention and the health promotion group, but did not differentiate the groups.

Taken together, these studies are moderately encouraging in their promise for AIDS prevention among women at risk. Results are most impressive for Likert-scale measures of condom use frequency—which may be more readily influenced by demand—and least for number of risk encounters, which some might argue are likely to be most clearly related to objective HIV risk. As is the case in risk-reduction studies with other populations, some studies do not report response rates, making it difficult to know how generalizable the sample might be, and others include in analysis only subjects who completed or nearly completed the intervention. However, these studies do illustrate that many inner-city women can reduce their behavioral risk for HIV infection to some degree after training in negotiation and condom use skills.

HELPING THE WOMEN MOST AT RISK

Although evidence is accumulating that some women are able to achieve behavior change, it is clear that even following participation in high-intensity risk-reduction programs, many women do not change their behavior to reduce their risk. This is not surprising since, despite the enormous strength and courage displayed by at-risk women in many areas of their lives, they also face considerable barriers to protection from HIV. Below, we consider some issues that we believe will be critical in this effort.

Many women at high risk for HIV infection are addicted to drugs, and these addictions militate heavily against their ability to protect themselves. Drug treatment programs may be a vital component of HIV prevention for many women, and these programs must be readily available and administered in humane ways (see Chapter 8). Beyond such programs, efforts must be made to provide supportive alternatives for women at risk for drug use or relapse. For example, former drug-using women who have been incarcerated appear considerably less likely to adopt their former life-styles if alternatives exist for housing, employment, and relationships (El-Bassel, personal communication).

Supportive services for women wishing to escape or to manage violence in their relationships without exacerbating their risk must be developed and made available. Some AIDS prevention researchers and providers have suggested the potential utility of "passive negotiation" techniques for women in abusive relationships. These involve giving reasons for condom use that do not have to do with disease per se (e.g., O'Leary, 1994) and that therefore obviate many potential partner objections such as questions regarding fidelity. The woman can claim that her health providers have recommended condoms because other contraceptive forms make her ill. Other reasons might include that she is allergic to semen or that condoms serve as a hygiene strategy to relieve persistent yeast infections. Recommending to women that they lie to their partners is a controversial strategy and may be seen as less desirable than other solutions such as encouraging such women to leave their partners. However, inclusion of such options in HIV prevention programs may be useful for some women. Interventions for couples, or at least ones that involve the male partner to some degree, may also be helpful to women. Development of woman-controlled and nondetectable prevention technologies (see Chapter 3) also deserves high priority in the effort to protect at-risk women in abusive relationships.

Many women desire to become pregnant, and this wish is likely to affect AIDS prevention efforts (De Bruyn, 1992; Kline, Kline, & Oken, 1992). Prevention efforts may need to include strategies for women to use to become pregnant in the safest possible way, e.g., by using joint testing with her partner.

Prevention efforts may not reach the women most in need, as many inner-city women are isolated and not attached to community agencies. Individualized outreach by trusted others is the most effective way to recruit disenfranchised women, particularly Latina women. When possible, integration of AIDS prevention intervention with ongoing trusted services already part of women's lives is likely to enhance maintenance of change. Emotional support for the client on the part of the change agent may be a crucial factor in promoting change (National Institute of Mental Health, 1992). Interventions have a greater chance of success if they are provided within community sources such as community-based organizations or neighborhood or tenant groups, and continuation of care may help to prevent return to risky behaviors following intervention.

As this epidemic continues to wreak its damage on humankind, it may be critically important that those of us involved in prevention efforts remain open to new ideas. Evidence that condom use predicts seroconversion in a positive direction (Detels *et al.*, 1989; McQuillan, Ezzati-Rice, Siller, Visscher, & Hurley, 1994; Nelson *et al.*, 1993) suggests that condoms *as used* (i.e., often inconsistently) may be ineffective relative to condoms as ideally used and suggests that a public health strategy that relies all but solely on condom recommendations may be inadequate. There is a need to document and study for effectiveness other behavioral changes that women (or men) may be using in the belief, correct or incorrect, that they may decrease risk. Such behaviors might include partner-selection strategies, use of withdrawal, antibody testing, and sexual-history-taking (O'Leary, Goodhart, Jemmott, & Boccher-Lattimore, 1992). We in this country also tend to value individual freedoms and rights to an extent that may eventually need to be rethought, as there are often trade-offs between individual freedoms and public health considerations (e.g., as regards partner notification and antibody testing policies). AIDS is a severe public health problem that has brought misery to the lives of millions and that shows no signs of abating. Behavior change remains our only hope for attenuating the epidemic's effects and will probably remain so for some time to come. We must use our resources and inventiveness to all possible advantage in this effort.

Acknowledgments. Work on this paper was supported by the National Research Council, by grant 5-U10-MH48013 from the National Institute of Mental Health to Ann O'Leary, and by grant 1-R01-NR03123 from the National Institute of Nursing Research to Loretta Sweet Jemmott. The authors wish to thank Ralph DiClemente for helpful comments on an earlier draft of this chapter.

REFERENCES

Amaro, H. (1988). Hispanic women and AIDS. *Psychology of Women Quarterly, 12,* 423–443.

Bandura, A. (1986). *Social foundations of thought and action: A social cognitive theory.* Englewood Cliffs, NJ: Prentice-Hall.

Brown, V. B., & Weissman, G. (1993). Women and men injection drug users: An updated look at gender differences and risk factors. In B. Brown & G. M. Beschner (Eds.), *Handbook on risk of AIDS: Injection drug users and their partners* (pp. 173–194). Westport, CT: Greenwood Press.

Catania, J. A., Dolcini, M. M., Coates, T. J., Kegeles, S. M., Greenblatt, R. M., Puckett, S., Corman, M., & Miller, J. (1989). Predictors of condom use and multiple partnered sex among sexually-active adolescent women: Implications for AIDS-related health interventions. *Journal of Sex Research, 26,* 514–524.

Cohen, J. B. (1991). Why women partners of drug users will continue to be at high risk for HIV infection. *Journal of Addiction Research, 10,* 99–110.

Corby, N. H., & Wolitski, R. J. (1992). Relationship between street sex workers' attitudes and condom use by type of partner. Paper presented at the Eighth International Conference on AIDS/Third STD World Congress, Amsterdam, July 1992.

De Bruyn, M. (1992). Women and AIDS in developing countries. *Social Science and Medicine, 34,* 249–262.

Detels, R., English, P., Visscher, B R., Jacobson, L., Kingsley, L. A., Chmiel, J. S., Dudley, J. P., Eldred, L. J., & Ginsburg, H. M. (1989). Seroconversion, sexual activity, and condom use among 2,915 HIV seronegative men followed for up to 2 years. *Journal of Acquired Immune Deficiency Syndromes, 2,* 77–83.

Ehrhardt, A. A. (1992). Trends in sexual behavior and the HIV pandemic. *American Journal of Public Health, 82,* 1459–1461.

El-Bassel, N., Gilbert, L., Schilling, R. F., Ivanoff, A., Borne, D., & Safyer, S. F. (1994). Correlates of crack abuse among drug-using incarcerated women: Trauma, social support and coping behavior. Unpublished manuscript. New York: Columbia University.

El-Bassel, N., & Schilling, R. F. (1992). Fifteen-month followup of women methadone patients taught skills to reduce heterosexual HIV transmission. *Public Health Reports, 107,* 500–504.

Flaskerud, J. H., & Nyamathi, A. M. (1990). Effects of an AIDS education program on the knowledge, attitudes and practices of low income black and Latina women. *Journal of Community Health, 15,* 343–355.

Fullilove, M., Fullilove, R. E., Haynes, K., & Gross, S. (1990). Black women and AIDS prevention: A view towards understanding the gender rules. *Journal of Sex Research, 27,* 47–64.

Harlow, L. L., Quina, K., Morokoff, P. J., Rose, J. S., & Grimley, D. M. (1993). HIV risk in women: A multifaceted model. *Journal of Applied Biobehavioral Research, 1,* 3–38.

Hobfall, S. E., Jackson, A. P., Lavin, J., Britton, P. J., & Shepherd, J. B. (1994). Reducing inner-city women's AIDS risk activities: A study of single, pregnant women. *Health Psychology, 13,* 397–403.

Ickovics, J. R., & Rodin, J. (1992). Women and AIDS in the United States: Epidemiology, natural history, and mediating mechanisms. *Health Psychology, 11,* 1–16.

Jemmott, J. B., III, Jemmott, L. S., & Fong, J. T. (1995). Reducing the risk of AIDS in black adolescents: Evidence for the generality of intervention effects. Unpublished manuscript. Princeton, NJ: Princeton University.

Jemmott, J. B., Jemmott, L. S., Spears, H., Hewitt, N., & Cruz-Collins, M. (1992). Self-efficacy, hedonistic expectancies, and condom-use intentions among sexually active black inner-city women: A social cognitive theory approach to AIDS risk behavior. *Journal of Adolescent Health, 13,* 512–519.

Jemmott, L. S., & Jemmott, J. B. (1992). Increasing condom-use intentions among sexually active black adolescent women. *Nursing Research, 41,* 273–278.

Kalichman, S. C., Hunter, T. L., & Kelly, J. A. (1992). Perceptions of AIDS susceptibility among minority and nonminority women at risk for HIV infection. *Journal of Consulting and Clinical Psychology, 60,* 725–732.

Kelly, J. A., Murphy, D. A., Washington, C. D., Wilson, T. S., Koob, J. J., Davis, D. R., Ledezma, G., & Davantes, B. (1994). HIV/AIDS prevention for women seen in primary health care clinics: Effects of intervention to change high-risk sexual behavior patterns. *American Journal of Public Health.*

Kline, A., Kline, E., & Oken, E. (1992). Minority women and sexual choice in the age of AIDS. *Social Science and Medicine, 34,* 447–457.

Levine, O. H., Britton, P. J., James, T. C., Jackson, A. P., Hobfall, S. E., & Lavin, J. P. (1993). The empowerment of women: A key to HIV prevention. *Journal of Community Psychology, 21,* 320–334.

LoConte, J. S., O'Leary, A., & Labouvie, E. (1993). Applying social–cognitive theory to the safety of sexual behavior of inner city African Americans. Paper presented at the Fourteenth Annual Meeting of the Society of Behavioral Medicine, San Francisco, March 1993.

Maibach, E., & Flora, J. (1993). Symbolic modeling and cognitive rehearsal: Using video to promote AIDS prevention self-efficacy. *Communication Research, 20,* 517–545.

Marin, G., & Marin, B. V. (1991). *Research with Hispanic populations.* Newbury Park, CA: Sage Publications.

McQuillan, G. M., Ezzati-Rice, T. M., Siller, A. B., Visscher, W., & Hurley, P. (1994). Risk behavior and correlates of risk for HIV infection in the Dallas County Household HIV Survey. *American Journal of Public Health, 84,* 747–753.

Moore, J. S., Harrison, J. S., & Doll, L. S. (1994). Interventions for sexually active, heterosexual women in the United States. In R. J. DiClemente & J. L. Peterson (Eds.), *Preventing AIDS: Theories and methods of behavioral interventions* (pp. 243–265). New York: Plenum Press.

National Institute of Mental Health (1992). Report of the working group on women. In Putting Knowledge to Work: HIV Prevention Research and Community Programs. Washington, DC, December 1992.

Nelson, K. E., Celentano, D. D., Suprasert, S., Wright, N., Eiumtrakul, S., Tulvatana, S., Matanasarawoot, A., Akaresewi, P., Kuntolbutra, S., Romyen, S., Sirisopana, N., & Theertranot, C. (1993). Risk factors for HIV infection among young adult men in Thailand. *JAMA, 270,* 955–960.

Nyamathi, A. M., Flaskerud, J., Bennett, C., Leake, B., & Lewis, C. (1994). Evaluation of two AIDS education programs for impoverished women. *AIDS Education and Prevention, 6,* 296–309.

Nyamathi, A. M., & Vasquez, R. (1989). Impact of poverty, homelessness, and drugs on Hispanic women at risk for HIV infection. *Hispanic Journal of Behavioral Sciences, 11,* 299–314.

O'Leary A. (1992). Self-efficacy and health: Behavioral and stress-physiological mediation. *Cognitive Therapy and Research, 16,* 229–245.

O'Leary, A. (1994). Factors associated with the sexual risk of AIDS in women. In J. R. Battjes, Z. Sloboda, & W. C. Grace (Eds.), *The context of HIV risk among drug users and their sexual partners* (pp. 64–81). National Institute on Drug Abuse Research Monograph No. 143, NIH Publication No. 94-3750. Washington, DC: U.S. Government Printing Office.

O'Leary, A., Celentano, D., Maibach, E., Weisman, C., McCormack, M., Raffaelli, M., Jemmott, J. B., & Lallange, L. (1993a). Social cognitive predictors of HIV preventive behavior among urban STD clinic patients. Paper presented at the Ninth International Conference on AIDS, Berlin, June 1993.

O'Leary, A., Goodhart, F., Jemmott, L. S., & Boccher-Lattimore, D. (1992). Predictors of safer sexual behavior on the college campus: A social cognitive theory analysis. *Journal of American College Health, 40,* 254–263.

O'Leary, A., Jemmott, L. S., Goodhart, F., Gebelt, J., & Boccher-Lattimore, D. (1994). Differences between male and female college students' responses to institutional AIDS prevention intervention. Proceedings of the American Public Health Association Annual Meeting, Washington, DC, November 1994.

O'Leary, A., Jemmott, L. S., Suarez-Al-Adam, M., AlRoy, C., & Fernandez, M. I. (1993b). Women and AIDS. In S. Matteo (Ed.), *American women in the 1990's: Today's critical issues* (pp. 173–192). Boston: Northeastern University Press.

Schilling, R. F., El-Bassel, N., Ivanoff, A., Gilbert, L., Su, K. H., & Safyer, S. M. (1994). Sexual risk behaviors of incarcerated, drug-using women. *Public Health Reports, 109,* 539–547.

Schilling, R. F., El-Bassel, N., Schinke, S. P., Gordon, K., & Nichols, S. (1991). Building skills of recovering women drug users to reduce heterosexual AIDS transmission. *Public Health Reports, 106,* 297–304.

Shayne, V. T., & Kaplan, B. J. (1991). Double victims: Poor women and AIDS. *Women and Health, 17,* 21–37.

Suarez-Al-Adam, M. (1995). Effects of psychological abuse, physical abuse, and machismo on Hispanic womens' ability to negotiate safer sex. Unpublished master's thesis. New Brunswick, NJ: Rutgers University.

Strauss, M. A., Gelles, R., & Steinmetz, S. (1980). *Behind closed doors: Violence in the American family.* New York: Doubleday.

Weissman, G., & Brown, V. (1995). Drug using women and HIV: Access to care issues. In A. O'Leary & L. S. Jemmott (Eds.), *Women and AIDS: Coping and care.* New York: Plenum Press (in press).

Worth, D. (1989). Decision making and AIDS: Why condom promotion among vulnerable women is likely to fail. *Studies in Family Planning, 20,* 297–307.

2

Interactions among HIV, Other Sexually Transmitted Diseases, Socioeconomic Status, and Poverty in Women

SEVGI O. ARAL and JUDITH N. WASSERHEIT

INTRODUCTION

AIDS has become the fourth leading cause of death among United States women aged 25–44 [Centers for Disease Control and Prevention (CDC), 1993]. Through June 1993, the CDC had received reports of 36,690 AIDS cases among United States adult and adolescent women. Although most AIDS cases in women have been reported among those who inject drugs, in 1992, for the first time, diagnosed cases attributed to heterosexual contact exceeded those attributed to injection-drug use. Annual reported AIDS cases among adult and adolescent women in the United States increased 9% between 1991 and 1992; among men, the increase during the same time period was 2.5%.

AIDS cases are disproportionately concentrated among women of racial/ethnic minorities. Although black and Hispanic women make up 21% of all women in the United States, they constitute 74% of United States women diagnosed with AIDS since 1981. According to the Survey of Childbearing Women, prevalence of HIV infection among childbearing women nationwide was 0.17% in 1991–1992. Seroprevalence was highest

SEVGI O. ARAL and JUDITH N. WASSERHEIT • Department of Health and Human Services, U.S. Public Health Service, Centers for Disease Control and Prevention, Atlanta, GA 30333.

Women at Risk: Issues in the Primary Prevention of AIDS, edited by Ann O'Leary and Loretta Sweet Jemmott. Plenum Press, New York, 1995.

among black women (CDC, 1994). The substantial role of heterosexual transmission in the epidemic of HIV infection among women, and particularly among racial/ethnic minority women, is further supported by its geographic distribution (Wasser, Guinn, & Fleming, 1993). HIV infection among women in the southern United States is largely attributable to heterosexual transmission, particularly in nonurban areas (Wasser *et al.*, 1993).

Risk of acquiring HIV infection through heterosexual transmission is not well recognized. Among persons diagnosed with AIDS, women compared to men, racial/ethnic minorities compared to the majority, and persons who have acquired HIV infection through heterosexual transmission compared to those who have acquired the infection through other modes of transmission tend to report "late-testing," i.e., being tested for HIV antibodies close to the time of onset of AIDS symptoms, more frequently (Wortley *et al.*, 1995).

Heterosexually acquired HIV infection presents a most rapidly growing and seriously neglected threat for women's health, particularly among racial/ethnic minority populations. Many sexually transmitted diseases (STDs) are concentrated in the same populations as is HIV. Infection with other STDs increases the likelihood of HIV transmission among those exposed to the virus (Wasserheit, 1992). The higher prevalence of other STDs among minority populations and the greater probability of male-to-female, compared to female-to-male, transmission of all STDs including HIV infection (Aral & Holmes, 1990) together define other STDs as the most important preventable risk factor for HIV infection and AIDS among particularly minority women.

Women in the United States apparently underestimate their risk for acquiring STDs, including HIV infection (American Medical Women's Association, 1994). According to a recent survey of a nationally representative sample of 1000 women aged 16–60, 73% of women think they are safe from STDs such as chlamydia, AIDS, and herpes. Fully two thirds of American women know "almost nothing" about STDs other than AIDS, and one third know "almost nothing" about AIDS; half of all American women in the age group surveyed think that monogamy protects against risk of sexual transmission, and fewer than one third use condoms during sex.

In this chapter, we discuss the complex interrelationships between HIV infection and the other STDs; the gender, race, and ethnicity differentials in STD rates; and the behavioral and societal determinants of these differentials. We conclude by considering needs in the areas of STD/HIV research and policy and the implications for STD/HIV prevention programs.

SEXUALLY TRANSMITTED DISEASES AND TRANSMISSION OF HIV INFECTION

In evaluating the available evidence to determine whether HIV transmission is increased in the presence of other STDs, it is important to consider at least four methodological problems. First, it is essential that analyses control for sexual behavior, since both HIV risk and risk for other STDs are associated with similar sexual behaviors. Second, such analyses must control for infection with other sexually transmitted pathogens due to the frequent co-occurrence of multiple STDs in the same individual. Third, prospective studies documenting temporal sequence are necessary to show that other STDs facilitate HIV transmission and are not simply markers for HIV-related immunosuppression. Fourth, the relationships between other STDs and HIV infection are probably not uniform; therefore, studies should examine these interactions stratified by gender and sexual preference.

Genital ulcer diseases (GUDs) may facilitate HIV transmission by a number of mechanisms. These STDs provide easy portals of entry and exit for HIV because they create breaks in the genital skin. In addition, GUDs result in an inflammatory response that includes the same kind of lymphocytes and macrophages that are HIV target cells. Finally, viral STDs like herpes may "turn on" HIV through molecular mechanisms that are still being elucidated (Wasserheit, 1992).

Currently available data that attempt to control for the potentially confounding effects of sexual behavior indicate that GUDs, including chancroid, syphilis, and genital herpes are risk factors for heterosexual transmission of HIV (Cameron *et al.,* 1989; Greenblatt *et al.,* 1989; Kreiss *et al.,* 1986; Plummer *et al.,* 1991; Simonsen *et al.,* 1988).

Much of the prospective data linking GUD with HIV transmission comes from heterosexual populations in developing countries in which the majority of GUD is caused by chancroid. These studies suggest that chancroid may increase HIV transmission 4- to 5-fold. A statistically significant relationship between serological evidence of the causative agent of chancroid (immunoglobulin G antibody to *Haemophilus ducreyi*) and HIV seropositivity has also been reported; however, the effects of sexual behavior and other STDs were not considered in this study (Piot, Van Dyck, Ryder, Nzila, & Laga 1989).

Case-controlled studies of the relationship between syphilis and HIV infection show a 2- to 9-fold increase in risk of HIV infection associated with syphilis (Cannon *et al.,* 1988, 1989; Chiphangwi, Dallabetta, Saah, Liomba, & Miott, 1990; Elifson, Soles, Sweet, & Darrow, 1989; Hayes *et al.,* 1990). Even after the potentially confounding effects of sexual behavior in prospective studies are controlled for, this relationship remains statistically significant with at least a 2- to 4-fold increase in risk of HIV transmission (Darrow *et al.,* 1987; Van Raden *et al.,* 1989).

Herpes simplex virus type 2 (HSV-2) infection may be associated with a similarly increased risk for HIV infection among homosexual men (Holmberg *et al.,* 1988a,b; Stamm *et al.,* 1988), but some studies did not confirm this association, and data from heterosexual cohorts remain limited (Van Raden, *et al.,* 1989; Kingsley, Armstrong, 1990; Rahman, Ho, & Rinaldo, 1990; Hayes et al., 1990).

Available data on the association between nonulcerative STDs, such as chlamydial infection, gonorrhea, and trichomoniasis, and HIV infection are more limited than those supporting the association between GUD and HIV infection. However, if nonulcerative STDs facilitate HIV transmission, they will account for greater proportions of HIV infection than GUDs because, in most communities, these STDs are more common than genital ulcers (Wasserheit, 1992). The most likely mechanism by which nonulcerative STDs facilitate HIV transmission is through the recruitment of HIV-susceptible or HIV-infected cells along with other inflammatory cells to form the discharge that is characteristic of these clinical syndromes.

Chlamydial cervicitis has been associated with 3- to 6-fold increases in the risk for HIV seroconversion in prospective studies among female prostitutes in Kinshasa and Nairobi (Laga *et al.,* 1990; Plummer *et al.,* 1991). Gonorrhea appears to be associated with a 3- to 9-fold increased HIV risk in cross-sectional studies of heterosexual populations and with risk estimates of 3.5–5.1 in prospective studies (Laga *et al.,* 1990; Kingsley *et al.,* 1990; Van Raden *et al.,* 1989). Female prostitutes followed prospectively in Kinshasa who developed trichomoniasis were also at 3 times greater risk of HIV seroconversion than those without trichomoniasis (Laga *et al.,* 1990).

Women with anogenital warts also appear to be more likely to have HIV infection than uninfected women (Chiphangwi *et al.,* 1990; Quinn *et al.,* 1988). However, no prospective studies that control for the potentially confounding effects of sexual behavior are available to suggest a causal association between human papillomavirus (HPV) infection and augmented transmission of HIV. It is likely that HIV-related immunosuppression leads to an increased expression of HPV infection, rather than that HPV infection facilitates transmission of HIV.

To summarize, with the exception of HPV infection, data support an important role for other STDs in HIV transmission. Risk estimates from studies of heterosexual populations appear to be similar for ulcerative and nonulcerative STDs and cluster in the range of a 3- to 5-fold increase in risk of HIV transmission in the presence of other STDs. The role of other

STDs may be somewhat greater in HIV transmission from women to men than in HIV transmission from men to women, but data are too sparse to be conclusive. Biologically, it is highly plausible that other STDs would facilitate the transmission of HIV (Wasserheit, 1992).

SEXUALLY TRANSMITTED DISEASES AND PROGRESSION OF HIV DISEASE

Only a handful of studies have addressed the role of other STDs in the progression of HIV disease. Furthermore, several methodological issues make studies of this question difficult. In studies focusing on the impact of STDs on HIV progression, it is important to control for duration of HIV infection, which requires prospective assessment of initially HIV-negative subjects. Adjustments for baseline immunological function and for age are also critical. More marked immunosuppression at enrollment may be associated with both accelerated progression of HIV disease and increased severity or frequency of recurrences of viral STDs. Age-related cohort effects in STD incidence and age-related differentials in rates of progression may create spurious correlations between STDs and accelerated progression of HIV disease. In addition, number of exposures to an STD pathogen may be a more appropriate variable than categorical presence or absence of any STD exposure for accelerated progression of HIV disease. If this is the case, the frequency of asymptomatic infection and the financial and compliance constraints on repeated testing may make it difficult to demonstrate this association (Wasserheit, 1992).

At this time, results regarding the effect of other STDs on the progression of HIV disease are inconclusive. Most studies of the impact of STDs on HIV progression are univariate analyses that do not control for the duration of HIV infection, baseline immunological status, or age (Wasserheit, 1992). Results of the few available studies suggest that HSV infection plays no role in HIV progression (Holmberg *et al.*, 1988a,b; Webster *et al.*, 1989; Kaslow *et al.*, 1989), while rectal gonorrhea may accelerate the disease process among homosexual men (Phair et al., 1992).

THE IMPACT OF HIV INFECTION ON OTHER SEXUALLY TRANSMITTED DISEASES

The impact of HIV infection on other STDs may further reinforce the role of STDs as risk factors for HIV transmission, especially at the community level. Theoretically, HIV infection might enhance susceptibility to other

STDs; lead to atypical presentations, including larger, more numerous, or more persistent lesions; or modify the natural history of STDs, resulting in more frequent recurrence or complications. HIV infection may also alter the accuracy of some STD detection methods or the response to standard therapy (Wasserheit, 1992). Such changes in the presentation, epidemiology, and effectiveness of diagnosis and treatment of STDs could further facilitate HIV transmission by increasing community-wide levels of these diseases.

Studies of these issues raise several of the same methodological concerns as those that are important in studies of the effect of STDs on HIV transmission. Sexual behaviors and infection with multiple STDs are, again, potential confounders, and prospective designs are necessary to tease apart whether STDs facilitate HIV transmission, whether HIV infection facilitates STD transmission, or whether both processes occur. In addition, consideration of health care behaviors such as response to STD symptoms or compliance with therapy may not only influence the course of STDs and their response to treatment, but also be related to whether an individual is HIV-infected. Finally, HIV-negative comparison groups are essential to interpretable studies of the effect of HIV infection on other STDs.

Unfortunately, much of our understanding of these issues still rests on case reports or case series and awaits confirmation from ongoing prospective studies. In the presence of HIV infection, atypical presentations of both chancroid and syphilis, including both larger and extragenital lesions, have been reported (Berger, Hensley, & Moskowitz, 1989; Caumes *et al.*, 1989; Latif, 1989; Quale, Tellitz, & Augenbraun, 1990). HIV infection also appears to augment the severity and frequency of recurrence of genital herpes and genital warts (Corey, 1990; Quinnan *et al.*, 1984; Sooy & Mills, 1988; Milburn *et al.*, 1988; Rudlinger *et al.*, 1988; Thomas *et al.*, 1990; McMillan & Bishop, 1989; Bishop, McMillan, & Fletcher, 1990). Preliminary data from studies of women with symptomatic pelvic inflammatory disease (PID) also suggest that HIV infection may increase the severity with which PID presents (Irwin *et al.*, 1993, Kamenga *et al.*, 1993).

Response to therapy may also be altered in the setting of HIV infection. For example, development of resistance may be promoted by the repeated need for antimicrobial agents (Youle *et al.*, 1988; Ehrlich *et al.*, 1989). Perhaps most important, HIV infection seems to result in decreased responsiveness to standard therapy among persons with chancroid (Cameron, Plummer, D'Costa, Ndinya-Achola, & Ronald, 1988). However, in contrast to initial impressions, HIV-negative and asymptomatic HIV-positive patients with early infection with syphilis (Berry, Hooton, & Collier, 1987; Duncan, 1989; Johns, Tierney, & Felsenstein, 1987; Rolfs *et al.*, 1993) or with PID (Irwin *et al.,* 1993; Kamenga *et al.,* 1993) appear to respond similarly to standard therapy.

Evidence that HIV infection may increase the incidence of serious STD complications has been particularly disturbing. HIV infection appears to facilitate progression of HPV infection to anogenital dysplasia or neoplasia (Feingold *et al.,* 1990; Schrager *et al.,* 1989; Schafer *et al.,* 1990; Muggiasca *et al.,* 1989; Goedert *et al.,* 1990; Frazer *et al.,* 1986; LaVigne *et al.,* 1990; Laga *et al.,* 1992). One study also suggests that the incidence of PID may be greater among positive women with gonorrhea than among their HIV-negative counterparts (Plummer *et al.,* 1989). It is noteworthy that the investigators did not find a similar HIV-related increase in the incidence of chlamydial PID.

In summary, HIV infection and other STDs are inextricably intertwined, particularly in heterosexual populations, and the relationships between HIV infection and other STDs appear to vary by specific STD. Three distinct patterns of relationships may occur (Wasserheit, 1992). GUDs and HIV infection appear to reinforce each other; GUDs facilitate HIV transmission, and thereby may increase HIV prevalence within the community. Simultaneously, HIV infection may prolong or augment the infectiousness of a person with GUD, thereby increasing the likelihood that the person will transmit the GUD. The discharge syndromes, including gonorrhea, chlamydial infection, and trichomoniasis, seem to promote HIV transmission without a synergistic increase in their own prevalence or incidence. HPV infection may represent a classic opportunistic infection, the expression and progression of which is augmented by HIV infection. These interrelationships mean that HIV infection and other STDs may amplify one another by establishing a mutually reinforcing spiral of infection. Clearly, this possibility suggests that in communities with high rates of STDs, augmented STD prevention and control efforts should be a central HIV prevention strategy.

GENDER, RACE, AND ETHNICITY DIFFERENTIALS IN SEXUALLY TRANSMITTED DISEASES

Historically, in the United States, rates of non-HIV STDs have varied by age, gender, race or ethnicity, and socioeconomic status (Aral & Holmes, 1990). Interactions among these variables, as well as their direct effects, determine the distribution of STD cases in the population. The age pattern of STD morbidity (and sexual behavior) tends to change little over time, and differences in the age pattern of STD incidence across gender and racial/ethnic groups tend to be small.

On the other hand, gender differentials and racial/ethnic differentials in STD incidence show marked changes over time. Gender differentials are greatest among Hispanics, followed by African Americans, and apparently have been decreasing in all racial/ethnic groups since 1960, with the gender gap closing much faster among whites than among members of any other group.

STDs disproportionately compromise the health of women. The "gender asymmetry" of STDs is the result of three factors:

1. Women are more likely than men to acquire STDs because the anatomy of the vagina facilitates prolonged exposure to infected secretions following intercourse and because few female-controlled technologies have demonstrated efficacy in prevention of STDs.
2. Women are less likely than men to seek care for STDs because, in contrast to men, the majority of STD-infected women are asymptomatic and therefore do not realize that they need care. Furthermore, in many communities, seeking care for STDs remains far more stigmatizing for women than for men.
3. Women are more difficult to diagnose than are men because the low sensitivity and specificity of clinical signs and symptoms in women necessitate use of laboratory tests that have traditionally required speculum examinations and expensive, technically sophisticated diagnostic procedures. Clinical diagnosis of STDs in men, on the other hand, is usually relatively accurate.

Moreover, women suffer more frequent and severe consequences of STDs than men because of many of the factors highlighted above and because of biological differences. These consequences include PID, involuntary infertility, potentially fatal ectopic pregnancy, other adverse outcomes of pregnancy (e.g., postpartum endometritis), and cervical cancer. Finally, the psychological and social consequences for women of STDs and complications such as infertility or adverse outcomes of pregnancy are just beginning to be appreciated.

Race/ethnicity differentials in STD incidence decreased during the 1960s and 1970s, reflecting, initially, increases in STD morbidity nationally among white women, followed by declines in incidence among members of racial/ethnic minorities. However, during the 1980s, this trend reversed itself; race/ethnicity differentials in STD incidence increased as syphilis incidence increased alarmingly, especially among heterosexual members of minority populations, and as gonorrhea incidence declined markedly among whites while either remaining stable or declining slightly among members of other racial/ethnic groups in most communities. The association between declining socioeconomic conditions for some members of racial/ethnic minorities and increasing race/ethnicity differentials in STD rates in the 1980s is remarkable.

Bacterial STDs: Gonorrhea, Syphilis, and Chlamydia

In the United States, the reported incidence of gonorrhea increased steadily at about 15% per year from 1962 through 1975, peaking at 473 per 100,000 in 1975, then declining at an accelerating pace to 275 per 100,000 in 1990. The gender-specific race/ethnicity differentials in overall gonorrhea incidence rates were greater in 1990 compared to 1981. Among men, the morbidity rate among African Americans was almost 56 times that among whites in 1990 and only 12 times that among whites in 1981; among women, the corresponding figures were 8 in 1990 and 12 in 1981. The differentials between Hispanic morbidity and white morbidity also increased during the 1980s, but to a lesser extent. Among men, the Hispanic morbidity rate was 4 times that of the white morbidity rate in 1990 and only 2 times that of the white rate in 1981; among women, the corresponding figures were 1.8 in 1990 and 1.4 in 1981. The greatest race/ethnicity differential was observed between African American and white men, both in 1981 and in 1990.

The gender-specific race/ethnicity differential for gonorrhea has consistently been highest among Hispanics and lowest among whites. In 1981, the male-to-female ratio of gonorrhea incidence rates ranged from 2.1 among Hispanics to 1.6 among African Americans and 1.56 among whites. The corresponding figures in 1990 were 1.73, 1.59, and 0.78. Thus, during the 1980s, the gender differential declined most among whites, followed by Hispanics, with no measurable change in the African American gender differential.

The incidence of primary and secondary syphilis had increased remarkably prior to 1965 to reach 12 per 100,000 in that year. Between 1965 and 1980, overall rates of primary and secondary syphilis were stable. As of 1981, the overall incidence rate for the United States was 13.4 per 100,000, with the highest rates being reported for African American men (96.1 per 100,000) and the lowest rates being reported for white women (1 per 100,000). The overall incidence of primary and secondary syphilis continued to increase through 1983, when the rate was 14.1 per 100,000, declined in 1984 and 1985 (11.3 per 100,000), and started to increase again in 1986. The rate had reached 20.4 per 100,000 in 1990, a 40-year high.

Interestingly, during the 1980s, most of the decline in syphilis incidence took place during the earlier part of the decade among white men, while most of the increase was during the later part of the decade among minority men and women. The greatest increases were observed among African Americans between 1985 and 1990, followed by Hispanic men (1984–1987) and Hispanic women (1982–1988). In 1981, the largest gender-specific race/ethnicity differentials were observed between African Americans and whites; the rate for African American men was 12 times that for white men, and the rate for African American women was 42 times that for white women. The corresponding figures for Hispanic men and women were 4 and 8. By 1990, most of these differentials had increased; the rate for African American men was 54 times that for white men, while the rate for African American women was 65 times that for white women. The primary and secondary syphilis incidence among Hispanic men was 8-fold that among white men, and the incidence among Hispanic women was 6 times that among white women.

In 1990, the pattern of gender differentials in primary and secondary syphilis rates was similar to the 1981 pattern in gonorrhea rates and was highest among Hispanics (a male-to-female ratio of 2.1), followed by whites (M:F = 1.6) and African Americans (M:F = 1.3). The gender differential declined in all three groups between 1981 and 1990; the 1981 M:F ratios had been 4.4 among Hispanics, 7.9 among whites, and 2.3 among African Americans.

Data on chlamydial infections are more limited than those on gonorrhea and syphilis. Indirect estimates indicate that chlamydial infections are more widely distributed in the population and show less pronounced differentials by racial/ethnic status and socioeconomic status (SES) (Aral & Holmes, 1990; W. M. McCormack, Rosner, McComb, Evrard, & Zinner, 1985; Schachter, Stoner, & Moncada, 1983).

Viral STDs

Data on incurable viral STDs are also limited. During the 1980s, however, improved tests were developed for type-specific serum antibody to HSV-2, the organism most commonly responsible for genital herpes. On the basis of the percentage of adults with serum antibody, women are more likely to have HSV-2 antibodies than men, HSV-2 antibody prevalence is higher among African Americans than among whites by approximately 3-fold, and is also higher among lower-SES individuals and inner-city residents than among whites. Race/ethnicity and SES were independent predictors of HSV-2 antibody prevalence (Johnson *et al.,* 1989).

Data on HPV infections are even more limited than those in HSV-2 infections. Technology that detects type-specific HPV DNA in epithelial cells has recently become available and will shed more light on race/ethnicity differentials in HPV infections in the future. At this time, some hypotheses regarding these differentials can be put forth, on the basis of indirect evidence. A potential complication of cervical HPV infection is cervical carcinoma. Cervical cytological screening allows early detection and treatment of cervical dysplasia, which may effectively prevent invasive cervical carcinoma. The higher incidence of cervical cancer among African American women than among white women may reflect a higher incidence of cervical HPV infection, or a lower frequency of cervical cytology screening, or both. Similarly, the higher rate for cervical cancer mortality among African American women compared to white women may reflect earlier diagnosis and treatment of invasive cancer among the latter (Aral & Holmes, 1990).

SES differentials in STD incidence and variations in such differentials over time and across racial/ethnic groups are difficult to describe. National STD morbidity data stratified by SES are not readily available over time. Nevertheless, both individual-level analyses and community-level analyses (Rothenberg, 1986; Potterat *et al.,* 1985) indicate a strong, inverse association between incidence of all STDs and all measures of SES, including education, income, residence, and occupation, at the individual level; and average income or percentage of population below poverty level associated with the zip code or census tract of residence, at the community level.

GENDER, RACE, AND ETHNICITY DIFFERENTIALS IN DETERMINANTS OF SEXUALLY TRANSMITTED DISEASE INCIDENCE

The higher prevalence and incidence of AIDS and other STDs among some members of African American and Hispanic populations cannot be accounted for by biases in reporting and do not appear to be related to biological differences. Determinants of STD incidence have been described at either the individual or the population level of analysis. At the individual level in epidemiological studies, various sociodemographic characteristics and sexual, health, and substance use behaviors emerge as risk factors for being infected with sexually transmitted pathogens (Aral, 1992). At the population or community level, comparisons of societies marked by high STD rates with those marked by lower STD rates reveal that various economic, demographic, organizational, and behavioral characteristics of populations may correlate strongly with STD incidence (Holmes & Aral, 1991). Both at the individual level and at the community level, determinants of STD risk tend to be strongly associated with each other and to mutually reinforce and magnify each others' effects. The overlap among high-risk behaviors of individuals is frequently noted in epidemiological studies that attempt to specify risk factors for AIDS and other STDs (e.g., Dryfoos, 1991; Penkower *et al.,* 1991).

Globally, societies marked by high STD rates and incidence of AIDS tend to be societies in which a youthful age composition coincides with low levels of economic development, per capita income, income equality, educational attainment, women's social status, and accessibility and utilization of health care services. These societies are also marked by high levels of poverty. These factors reinforce one another, although detailed discussion of the mechanisms of synergy among these societal properties is beyond the scope of this chapter. Finally, it is important to note that the societal context in which a person lives is determined, to an important extent, by that person's sociodemographic characteristics and, in turn, affects both the risk behaviors in which he engages and the magnitude of risk to which he is exposed as a result of engaging in those behaviors (Aral, Fullilove, & Coutinho, 1991a). In this section, we briefly review the available evidence on these determinants and the extent to which they vary by racial/ethnic minority status.

Behavioral Determinants of STD Incidence

Sexual Behaviors

The dimensions of sexual behavior that increase risk for infection with curable bacterial and incurable viral STDs include early age at sexual debut, large numbers of lifetime and current sex partners, nondiscriminating sex partner recruitment patterns, high-risk characteristics of sex partners, specific sexual practices such as anal intercourse, and frequency and timing of sexual intercourse (Aral, 1992). More recently, sexual abuse during childhood has been associated with increased risk for HIV infection (Zierler *et al.,* 1991).

Age at sexual debut is an important risk factor for STDs, especially among women. The race/ethnicity differentials in age at sexual debut were limited by the end of the 1980s, following two decades of declining differentials that helped close the gap between the initial sexual experience of the majority and that of the racial/ethnic minority women. In 1988, the percentage of women aged 15–19 years who had ever had sexual intercourse was 52.4% among non-Hispanic whites, 60.8% among non-Hispanic blacks, and 48.5% among Hispanics. In 1982, the corresponding figures were 44.5%, 59.0%, and 50.8% respectively. The decline in the race/ethnicity differential was clearly attributable to increases in the percentage of non-Hispanic white adolescents who had initiated intercourse (Forrest & Singh, 1990).

Sexual activity levels among 15- to 19-year-old young men also vary by racial/ethnic background (Sonenstein, Pleck, & Ku, 1989). In 1988, based on a survey of a nationally representative sample, 60% of young men aged 15–19 reported having had sexual intercourse with a girl at least once. The proportion of sexually experienced young men was highest among African Americans (81%) and lower among Hispanic (60%) and white young men (57%).

The differential between poor and nonpoor teenagers with respect to age at sexual debut also declined during the 1980s and was not great by 1988. In 1982, 55.5% of 15- to 19-year-old women living in families with incomes of less than 200% of the poverty[1] level had sexual intercourse, while only 39.7% percent of those living in families with incomes above 200% of the poverty level reported this experience. During the 1980s, teenagers with higher family incomes experienced a 25% increase in the proportion of sexually experienced in their category. Thus, in 1988, the percentage of 15- to 19-year-old women who had ever had intercourse was 56.5% among the poor and 50.1% among the nonpoor (Forrest & Singh, 1990). Having multiple sexual partners is another dimension of sexual behavior that is affected by a person's race/ethnicity status. On the basis of the most recent national survey of sexual behavior, people are more likely to report multiple sexual partners if they are African American ($OR = 1.5$) or white ($OR = 1.4$) relative to Hispanic ($p = 0.01$) (Catania *et al.*, 1992). Of the dimensions of SES, education was the only one that emerged as statistically significantly associated with having multiple sexual partners in multivariate analyses of these data; persons who had received education beyond high school were more likely ($OR = 1.3$) to report multiple sexual partners compared to those who had not received a high school education.

Analysis of data reported by teenage women reveals somewhat different findings. The proportion reporting four to five or six or more partners appears to have increased significantly between the 1970s and the late 1980s. The proportions with multiple partners differ little by race (30% among African Americans and 31% among whites), and the time trends appear to hold equally among both whites and African Americans aged 15–19 (Kost & Forrest, 1992).

Among adolescent males aged 17–19, trends may be similar; the average number of partners in the previous 12 months was 2.6 in 1991, compared to 2.0 in 1988. In 1991, 11% reported at least five partners in the previous

[1]Poverty is defined in accordance with the definition adopted for official government use by the Office of Management and Budget and consists of a set of money income thresholds that vary by family size and composition.

12 months, compared to 6% in 1988 (Sonenstein, unpublished manuscript). Among 17- to 22-year-olds in 1990–1991, the mean number of sex partners in the past 12 months was highest among African Americans (3.6), followed by white Americans (2.3) and Hispanic Americans (Ku, Sonenstein, & Pleck, 1992).

Nondiscriminating sex partner recruitment patterns are reflected in part in having sexual intercourse with risky partners (partners who engage in high-risk behaviors). In the recent national survey of sexual behavior mentioned above, people with low incomes (< $10,000 per year) compared to those with high incomes (> $40,000 per year) ($OR$ = 1.9), and women relative to men (OR = 1.5), were more likely to report having risky sex partners. Racial/ethnic background did not emerge as a statistically significant correlate of having risky partners. However, these results may be an artifact of the particular manner in which the multivariate analysis was conducted; i.e., the risk factors were hierarchically defined and assumed to be mutually exclusive (Catania *et al.,* 1992).

Data on prevalence and distribution, by race/ethnicity or SES, of specific sexual practices that increase risk for STDs, such as anal intercourse and dry sex (i.e., sexual intercourse that follows the removal of vaginal lubricants either mechanically by wiping or chemically through the insertion of certain plants), are more limited. Anecdotal information suggests that anal intercourse may be more frequently practiced by Hispanic Americans, and dry sex may be preferred by a greater proportion of African Americans. The only available national data were collected in the National Survey of Adolescent Males; in 1990–1991, among young men aged 17–22, heterosexual anal intercourse (ever) was reported by 12.9% of Hispanic Americans, 11.7% of African Americans, and 8% of white Americans (Ku *et al.,* 1992). Similarly, on the basis of anecdotal information that persons of higher SES engage in a greater variety of sexual practices, it may be hypothesized that frequency of anal intercourse increases with increasing SES. No national data are available to test this hypothesis.

Frequency of sexual intercourse was reportedly higher among white women compared to women of other race/ethnicity groups in 1982 (Aral & Cates, 1989). No analyses of SES variations in frequency of sexual intercourse are available at this time. Similarly, no published data are available on the timing of sexual intercourse or the population prevalence of sexual intercourse during menses or its distribution by race/ethnicity or SES. Unpublished data indicate that sexual intercourse during menses is practiced by a greater proportion of white Americans (27.7%) and Hispanic Americans (25.9%) than by African Americans (17.6%). This practice is also reported more frequently by those with higher income and education (Tanfer *et al.,* unpublished).

Health Behaviors

Health behaviors, including condom and other contraceptive use, vaginal douching, and male circumcision, affect a person's risk for STDs. While consistent and proper condom use and male circumcision decrease STD risk, vaginal douching is associated with increased risk for STD-related syndromes, including PID, ectopic pregnancy, and cervical cancer (Aral 1992; Aral, Mosher, & Cates, 1992). Timely health care seeking and compliance with therapy and behavioral recommendations, including abstaining from sexual intercourse when one (or one's partner) has symptoms of STDs, are behaviors that decrease risk for STDs.

Regarding condom use, a preventive behavior, data on racial/ethnic status differentials are inconsistent with data on SES differentials. Many studies conducted on selective samples indicated greater reporting of condom use by people at higher risk of exposure to HIV and other STDs; thus, people of racial/ethnic minority backgrounds reported more condom use (e.g., Soskolne, Aral, Magder, & Bowen, 1991). However, the recent sexual behavior survey mentioned above revealed no differences by racial/ethnic background in the use of condoms in multivariate analysis. The same survey found condom use to be related to socioeconomic status as reflected in educational attainment; those who had completed high school were more likely to report condom use ($OR = 1.6$) compared to those who had not (Catania *et al.,* 1992).

Another study that was conducted on a population-based sample of unmarried adults focused on beliefs regarding condoms. The results showed that among women, 77% of whites, 71% of African Americans, and 52% of Hispanics believed that condoms were effective protection against transmission of HIV. Among men, these proportions were 76%, 64%, and 55%, respectively. Thus, belief in the effectiveness of condoms as prophylaxis against infection is most widespread among whites and least among Hispanics (Kegeles *et al.,* 1991).

In the survey of a nationally representative sample of young men conducted in 1988, 57% of young, sexually active men reported having used condoms the last time they had intercourse. Reported rates of condom use during last intercourse were higher among African Americans (66%) compared to whites (54%) and Hispanics (53%) (Sonenstein *et al.,* 1989). Data from the National Survey of Adolescent Men also suggest that consistency of condom use is greatest among African Americans, who report using condoms 61.4% of the time, followed by white Americans (54.4%) and Hispanic Americans (51.1%) (Ku *et al.,* 1992).

Racial background is strongly associated with vaginal douching. In a national survey conducted in 1988, two thirds of African American women compared to only one third of white women reported douching. Douching was also more common among women who lived in poverty (50%) compared to those who did not (28%). The synergistic effects of poverty and minority racial status are observed in patterns of vaginal douching; 70% of African American women living in poverty reported vaginal douching (Aral *et al.,* 1992).

National data on prevalence of male circumcision or its distribution by race/ethnicity and SES are not available. Anecdotal data suggest that male circumcision may be more prevalent among white Americans compared to other racial/ethnic groups.

Health-care seeking behaviors, another determinant of STD incidence at the individual level, also vary by racial/ethnic status (Darrow, 1979). In one clinic-based study, the higher rates of gonorrhea among African Americans compared to whites and Hispanics were attributed in part to longer delay on the part of African Americans in seeking care when STD symptoms appeared (Darrow, 1976). Congenital syphilis was more prevalent among babies of African American and Hispanic women in Texas and was associated with a relative lack of prenatal health care utilization in these groups (Mascola *et al.,* 1984). Conversely, another STD-clinic-based study reported more timely and appropriate health care behaviors among members of African American populations than among whites (Kramer, Aral, & Curran, 1980). While it is clear that race/ethnicity differences exist in health service utilization, health care seeking, and compliance with therapy recommendations (Radecki & Bernstein, 1989), depending on the population studied, the direction of these differentials changes. Data on SES differentials in STD-related health care seeking, and SES–race/ethnicity interactions as they affect health care seeking, are unavailable. Thus, it is difficult to interpret the existing differences. At this time, data are inconclusive regarding the extent to which race/ethnicity differentials in STD morbidity are due to differentials in health behaviors.

Patterns of testing and screening for STDs reflect the combined effect of health care providers' behaviors and health-care-seeking behaviors of the patient population. In 1982 and in 1988, reproductive-age women reported a higher frequency of testing for STDs among African Americans compared to white Americans (Aral, Mosher, Horn, & Cates, 1986; Mosher & Aral, 1991). In 1988, African American women were twice as likely to report having been tested for STDs during the previous 12 months as were white American women (47% and 23%, respectively). Patterns of testing and screening for STDs also reflected SES differentials. Women with lower income were more likely to report having been tested for STDs during the previous 12 months (35%) compared to women with higher income (23%).

Substance Use

Intravenous-drug use has been an increasingly important risk factor for HIV infection through the 1980s. Drug use in general, and crack cocaine use in particular, constitute risk factors for sexual transmission of all sexually transmitted pathogens. Drug use is associated with anonymous sex and sex in exchange for drugs or money; it also reduces the likelihood that safer sex will be practiced. Recent data from a representative survey of households have pointed to an additional substance-use-related risk factor for STDs (Ericksen & Trocki, 1992). Female problem drinkers were $4\frac{1}{2}$ times more likely (adjusted $OR = 4.65$) than other women to have had STDs, independent of the effects of age, race, age at sexual debut, and number of partners.

Most studies indicate that both intravenous and other drug use, including use of crack cocaine, is more frequent among African Americans and Hispanic Americans than among white Americans. For example, the 1988 National Household Survey on Drug Abuse (NHSDA) revealed that lifetime use of crack cocaine was twice as high for African Americans and Hispanic Americans as for white Americans (NIDA, 1990). In addition, most studies suggest an inverse relationship between SES and drug use (Marx, Aral, Rolfs, Sterk, & Kahn, 1991). Other studies have reported an association between higher prevalence of crack cocaine use among racial/ethnic minority adolescents and increased incidence of gonococcal infection (Fullilove, Fullilove, Bowser, & Gross, 1990). In addition, most studies suggest an inverse relationship between SES and drug use (Marx *et al.*, 1991). Published data on alcohol use paint a different picture of race/ethnicity differentials (Grant *et al.*, 1991). Prevalence of alcohol abuse and dependence is apparently greater among white Americans compared to Americans of color. This pattern is valid for both genders and most age groups, for total alcohol dependence and abuse (13.9% among white men and 4.7% among white women compared to 9.3% among men of color and 2.5% among women of color), for alcohol abuse only, for alcohol dependence only, and for combined alcohol dependence with abuse. Alcohol abuse appears inversely related to SES.

The meaning of these reported racial and ethnic group differences in prevalence of drug use is less clear. A more recent reanalysis of the NHSDA data mentioned above, which adjusted for the effects of social and environmental factors, showed that once respondents were grouped into neighborhood clusters, the relative odds of crack use did not differ significantly for African Americans ($RO = 0.85$; CI 0.37–1.93) or Hispanic Americans ($RO = 0.88$; CI 0.47–1.67) compared with white Americans (Lillie-Blanton, Anthony, & Schuster, 1993). This finding is important because it clearly documents the overlapping effects of racial/ethnic status and social context that often cannot be (or are not) differentiated during data analysis and that may result in misinterpretation and misguided targeting of prevention efforts.

The reanalysis by Lillie-Blanton and colleagues also showed that neighborhoods with at least one crack cocaine smoker did not differ greatly in their distributions by education and income than neighborhoods that did not have any crack cocaine smokers. This analysis also raises questions regarding racial/ethnic differences in other risk factors for STDs, which were discussed above. We would expect analyses adjusted for environmental factors to result in significant reductions in race/ethnicity differentials in many behavioral risk factors. Next, we turn our attention to some contextual, environmental, or social factors that may affect STD rates among African Americans and Hispanic Americans.

Societal Determinants of STD Incidence

Determinants of STD rates at the population level include age and gender composition of the population; level of urbanization, volume of internal and external migration; economic change resulting in unemployment, poverty levels; societal upheaval resulting from political conflict and war; sexual mixing patterns, and social status of women (Aral & Holmes, 1991; Holmes & Aral, 1991). In addition, establishment and effective implementation of STD prevention and control programs and availability and accessibility of health services affect incidence of STDs at the population level.

In the United States, both historically and currently, the age and gender composition of African American and Hispanic populations are more conducive to higher STD rates than is that of the white population (Ehrhardt & Wasserheit, 1991; Aral, Johnson, Zaidi, Fichter, & Reynolds, 1983). Both minority racial/ethnic groups have more youthful populations than white Americans. In addition, especially among African Americans, the gender composition of the population is marked by a clear imbalance—an excess of women over men in young, sexually active age groups. The relative scarcity of young men, and particularly economically self-sufficient young men (termed "the male marriageable pool index"), leads to these young men having relatively greater numbers of female partners and is strongly correlated with teenage pregnancy and proportion of female-headed households (Wilson, 1987).

African American and Hispanic populations in the United States are also more concentrated in urban areas, more subject to politically and economically motivated migration, and to a greater extent subject to poverty when compared to the white majority population (U.S. Department of Commerce, 1992a,b). According to Census Bureau estimates, in 1990–1991, 23.4% of Hispanic Americans, 18.4% of African Americans, and 16.6% of white Americans moved. Migration is also associated with SES; 28.7% of the unemployed compared to 18.2% of the employed, and 33.6% of those who rented their homes compared to 8.8% of those who owned their homes, moved in 1990–1991 (DeAre, 1992). In addition, both members of racial/ethnic minority groups and persons with lower SES have a greater likelihood of living in neighborhoods marked by crime and violence. The social status of women tends to be relatively lower among persons of lower SES and among Hispanic Americans, but not African Americans. Availability of health care services is in general greater for persons of higher SES and white Americans. The health care accessibility gap between white Americans and African Americans has been declining significantly in recent years (J. Williams & Torrens, 1988). Hispanic Americans apparently have the least access to health care services. This lack of access to health care is particularly marked among those living below the poverty level. In 1991, among poor persons, those of Hispanic origin were more likely to be uninsured (40.5%) than whites (31.2%) or African Americans (22.6%) (U.S. Department of Commerce, 1992b).

In the case of sexually transmitted infections, membership in racial/ethnic minority groups, to a large extent, influences the pool of potential sex partners from which one may choose. Similarly, SES probably affects the pool of potential sex partners (Ramstedt, Giesecke, Forssman, & Granath, 1991). A sex partner pool is marked by a given prevalence of specific STDs and therefore determines the frequency with which persons choosing sex partners from that particular pool are exposed to sexually transmitted pathogens. Thus, some persons who do not engage in risky sexual behaviors may in fact be at high risk for STDs because their partners come from high-prevalence partner pools. For example, even though the incidence of both bacterial and viral STDs is higher among African Americans compared to whites, African American women do not report greater numbers of current partners than do white women (Seidman, Mosher, & Aral, 1992). Nevertheless, the probability of exposure to a sexually transmitted pathogen per sexual encounter is higher among African American women than among white women. African American women who have two or three lifetime sex partners have a 100% increased likelihood of developing acute PID compared to those with one lifetime partner; the increased risk is only 50% among white women (Aral et al., 1991b). This finding suggests that for many African American women, an especially important risk factor for STDs may be the high prevalence of infection among their sex partners, largely African American men (Seidman & Aral, 1992).

Finally, racial/ethnic status by itself is probably less meaningful than racial/ethnic status in combination with other sociodemographic characteristics in influencing sexual behavior and STD risk. The effects of race/ethnicity on sexual behavior and STD risk may be conditional on the values of other parameters with which it is combined. For example, among women, being white (compared to African American) may be associated with having more or fewer sex partners, depending on level of educational attainment (Seidman *et al.,* 1992). Similarly, the effects of race/ethnicity on sexual behavior may depend on gender. In one study of STD clinic attendees, men's sexual behavior varied by age, but not by race; younger men had more partners and were less discriminating in their partner recruitment. In the same population, women's sexual behavior varied by race, but not by age; African American women had fewer partners and were more discriminating in partner selection (Aral et al., 1991c). It is conceivable that measurement of individual characteristics and comparisons across individuals, which comprise an overwhelming majority of studies in STDs and HIV infection, do not adequately reflect the complex and powerful effects of sociopolitical environment on health in their entirety (Rose, 1985). Analyses conducted at the population level may indicate that effects of environments of poverty, social disadvantage, powerlessness, and racial/ethnic minority status may interact synergistically in producing negative health effects. Population-level approaches show that as socioeconomic conditions in a population deteriorate, rates of infectious diseases rise (McKeown, 1976, 1979; Fahs, 1991). In the United States, in the past decade, rates of poverty have increased and rates of infectious diseases, and especially STDs, including AIDS, have risen dramatically in populations in poverty (Swenson, 1992).

Interactions among Gender, Race/Ethnicity, and Poverty as Determinants of STD Incidence

The number of persons below the official government poverty level was 35.7 million in 1991, a figure 2.1 million higher than the 33.6 million poor in 1990. The poverty rate was 14.2% in 1991, significantly higher than the 13.5% poverty rate in 1990 (U.S. Department of Commerce, 1992b).

Children are overrepresented among the poor, and the elderly are underrepresented; children under 18 years of age comprised 40.2% of the poor in 1991. The poverty rate for children under 18 was 21.8% in 1991, higher than the poverty rate for other age groups. Compared to the age composition of the nonpoor population, the age composition of the poor population is remarkably more youthful, a characteristic of populations that is conducive to higher STD rates.

The age composition of the population below the poverty level varies by race/ethnicity. In the United States, the population of Hispanic origin is the most youthful of all racial/ethnic groups, with 34% below age 18 and 47% below age 25. In comparison, 48% of the Hispanic population below the poverty level is below age 18 and 60% is below age 25. Similarly, 33% of African Americans in the United States are below age 18 and 44% are below age 25. The corresponding figures for the African American population below the poverty level are 46% and 57%, respectively. The least youthful of United States populations is the white majority, with 24% below age 18 and 34% below age 25; the white population below the poverty level is more youthful, however, with 37% below age 18 and 43% below age 25. Thus, while populations in poverty and racial/ethnic minority populations are both characterized by youthful compositions, the joint distribution of poverty and race/ethnicity tends to magnify each of these patterns. Racial/ethnic minority populations below poverty level have the most youthful age compositions that are most conducive to high STD rates.

The gender composition of the population below the poverty level is of relevance as well. The poverty rate is higher among women (16%) than men (12.3%). In the United States, the number of men of Hispanic origin equals the number of women of Hispanic origin; thus, the sex ratio of the Hispanic population is 1.00. Conversely, both the African American population and the white population are marked by a relative scarcity of men. The African American sex ratio is 0.88 and the white sex ratio is 0.95. The sex ratio for the American population as a whole is 0.95, indicating a slight excess of women. In contrast, the sex ratio of the population below the poverty level is 0.73, indicative of a much greater excess of women in poverty. Such gender imbalance usually correlates with high STD rates. The gender imbalance of the African American population in poverty is particularly marked, and a sex ratio of 0.69, compared to a sex ratio of 0.73 among whites below the poverty level and 0.84 among Hispanics below the poverty level. Thus, the joint distributions in the population of age, gender, and poverty create a sizable excess of poor, young, minority women, especially poor, young, African American women, over men.

CONCLUSIONS

An important factor that contributes to increasing levels of HIV infection among women is other STDs. Infections with other sexually transmitted pathogens also contribute to higher levels of HIV prevalence among women of racial/ethnic minorities compared to white women, and among women of lower socioeconomic status compared to women of higher income and education. Current HIV seroprevalence rates are highest among minority women, particularly in the southeastern United States. Rates of STD are also highest in these same population groups. Available data on gender and race ethnicity differentials in behavioral determinants of HIV infection and other STDs paint an incomplete picture. Overall, women are increasingly burdened by STDs, including HIV infection, even though prevalence of risk behaviors is lower among women than among men. Some individual behaviors that increase STD risk such as multiple partners and drug use are observed more frequently among African Americans and Hispanic Americans, and among persons of lower SES, while other risk behaviors such as higher frequency of sexual intercourse, problem drinking, sexual intercourse during menses, and alcohol use during sexual intercourse are observed more frequently among white Americans. Similarly, some preventive behaviors that decrease STD risk, such as condom use, are reported by a greater proportion of African Americans, and of white Americans, than of Hispanic Americans, and by persons of higher SES, while other preventive behaviors such as male circumcision are most frequent among white Americans. In most cases, the risk and preventive behaviors that are more frequently reported by persons of minority racial/ethnic status are also more frequently reported by persons of lower SES.

Race/ethnicity and SES differentials in the societal factors that influence STD incidence paint a relatively more complete and consistent picture. All societal factors that increase STD incidence, including youthful age composition, sex ratio imbalance, and lower social status of women, are observed to a greater extent in African American and Hispanic American populations and in the population below the poverty level. Of the societal factors that decrease STD incidence in the population, those on which we have data, such as availability of health care, characterize the white American population and the population above the poverty level to a much greater extent than the African American or Hispanic American populations or the population below the poverty level.

These observations suggest a three-tiered programmatic approach to the control of HIV infection among women and particularly among minority women. In the short term, significantly expanding access to nonstigmatizing STD prevention services may have the greatest impact. These services should include timely diagnosis and treatment of STDs, notifying and treating exposed partners, increasing condom availability, and providing information about the links between STDs and severe complications, such as increased risk of HIV infection. In the medium term, developing and implementing effective community-based interventions to reduce risk behaviors of individuals, including male partners, and to increase their preventive behaviors, is essential. In the long term, societal changes to reduce the levels of poverty, inequity, and gender and racial/ethnic discrimination are needed. Changes at this level are the most difficult to accomplish, but probably they are the most important to realize, in that they will have the greatest positive impact not only on levels of HIV infection and other STDs, but also on the overall health and well-being of men and women and of minority *and* majority populations.

REFERENCES

American Medical Women's Association (1994). Women unconcerned about STDs. Reuters and UPI, February 14, 1994.

Aral, S. O. (1992). Sexual behavior of women as risk factor for reproductive tract infections. In A. Germain, J. N. Wasserheit, P. Piot, & K. K. Holmes (Eds.), *Reproductive tract infections in the third world: National and international policy implications* (pp. 185–198). New York: Plenum Press.

Aral, S. O., & Cates, W., Jr. (1989). The multiple dimensions of sexual behavior as a risk factor for STD: The sexually experienced are not necessarily sexually active. *Sexually Transmitted Diseases, 16*(4), 173–177.

Aral, S. O., Fullilove, R., & Coutinho, R. (1991a). Societal factors affecting STD risk behaviors. In J. N. Wasserheit, S. O. Aral, & K. K. Holmes (Eds.), *Research issues in human behavior and STD in the AIDS era* (pp. 161–176). Washington, DC: American Society of Microbiology Publications.

Aral, S. O., & Holmes, K. K. (1990). Epidemiology of sexual behavior and sexually transmitted diseases. In K K. Holmes, P.-A. Mardh, P. F. Sparling, P. J. Wiesner, W. Cates, S. M. Lemon, & W. E. Stamm (Eds.), *Sexually transmitted diseases,* Vol. 2 (p. 31). New York: McGraw-Hill.

Aral, S. O., & Holmes, K. K. (1991). Sexually transmitted diseases in the AIDS era. *Scientific American, 1991,* 62–69.

Aral, S. O., Johnson, R. E., Zaidi, A., Fichtner, R., & Reynolds, G. (1983). Demographic effects on sexually transmitted diseases in the 70s: The problem could be worse. *Sexually Transmitted Diseases, 10*(2), 100–101.

Aral, S. O., Mosher, W. D., & Cates, W., Jr. (1991b). Self-reported pelvic inflammatory disease among women of reproductive age: United States, 1982–1988. *JAMA, 266*(18), 2570–2573.

Aral, S. O., Mosher, W. D., & Cates, W., Jr. (1992). Vaginal douching among reproductive age women in the United States, 1988. *American Journal of Public Health, 82*(2), 210–214.

Aral, S. O., Mosher, W. D., Horn, M., & Cates, W., Jr. (1986). Screening for sexually transmitted diseases by family planning providers: Is it adequate and appropriate? *Family Planning Perspectives, 18*(6), 255–258.

Aral, S. O., Soskolne, V., Joesoef, R. M., & O'Reilly, K. R. (1991c). Sex partner selection as risk factor for STD: Clustering of risky modes. *Sexually Transmitted Diseases, 18*(1), 10–17.

Berger, J. R., Hensley, G., & Moskowitz, L. (1989). Syphilitic myelopathy with human immunodeficiency virus: A treatable cause of spinal cord disease (abstract W.B.P.51). Fifth International AIDS Conference, Montreal.

Berry, C. D., Hooton, T. M., & Collier, A. C. (1987). Neurologic relapse after benzathine penicillin therapy for secondary syphilis in a patient with HIV infection. *New England Journal of Medicine, 316,* 1587–1589.

Bishop, P. E., McMillan, A., & Fletcher, S. (1990). Immunological study of condylomata acuminata in men infected with the human immunodeficiency virus. *International Journal of STD and AIDS, 1,* 28–31.

Cameron, D. W., Lourdes, J. D., Gregory, M. M., Simonsen, J. N., D'Costa, L. J., Ronald, A. R., Maitha, G. M., Gakinya, M. N., Cheang, M., Ndinya-Achola, J. O., Piot, P., & Brunham, R. C. (1989). Female-to-male transmission of human immunodeficiency virus type 1: Risk factors for seroconversions in men. *Lancet, 2,* 403–407.

Cameron, D. W., Plummer, F. A., D'Costa, L. J., Ndinya-Achola, J. O., & Ronald, A. R. (1988). Prediction of HIV infection by treatment failure for chancroid, a genital ulcer disease (abstract 7637). Fourth International AIDS Conference, Stockholm.

Cannon, R. O., Hook, E. W., Nahmias, A. J., Lee, F. K., Glasser, D., & Quinn, T. C. (1988). Association of herpes simplex virus type 2 with HIV infection in heterosexual patients attending sexually transmitted disease clinics (abstract 458). Fourth International AIDS Conference, Stockholm.

Cannon, R. O., Quinn, T., Rompalo, A., Glasser, D., Groseclose, S., & Hook, E. (1989). Syphilis is strongly associated with HIV infection in Baltimore STD clinic patients independent of risk group (abstract Th.A.O. 18). Fifth International AIDS Conference, Montreal.

Catania, J. A., Coates, R. J., Stall, R., Turner, H., Peterson, J., Hearst, N., Dolcini, M. M., Hudes, E., Gagnon, J., Wiley, J., & Groves, R. (1992). Prevalence of AIDS related risk factors and condom use in the United States. *Science, 258,* 1101–1106.

Caumes, E., Janier, M., Janseen, F., Rybojad, M., Dallot, A., & Morel, P. (1989). Atypical secondary syphilis in HIV seropositive patients (abstract W.B.P. 49). Fifth International AIDS Conference, Montreal.

Centers for Disease Control and Prevention (1993). Facts about women and HIV/AIDS, October 1993. Atlanta: Office of the Associate Director, HIV/AIDS, Centers for Disease Control and Prevention.

Centers for Disease Control and Prevention (1994). National HIV serosurveillance summary: Results through 1992, Vol. 3. Atlanta: U.S. Department of Health and Human Services.

Chiphangwi, J., Dallabetta, G., Saah, A., Liomba, G., & Miott, D. (1990). Risk factors for HIV-1 infection in pregnant women in Malawi (abstract Th.C. 98). Sixth International AIDS Conference, San Francisco.

Corey, L. (1990). Genital herpes. In K. K. Holmes (Ed.), *Sexually transmitted diseases* (pp. 391–413). New York: McGraw-Hill.

Darrow, W. W. (1976). Venereal infections in three ethnic groups in Sacramento. *American Journal of Public Health, 66,* 446–450.

Darrow, W. W. (1979). Social stratification, sexual behavior, and the sexually transmitted diseases. *Sexually Transmitted Diseases, 6,* 228–230.

Darrow, W. W., Echenberg, D. F., Jaffe, H. W., O'Malley, P. M., Byers, R. H., Getchell, J. P., & Curran, J. W. (1987). Risk factors for human immunodeficiency virus (HIV) infections in homosexual men. *American Journal of Public Health, 77,* 479–483.

DeAre, D. (1992). Geographical mobility: March 1990–March 1991 current population reports, population characteristics, P20–463. Washington, DC: Economics and Statistics Administration, Bureau of the Census, U.S. Department of Commerce.

Dryfoos, J. G. (1991). Preventing high risk behavior. *American Journal of Public Health, 81*(2), 157–158.

Duncan, W. C. (1989). Failure of erythromycin to cure secondary syphilis in a patient infected with the human immunodeficiency virus. *Archives of Dermatology, 125,* 82–84.

Ehrhardt, A. A., & Wasserheit, J. N. (1991). Age, gender, and sexual risk behaviors for sexually transmitted diseases in the United States: Principles of sexual behavior over the life cycle: Effects of age and gender. In J. N. Wasserheit, S. O. Aral, & K. K. Holmes (Eds.), *Research issues in human behavior and sexually transmitted diseases in the AIDS era* (pp. 97–121). Washington, DC: American Society for Microbiology.

Elifson, K., Soles, J., Sweet, H., & Darrow, W. (1989). Risk factors for HIV infection among male prostitutes in Atlanta (abstract W.A.P. 38). Fifth International AIDS Conference, Montreal.

Ericksen, K. P., & Trocki, K. F. (1992). Behavioral risk factors for sexually transmitted diseases in American households. *Social Science and Medicine, 34*(8), 843–853.

Ehrlich, K., Mills, J., Chatis, P., Mertz, G. J., Busch, D. F., Follansbee, S. E., Grant, R. M., & Crumpacker, C. S. (1989). Acyclovir-resistant herpes simplex virus infections in patients with the acquired immunodeficiency syndrome. *New England Journal of Medicine, 320,* 293–296.

Fahs, M. C. (1991). The economic consequences of inaction. In Kevin M. Cahil, (Ed.), *Imminent peril: Public health in a declining economy* (pp. 65–80). New York: Twentieth Century Fund Press.

Feingold, A. R., Vermund, S. H., Burk, R. D., Kelley, K. F., Schrages, L. K., Schreiber, K., Munk, G., Friedland, G. H., & Klein, R. S. (1990). Cervical cytologic abnormalities and papillomavirus in women infected with human immunodeficiency virus. *Journal of Acquired Immune Deficiency Syndromes, 3,* 896–903.

Forrest, J. D., & Singh, S. (1990). The sexual and reproductive behavior of American women, 1982–1988. *Family Planning Perspectives, 22*(5), 206–212.

Frazer, I. H., Medley, G., Crapper, R. M., Brown, T. C., & Mackay, I. R. (1986). The association between anorectal dysplasia, human papillomavirus, and human immunodeficiency virus infection in homosexual men. *Lancet, 2,* 657–660.

Fullilove, R. E., Fullilove, M. T., Bowser, B. P., & Gross, S. A. (1990). Risk of sexually transmitted disease among black adolescent crack users in Oakland and San Francisco, Calif. *JAMA, 263,* 851–855.

Greenblatt, R. M., Lukehart, S. A., Plummer, F. A., Quinn, T. C., Critchlow, C. W., Ashley, R. L., D'Costa, L. J., Ndinya-Achola, J. O., Corey, L., & Ronald, A. R. (1989). Genital ulceration as a risk factor for human immunodeficiency virus infection. *AIDS, 2,* 47–50.

Hayes, C. G., Manaloto, C. R., Basaca-Sevilla, V., Padre, L. P., Laughlin, L. W., O'Rourke, T. K., Espinosa, G. E., Andrada, A. B., Mejia, P., & Cano, P. (1990). Epidemiology of HIV infection among prostitutes in the Philippines. *Journal of Acquired Immune Deficiency Syndromes, 3,* 913–920.

Holmberg, S. D., Stewart, J. A., Gerber, A. R., Byers, R. H., Lee, F. K., O'Malley, P. M., & Nahmias, A. J. (1988b). Prior herpes simplex virus type 2 infection as a risk factor for HIV infection. *JAMA, 259,* 1048–1050.

Holmes, K. K., & Aral, S. O. (1991). Behavioral interventions in developing countries. In J. N. Wasserheit, S. O., Aral, & K. K. Holmes, (Eds.), *Research issues in human behavior and STD in* the AIDS era (pp. 318–344). Washington, DC: American Society of Microbiology Publications.

Irwin, K., Rice, R., O'Sullivan, M., Sperling, R., Brodman, M., Moorman, A., & the Multicenter HIV and PID Study Group (Centers for Disease Control and Prevention, Atlanta; University of Miami; Mt. Sinai Medical Center, New York) (1993). The clinical presentation and course of pelvic inflammatory diseases in HIV^+ and HIV^- women: Primary results of a multicenter study. Ninth International Conference on AIDS, Berlin.

Johns, D. R., Tierney, M., & Felsenstein, D. (1987). Alteration in the natural history of neurosyphilis by concurrent infection with the human immunodeficiency virus. *New England Journal of Medicine, 316,* 1569–1572.

Johnson, R. E., Natmias, A. J., Magder, L. S., Lee, F. K., Brooks, C. A., & Snowden, C. B. (1989). A seroepidemiologic survey of the prevalence of herpes simplex virus type 2 infection in the U.S. *New England Journal of Medicine, 321,* 7–12.

Kamenga, M., Toure, C. K., N'gbichi, J. M., Kreiss, J., St. Louis, M., & DeCock, K. (1993). Projet SIDA, Kinshasa, Zaire (University of Washington, Seattle: CIIU de Treichville, Abidjan, Côte d'Ivoire); Projet Retro-CI, Abidjan, Côte d'Ivoire (Centers for Disease Control and Prevention, Atlanta). Ninth International Conference on AIDS, Berlin.

Kaslow, R. A., VanRaden, M., DeLoria, M., Zeger, S., Dudley, J., Alwood, K., Wolinski, S., & Ho, M. (1989). Do clinical herpes simplex virus (HSV) and varicella-zoster (VSV) infections accelerate HIV-1-induced immunodeficiency? (abstract Th.A.P. 100). Fifth International AIDS Conference, Montreal.

Kegeles, S., Catania, J., Peterson, J., Marin, B., Fullilove, M., Hulley, S., & Coates, T. (1991). *What about condoms?: Black, Hispanic, and white views from a population-based sample.* San Francisco: UCSF Center for AIDS Prevention Studies (CAPS).

Kingsley, L. A., Armstrong, J., Rahman, A., Ho, M., & Rinaldo, C. R. (1990). No association between herpes simplex virus type-2 seropositivity or anogenital lesions and HIV seroconversion among homosexual men. *Journal of Acquired Immune Deficiency Syndromes, 3,* 773–779.

Kost, K., & Forrest, J. D. (1992). American women's sexual behavior and exposure to risk of sexually transmitted diseases. *Family Planning Perspectives, 24*(6), 224–254.

Kramer, M., Aral, S. O., & Curran, J. C. (1980). Self reported behavior patterns of STD patients. *American Journal of Public Health, 70,* 997.

Kreiss, J. K., Koech, D., Plummer, F. A., Holmes, K. K., Lightfoote, M., Piot, P., Ronald, A. R., Ndinya-Achola, J. O., D'Costa, L. J., & Roberts, P. (1986). AIDS virus infection in Nairobi prostitutes. *New England Journal of Medicine, 314,* 414–418.

Ku, L., Sonenstein, F. L., & Pleck, J. H. (1992). HIV and STD risk behaviors of young men: 1988–1991. Paper presented at the Annual Meeting of the Population Association of America, Denver, May 1992.

Ku, L., Sonenstein, F. L., & Pleck, J. H. (1993). Young men's risk behaviors for HIV infection and sexually transmitted diseases, 1988 through 1991. *American Journal of Public Health, 83*(11), 1609–1615.

Laga, M., Icenogle, J. P., Marsella, R., Manoka, A. T., Nzila, N., Ryder, R., Vermund, S. H., Heyward, W. L., Nelson, A., & Reeves, W. C. (1992). Genital papillomavirus infection and cervical dysplasia—opportunistic complications of HIV infection. *International Journal of Cancer, 50,* 45–48.

Laga, M., Nzila, N., Manoka, A. T., Malele, M., Bush, T. J., Behets, F., Heyward, W. L., Piot, P., & Ryder, R. (1990). Non ulcerative sexually transmitted diseases (STD) as risk factors for HIV infection (abstract Th.C. 97). Sixth International AIDS Conference, San Francisco.

Latif, A. S. (1989). Epidemiology and control of chancroid (abstract 66). Eighth Conference of the International Society for Sexually Transmitted Disease Research, Copenhagen.

LaVigne, J., Thomas, G., Geraci, A., & Levy, M. (1990). Occurrence of malignancy in the setting of anogenital warts in the gay male population (abstract S.B. 520). Sixth International AIDS Conference, San Francisco.

Lillie-Blanton, M., Anthony, J. C., & Schuster, C. R. (1993). Probing the meaning of racial/ethnic group comparisons in crack cocaine smoking. *JAMA, 269*(8), 993–997.

Marx, R., Aral, S. O., Rolfs, R. T., Sterk, C. E., & Kahn, J. G. (1981). Crack, sex, and STD. *Sexually Transmitted Diseases, 18*(2), 92–101.

Mascola, L., Pelosi, R., Blount, J. H., Binkin, N. J., Alexander, C. E., & Cates, W. (1984). Congenital syphilis, why is it still occurring? *JAMA, 252,* 1719–1722.

McCormack, W. M., Rosner, B., McComb, D. E., Evrard, J. R., & Zinner, S. H. (1985). Infection with *Chlamydia trachomatis* in female college students. *American Journal of Epidemiology, 121,* 107–115.

McKeown, T. (1976). *The modern rise of population.* New York: Academic Press.

McKeown, T. (1979). *The role of medicine.* Princeton, NJ: Princeton University Press.

McMillan, A., & Bishop, P. E. (1989). Clinical course of anogenital warts in men infected with human immunodeficiency virus. *Genitourinary Medicine, 65,* 225–228.

Milburn, P. B., Brandsma, J. L., Goldsman, C. I., Teplitz, E. D., & Heilman, E. I. (1988). Disseminated warts and evolving squamous cell carcinoma in a patient with acquired immunodeficiency syndrome. *Journal of the American Academy of Dermatology, 19,* 4019–4105.

Mosher, W. D., & Aral, S. O. (1991). Testing for sexually transmitted diseases among women of reproductive age: United States, 1988. *Family Planning Perspectives, 23*(5), 216–221.

Muggiasca, M. L., Conti, E., Ravasi, L., Imperiale, D., Agarossi, A., & Conti, M. (1989). Human immunodeficiency virus and human papilloma virus in the development of cervical intraepithelial neoplasia (CIN) in past intravenous drug abusers (PIVDA) women (abstract M.B.P. 56). Fifth International AIDS Conference, Montreal.

NIDA (National Institute on Drug Abuse) (1990). *NIDA national survey on drug abuse: Main findings in 1988.* Washington, DC: National Institute on Drug Abuse, U.S. Department of Health and Human Services Publication No. ADM 90–1692.

Penkower, L., Dew, M. A., Kingsley, L., Becker, J. T., Satz, P., Schaerf, F. W., & Shendar, K. (1991). Behavioral, health, and psychosocial factors and risk for HIV infection among sexually active, homosexual men: The Multicenter AIDS Cohort Study. *American Journal of Public Health, 81*(2), 194–196.

Phair, J., Jacobson, L., Detels, R., Rinaldo, C., Saah, A., Schrager, L., & Munoz, A. (1992). Acquired immune deficiency syndrome occurring within 5 years of infection with human immunodeficiency virus type-1: The Multicenter AIDS Cohort Study. *Journal of Acquired Immune Deficiency Syndromes, 5,* 490–496.

Piot, P., Van Dyck, E., Ryder, R. W., Nzila, N., & Laga, M. (1989). Serum antibody to *Haemophilus ducreyi* as a risk factor for HIV in Africa, but not in Europe (abstract M.A.O. 32). Fifth International AIDS Conference, Montreal.

Plummer, F. A., Simonsen, J. N., Cameron, D. W., Ndinya-Achola, J. O., Kreiss, J. K., Gakinya, M. N., Waiyaki, P., Cheang, M., Piot, P., & Ronald, A. R. (1991). Co-factors in male-to-female transmission of HIV. *Journal of Infectious Diseases, 163,* 233–239.

Plummer, F. A., Simonsen, J. N., Chubb, H., Slaney, L., Kimata, J., Bosire, M., Ndinya-Achola, J. O., & Ngugi, E. N. (1989). Epidemiological evidence for the development of serovar-specific immunity after gonococcal infection. *Journal of Clinical Investigation, 83,* 1472–1476.

Potterat, J. J., Rothenberg, R. B., Woodhouse, D. T., Muth, J. B., Pratts, C. J., & Fogle, J. S. (1985). Gonorrhea as a social disease. *Sexually Transmitted Diseases, 12,* 25–32.

Quale, J., Tellitz, E., & Augenbraun, M. (1990). Atypical presentation of chancroid in a patient infected with the human immunodeficiency virus. *American Journal of Medicine, 88*(5), 43N–44N.

Quinn, T. C., Glasser, D., Cannon, R. O., Matuszak, D. L., Dunning, R. W., Campbell, C. H., Israel, E., Fauci, L. S., & Hook, E. W. (1988). Human immunodeficiency virus infection among patients attending clinics for sexually transmitted diseases. *New England Journal of Medicine, 318,* 197–204.

Quinnan, G. V., Masur, H., Rook, A. H., Armstrong, G., Frederick, W. R., Epstein, J., Manischewitz, J. F., Macher, A. M., Jackson, L., & Ames, J. (1984). Herpes virus infections in the acquired immune deficiency syndrome. *JAMA, 252,* 72–77.

Radecki, S. E., & Bernstein, G. S. (1989). Use of clinic versus private family planning care by low income women: Access, cost, and patient satisfaction. *American Journal of Public Health, 79*(6), 692–697.

Ramstedt, K., Giesecke, J., Forssman, L., & Granath, F. (1991). Choice of sexual partners according to rate of partner change and social class of the partners. *International Journal of STD and AIDS, 2,* 428–431.

Rolfs, R., Hindersho, E., Hackett, K., Augerber, M., Bolan, G., Johnson, S., Wagner, K., Brady, W., Joseph, M., Larson, S., & the Syphilis & HIV Study Group (1993). Treatment of early syphilis in HIV-infected and HIV-uninfected patients—Preliminary report of the Syphilis & HIV Study Group (Centers for Disease Control and Prevention, Atlanta, Philadelphia, Baltimore, Brooklyn, San Francisco, and Bethesda, MD).

Rose, G. (1985). Sick individuals and sick populations. *International Journal of Epidemiology, 14,* 32–33.

Rothenberg, R. (1986). The geography of syphilis: A demonstration of epidemiological diversity. In R. Marriset & E. Kusstah (Eds.), *Advances in sexually transmitted diseases: Diagnosis and treatment* (pp. 125–133). Utrecht: VNU Science Press.

Rudlinger, R., Grob, R., Buchmann, P., Christen, D., & Steiner, R. (1988). Anogenital warts of the condyloma acuminatum type in HIV-positive patients. *Dermatologica, 176,* 277–288.

Schachter, J., Stoner, E., & Moncada, J. (1983). Screening for chlamydial infections in women attending family planning clinics. *Western Journal of Medicine, 138,* 375–379.

Schafer, A., Wolfgang, F., Mielke, M., Schwartlander, B., & Koch, M. A. (1990). Increased frequency of cervical dysplasia/neoplasia in HIV-infected women is related to the extent of immunosuppression (abstract S.B. 519). Sixth International AIDS Conference, San Francisco.

Schrager, L. K., Friedland, G. H., Maude, D., Schreiber, K., Adachi, A., Pizzuti, D. J ., Koss, L. A., & Klein, R. S. (1989). Cervical and vaginal squamous cell abnormalities in women infected with human immunodeficiency virus. *Journal of Acquired Immune Deficiency Syndromes, 2,* 570–575.

Seidman, S. N., & Aral, S. O. (1992). Sub-population differentials in STD transmission (letter to editor). *American Journal of Public Health, 82*(9), 1297.

Seidman, S. N., Mosher, W. D., & Aral, S. O. (1992). Women with multiple sexual partners: USA, 1988. *American Journal of Public Health, 82,* 1388–1394.

Simonsen, J. N., Cameron, D. W., Gakinya, M. N., Ndinya-Achola, J. O., D'Costa, L. J., Karasira, P., Cheang, M., Ronald, A. R., Piot, P., & Plummer, F. A. (1988). Human immunodeficiency virus infection among men with sexually transmitted diseases. *New England Journal of Medicine, 319,* 274–278.

Sonenstein, F. L., Pleck, J. H., & Ku, L. C. (1989). Sexual activity, condom use, and AIDS awareness among adolescent males. *Family Planning Perspectives, 21*(4), 152–158.

Sooy, C. D., & Mills, J. (1988). Herpes virus infection presenting as giant herpetic nasal ulcers in AIDS (abstract 7096). Fourth International AIDS Conference, Stockholm.

Soskolne, V., Aral, S. O., Magder, L. S., & Bowen, G. S. (1991). Condom use with regular and casual sex partners: Women attending family planning clinics. *Family Planning Perspectives, 23,*(5), 222–225.

Stamm, W. E., Handsfield, H. H., Rompalo, A. M., Ashley, R. L., Roberts, P. L., & Corey, L. (1988). The association between genital ulcer disease and acquisition of HIV infection in homosexual men. *JAMA, 260,* 1429–1433.

Swenson, R. M. (1992). The lessons of Belle Glade. *Annals of Internal Medicine, 116,* 343–346.

Tanfer, K., & Aral, S. O. (1995). Sexual intercourse during menses: Risk factor for STD (in preparation).

Thomas, G., Geraci, A., Lavigne, J., & Levy, M. (1990). Recurrent anogenital warts and HIV status (abstract Th.B. 362). Sixth International AIDS Conference, San Francisco.

U.S. Department of Commerce (1992a). Money income of households, families, and persons in the United States: 1991. In *Current population reports on consumer income, August 1992* (pp. 60–180). Washington, DC: Economics and Statistics Administration, Bureau of the Census, U.S. Department of Commerce.

U.S. Department of Commerce (1992b). Poverty in the United States: 1991. In *Current population reports of consumer income, August 1992* (pp. 60–181). Washington, DC: Economics and Statistics Administration, Bureau of the Census, U.S. Department of Commerce.

Van Raden, M., Kaslow, R., Kingsley, L., Detels, R., Narer, J., Murphy, R., & Liang, K. Y. (1989). The Multicenter AIDS Cohort Study: The role of ulcerative genital diseases in promoting acquisition of HIV-1 by homosexual men (abstract Th.A.O. 17). Fifth International AIDS Conference, Montreal.

Wasser, S. C., Guinn, M., & Fleming, P. (1993). Urban–nonurban distribution of HIV infection in childbearing women in the United States. *Journal of Acquired Immune Deficiency Syndromes, 6*(9), 1035–1042.

Wasserheit, J. N. (1992). Epidemiological synergy: Interrelationships between human immunodeficiency virus infection and other sexually transmitted diseases. *Sexually Transmitted Diseases, 19*(2), 61–77.

Webster, A., Grundy, J. E., Lee, C. A., Cook, D. G., Emergy, V. C., Kernoff, P. B., & Griffiths, P. B. (1989). Cytomegalovirus infection and progression to AIDS [letter, comment]. *Lancet, 2,* 681.

Williams, J., & Torrens, P. R. (1988). *Introduction to health services.* Albany, NY: Delmar Publishers.

Wilson, J. W. (1987). *The truly disadvantaged: The inner city, the underclass, and public policy.* Chicago: University of Chicago Press.

Wortley, P. M., Chu, S. Y., Diaz, T., Ward, J. W., Doyle, B., Davidson, A. J., Checko, P. J., Herr, M., Conti, L., Fann, S. A., Sorvillo, F., Mokotoff, E., Levy, A., Hermann, P., & Norris-Walczak, E. (1995). HIV testing patterns: Where, why and when were persons reported with AIDS tested for HIV? *AIDS, 9*(5), 487–492.

Youle, M. M., Hawkins, D. A., Collins, P., Shanson, D. C., Evans, R., Oliver, N., & Lawrence, A. (1988). Acyclovir-resistant herpes in AIDS patients treated with Foscarnet. *Lancet, 2,* 341–342.

Zierler, S., Feingold, L., Laufer, D., Valentgas, P., Kantrowitz-Gordon, J., & Mayer, K. (1991). Adult survivors of childhood sexual abuse and subsequent risk of HIV infection. *American Journal of Public Health, 81,* 572–575.

3

Women-Centered Prevention Techniques and Technologies

ERICA L. GOLLUB

INTRODUCTION

> The experience with the [female condom] allowed us to re-assess our decision-making capacity, our right to health services, the importance of our bodies as our work tool, the importance of self-care and the perception of risk as key factors to move ourselves towards self-protection and prevention. This device is of great help to prevent HIV infection, but more important, it can help liberate that woman who is now a victim of machismo, infected not only with the virus, but also mentally and spiritually with a selfishness that has no place in a couple's relationship (Colimoro, 1993).

> . . . AIDS or not, more women have joined the game, as poverty and unemployment continue to grow. Governments or anybody else who is serious about protecting prostitutes from AIDS, need to address women's economic problems, so that women can afford to walk out of a job on the issue of condoms, or walk out of the game altogether (English Collective of Prostitutes, 1992).

> Meanwhile, being a male of my culture, he was very macho: no condoms. I was his woman, his wife, his property—testimony of Ana, a New York City woman living with HIV, before the U.S. Food and Drug Administration on the female condom, December 1992.

The meaning of AIDS for women has been expressed in different voices, by women of greatly diverse backgrounds and cultures. Yet this epidemic in women will always represent for us one of the most tangible signs of our oppression. This chapter is written with a sense of urgency and in the spirit of unity. Urgency because, while behavioral intervention

ERICA L. GOLLUB • AIDS Activities Coordinating Office, Department of Public Health, Philadelpha, PA 19146.

Women at Risk: Issues in the Primary Prevention of AIDS, edited by Ann O'Leary and Loretta Sweet Jemmott. Plenum Press, New York, 1995.

efforts—encouraging abstinence, monogamy, and male condom use—directed at men and women continue unabated, there have been only modest advances in the actual level of protection achieved for the population. The success stories are usually limited to highly labor-intensive programs that will be difficult if not impossible to support on a wide scale both in the United States and around the world. The most recent surveys from the United States and Europe indicate that, among heterosexuals, condoms are used consistently by 10% or fewer of individuals, with slightly larger percentages reporting occasional condom use (Moatti, Bajos, Durbec, Menard, & Serrand, 1991; Campbell & Baldwin, 1991; Catania et al., 1992; Spira, Bajos, & the ACSF Investigators, 1992; Leigh, Temple & Trocki, 1993). It is clear that in most settings around the world, major political and social changes must occur to increase the level of control a woman has over her own well-being and to support men in making fundamental changes in their social and sexual behaviors that put women at risk from AIDS and other sexually transmitted infections (Worth, 1989; Stein, 1990; Hankins, 1990). Indeed, some suggest dismissing entire governments for their lack of attention and action in this area (Zewdie, 1994).

Yet this chapter also appeals to the reader in a spirit of unity and cooperation, because behavioral, social, and political changes that have been realized, no matter how small-scale, are laudable. Without the collective action on the part of small groups and, indeed, individuals, the slow evolution of changes leading to increasing empowerment of women in society will not occur. Work among heterosexual men must expand. In fact, concentrating exclusively on women's options for prevention of AIDS and other sexually transmitted diseases (STDs) may have the unintended effect of stigmatizing women and placing all responsibility on them for protecting the health of their sexual partnerships (Strebel, 1993). This situation has already arisen in the case of male condom use, where women have often been indirectly blamed for not effectively persuading their partners to practice safe sex. Thus, the time is ripe for a multitude of strategies confronting women's institutionalized oppression and consequent vulnerability to reproductive tract infection and other poor health outcomes. Such a strategic approach necessarily involves, on one front, the development of actual tangible protection methods women control with their own hands and, on another, the rigorous pursuit of longer-term behavioral and societal change.

This chapter reviews the data pertaining to barrier methods and other protective strategies now available for use by women. Although contraception is probably not necessary for AIDS prevention, all current barrier methods are contraceptives. This overlap has posed in fact an important obstacle to many women, worldwide—the inability to conceive while practicing STD/AIDS prevention. But mounting scientific evidence suggests that conception and disease prevention may be separable phenomena, able to be practiced independently of each other. Therefore, future barrier technologies for disease prevention should aim to provide women with the choice of conception.

A second outcome of the overlap between disease prevention and the contraceptive function of barriers has been an undeniable tension between the family planning and AIDS/STD camps. Family planning workers have expressed concerns that promoting HIV/STD prevention will entail a return to "less effective" methods of contraception (i.e., condoms and women's barrier methods, as opposed to the Pill), whereas AIDS workers and women's health activists have been alarmed by the lack of attention given to HIV/STD counseling in family planning settings and to many women's belief that a pill, injection, or implant can provide "all-around" protection.

The result of family planning efforts over the past few decades has been poor overall confidence in the male condom. The mission of AIDS educators, then, in the case of male condoms, has been to encourage their use as an adjunct to women's contraceptive use (so-called "dual protection"). In the case of women's barriers, however, the situation is quite a bit more complex. Here, the fear expressed by family planners is that anti-AIDS efforts will provide direct competition with their programs, since, they claim, women will not readily take up two methods of protection, one for contraception and one for HIV/STD protection, particularly since both require the woman to take the initiative. This conflict has led to the unconscionable and risky practice of weighing the health risk considered to be *most* important for a given population of women (i.e., pregnancy vs. HIV)—this weighing being done not by the women themselves, but by policy makers or service providers.

But the premise that women will not jointly use a women's barrier and a non-barrier method has not been tested. Studies of the uptake of joint male condom and hormone use have not been conclusive and may not apply to this question. Furthermore, women's attitudes toward their own barrier methods—and thus the effectiveness demonstrated by women's use of barrier methods—have been confounded by a profoundly negative portrayal of these methods as contraceptives and a historic lack of effective teaching/counseling programs directed at women. If women were to demonstrate highly effective use of these methods (which many argue would occur with adequate education and provider support), the tension between family planning and AIDS workers would be greatly reduced, since when barrier methods are used consistently, they provide a very high level of contraception (as well as protection from disease). Indeed, evidence already exists that some adolescent women may have greater success with partner negotiation on the issue of male condom use than they have with practicing birth-control-pill use, underscoring the utility of and need for "dual-method" counseling (Weisman, Plichta, Nathanson, Ehsminger & Robinson, 1991).

In a more general context, the tension between family planners and AIDS/STD workers maybe considered but one symptom of what many feel to be a "piecemeal" approach to women's health needs. Indeed, the point of contact in the healthcare system that is most oriented toward prevention counseling for women is often the family planning center, while STD care continues to be treatment-based. It is critical, therefore, that this occasion be dedicated toward serving a broader set of public health goals.

There has existed for sometime now a call for the provision of integrated reproductive health services for women, services that will combine many aspects of the presently fractured approach (Bruce, 1987; Hardon, 1992; Germain, 1993; Sen & Snow, 1994).

Although the response to this growing movement was slow to develop, in recent years a keen interest in setting a new action agenda that subsumes family planning goals under a broader reproductive health approach has been shown on the part of some family planning organizations concerned with developing countries (Elias, 1995). Preliminary trial research projects suggest that such integrated models of service delivery may be attainable in the short run (Vernon, 1990), although "hard" evidence of a resulting decrease in HIV/STD or other reproductive tract infections (RTIs) is not yet available. This research found that dedication of 20% of field workers' time to activities aimed at preventing STD/HIV did not cause contraceptive sales to decline and resulted in greater condom sales and more information conveyed to clients overall. Work of this nature must expand internationally as well as nationally, where many women are also at high risk of HIV and RTI (Persson, 1991). Program evaluation must also include the assessment of a "dual-method" approach as it applies to concurrent use of two *women's* methods (women's barrier plus non-barrier contraceptive method).

A final and quite serious issue complicating an integrated approach to women's reproductive health among family planning and AIDS/STD workers is the potential for a direct increased risk of infection through use of the long-acting family planning methods. This issue, for which data are still preliminary, is discussed in more detail later. It is mentioned here as an additional justification for dialogue between those working in the family planning and AIDS arenas. The aim of this dialogue should be to develop a cooperative and comprehensive approach that maximizes women's *choice* for women facing risks of unintended pregnancy and life-threatening infection.

The following sections first discuss issues of effectiveness and acceptability for various physical and chemical barriers that have demonstrated their ability to reduce the risk of sexually transmitted infections, such as chlamydia and gonorrhea. Evidence is now accumulating that these methods may also be expected to help reduce the risk of HIV. Next, practices that may increase women's vulnerability to HIV and other sexually transmitted organisms are considered. A summary of research areas for the future includes the issue of the as yet unavailable "microbicide," as well as that of the integration of STD prevention and family planning services into a reproductive health care approach to women's health needs. The closing section delivers an appeal for solidarity among women of all disciplines and backgrounds who are working to put an end to this epidemic.

REVIEW OF DATA ON WOMEN'S METHODS

Spermicides

Spermicidal formulations of nonoxynol-9 (N9) or octoxynol-9 (O9) have been available for women as contraceptive preparations that can be purchased without prescription [i.e., over-the-counter (OTC)] for contraception for at least 40 years (Population Reports, 1979; Sciarra, 1980) and have been used by millions of sexually active women, either alone or in conjunction with a diaphragm, cervical cap, or male condom. In 1972, an independent advisory panel to the United States Food and Drug Administration (FDA) undertook a review of all OTC drugs, leading to an eventual "proposed rule" that N9 and O9 be certified as "generally safe and effective" (USDHHS, 1980). Spermicides containing mercury were dropped from the United States market at this time.

In laboratory studies, N-9 inactivates HIV within 60 seconds at a concentration of 0.05% or greater, a concentration that is much lower than that of available spermicidal products (Hicks, Martin, Getchell, Health, Francis, McDougal, Curran, & Voeller, 1985; Voeller, 1986). N9 also inhibits growth of many other STD pathogens tested in most lab studies conducted to date, including those responsible for gonorrhea, syphilis, trichomonas, herpes, hepatitis B, and chlamydia (although one study of four showed no effect against c. trachomatis) (Stone, 1986, 1990). N9 does not inhibit human papillomavirus in the laboratory, a few strains of which are implicated in the development of cervical cancer (Hermonat, Daniel, & Shah, 1992). However, clinical studies tend to support a protective effect of spermicides against cervical cancer (see below). While lab results on spermicide are encouraging, these data can not substitute for actual use-experience with the product, where a multitude of other variables affect its dispersion and potency, and therefore, its efficacy.

Numerous clinical studies on N9- and O9-containing spermicides, which have sought to assess the protection they afford against STD, have been conducted since the 1970s. Most of these studies produce estimates of "use-effectiveness" (Rosenberg & Gollub, 1992), or the performance of the product among a population of various kinds of users—including those who may not use the product at every intercourse or may not employ correct use. (This has been referred to as "typical use" effectiveness in the family planning literature; see Hatcher, Trussell, Stewart, Kowal, Guest, Cates & Policar, 1994.) Depending on the population studied and the study setting, use-effectiveness rates will vary. Another useful index is "method-effectiveness" (or "perfect use" effectiveness), which may be estimated in studies in which subjects' use patterns have been carefully selected or strongly influenced (such as in clinical trials, in which a strong emphasis is placed on consistent and correct use). Method-effectiveness refers to the performance of the product under ideal use circumstances. Knowledge of this rate can help in counseling intended to motivate a client to initiate or maintain consistent use of a method, as well as in planning and evaluating educational interventions aimed at narrowing the gap between use-effectiveness and method-effectiveness.

Controlled clinical trials have resulted in a wide range of estimates for the reduced risk for bacterial STDs, with consistent use of spermicides, of between (approximately) 25% and 70%, when compared to women not using these compounds (Louv, Austin, Alexander, Stagno, & Cheeks, 1988; Rosenberg, Feldblum, Rojanapithayakorn, & Sawasdivorn, 1987; Niruthisard, Roddy, & Chutivongse, 1992). (See also Chapter 2, this volume). The variability is due in part to different study settings, populations, and protocols and in part to the differences in the product studied (i.e., gel vs. soluble film, for example). A summary rate of protection of 50% over all spermicidal products has been proposed, given the present lack of precision about these estimates (Rosenberg & Gollub, 1992; Rosenberg, Holmes, & WHO working group, 1993). Some observational studies (which follow women who have chosen to use these products instead of randomly assigning their use) have demonstrated reduced risks of above 75% and indicate that, under nonexperimental conditions, women tend to obtain better protection against STDs—gonorrhea, chlamydia, trichomonas, and cervical cancer, which acts like an STD—with spermicides, whether used alone or with a diaphragm, than with a male condom (Rosenberg & Gollub, 1992). That is to say, the relatively low prevalence of male condom use often translates into a low use-effectiveness. (The higher rates usually attributed to male condoms—i.e., 95% or higher—refer to method-effectiveness, or male condoms in the ideal.)

Though it is often stated as a conclusion of such studies, it is still not yet widely appreciated that, with all these protective barriers, regular and correct use play the most important role in ensuring the highest levels of anti-STD effectiveness. Indeed, inconsistent use of barriers has, in some studies, provided no more protection, statistically speaking, than use of no method at all (Saracco *et al.,* 1993).

Studies on HIV

The role of spermicides in HIV prevention is controversial. The protection spermicides afford for gonorrhea, chlamydia, and, perhaps, trichomonas and cervical cancer translates into an immediate, indirect benefit vis-à-vis the risk of HIV/AIDS, since these STDs have been associated with a raised risk of HIV infection (Wasserheit, 1992; Laga, 1993; Alexander, 1990). (See also Chapter 2, this volume). For women already infected with HIV, spermicides can help reduce the risk of contracting other STDs that tend to produce more serious symptoms and be more resistant to treatment in the presence of HIV infection (Wassherheit, 1992).

However, some investigators have raised concerns about the theoretical adverse effects of spermicides in the prevention of HIV infection. These concerns stem from the observation of vaginal irritation in some users, particularly those with a high frequency of use or exposure to a large cumulative dose or both.

Evidence Against a Role for Spermicides in HIV Risk Reduction

The first attempt to study the direct role of spermicides in HIV prevention was a randomized clinical trial conducted among Nairobi prostitutes, half of whom used the spermicide-impregnated "Today" sponge and half (so-called "controls") who used either a nonspermicidal cream or insert. All women were also provided with male condoms (Kreiss *et al.,* 1992).

The women reported an average of 42 partners per week. The authors found no reduced risk of HIV infection among sponge users. In addition, they found an increase in genital ulcers among sponge users, a finding that they speculated may have been owed to the irritating qualities of spermicides (see Table 1). Although this study was immediately taken as evidence against a protective role for N9, the study was beset by a number of serious methodological problems, making definite conclusions about the value of N9 in HIV prevention impossible (Gollub and Stein, 1992). First, the two groups of women compared at the end of the study were unequal at the study's outset in the prevalence of genital ulcers; the sponge group had more genital ulcers even before they began to use the sponge. Also, sponge users demonstrated a significant increase in lesions on the vulva, but not in the vagina or on the cervix, biologically an unlikely side effect of sponge use, and one that has neither previously (Rosenberg *et al.,* 1987) nor subse-

Table 1. Studies of Nonoxynol-9 and HIV

			Results[a]		
Setting	Study design	Formulation	Condoms	Spermicide	Comments
Nairobi, 138 sex workers (42 partners/week)[b]	Randomized controlled trial	"Today" sponge (1000 mg N9)	(Not given)	No protection observed ($RR = 1.7$). Suggestion of possible raised risk.	Excess of vulvar ulcers in sponge group (16% vs. 3%). Study had no placebo sponge controls; unequal allocation of ulcers at start of study; exposure >1000 mg/day N9.
Cameroon, 273 sex workers (3.2 partners/week)[c,d]	Prospective follow-up	Suppositories (100 mg N9)	High-level protection observed in more detailed analysis ($RR = 0.3$).[d]	High-level protection observed ($RR = 0.2$–0.4).	No evidence of increased risk of ulcers with N9.
Zambia, 110 HIV-discordant couples[e]	Prospective follow-up	Suppositories (100 mg N9), film (70 mg N9), gel (100 mg N9)	High-level protection observed for both male and female partners ($RR = 0.2$).	No protection observed when controlled for condom use consistency	No evidence of increased risk of ulcers with N9; insufficient statistical power to observe spermicide effect (78% episodes involved condoms).

[a]Crude relative risks (before adjustment for confounders) are given unless indicated.
[b]Kreiss et al. (1992).
[c]Zekeng et al. (1993).
[d]Feldblum and Weir (1995).
[e]Feldblum et al. (1992).

quently (see below) been associated with the sponge. A third problem was that those women using the sponges were instructed to change them a few times a day (after every 2 or 3 partners), thereby exposing the women to unusually high doses of spermicide. This practice further complicated the interpretation of study results, since the sponge is purposely designed with a large quantity of spermicide (1000 mg N9) to accommodate continuous wear for 24 hours.

Thus, the harmful effect attributed to the sponge in this study—increased presence of vulvar ulcers—may be attributable to behaviors that were not adequately measured during the study (douching, dry washing, or the insertion of organic or synthetic substances into the vagina to make it tighter and drier) or to the failure of the study's randomization procedure. It has been pointed out that the rate of genital ulcer development is very high in this area of Africa, as demonstrated by a concurrent study in the same geographic region among women not using N9, in which the prevalence of genital ulcers among the women was comparable to that for the sponge group in the study by Kreiss and co-workers (Roddy, Cordero, Cordero, & Fortney, 1993).

The reason for the absence of a protective effect of N9 in the Nairobi study is difficult to interpret. The relative contributions of the spermicide component vs. the sponge component of the product cannot be teased out due to the lack of a proper placebo sponge control group. Some have argued that physical qualities of the sponge (such as drying) may have undermined any potential beneficial effects of N9. On the other hand, the spermicidal sponge has previously been shown to reduce the risk of other STDs (Rosenberg *et al.,* 1987). Alternatively, the excess vulvar ulcers found among the sponge group in Nairobi may have contributed to the absence of protection observed for this group.

Given the many flaws of the Nairobi study, a conservative interpretation might be that a preparation like the sponge could have a place in prevention for many women, but not for sex workers. However, this study clearly raised more questions than it answered (Stone & Peterson, 1992; Stein, 1992; Cates, Stewart, & Trussell, 1992).

Subsequent studies on N9 have failed to replicate the finding of an increased risk of vulvar ulcers. Two small studies of women inserting spermicides but required to abstain from sex have been completed. These studies were designed to explore further the proposition that N9 could have irritating effects on the vaginal and cervical epithelium. In the first, 14 women inserted suppositories (150 mg N9) up to four times a day for up to 2 weeks (Niruthisard, Roddy, & Chutivongse, 1991). Almost half the study group demonstrated signs of epithelial disruption when examined with a colopo-scope. (No control group was available for comparison.) The results suggested that epithelial damage was possible under the conditions of the experiment.

In the second study, women inserting suppositories (150 mg N9) more frequently than every other day experienced a higher rate of epithelial breakage than did controls who inserted placebos (Roddy *et al.*, 1993). Self-reported irritation (including burning, itching, or painful urination) from spermicides did not correlate well with actual epithelial damage (epithelial disruption or bleeding) as determined by colposcopic examination. The cervix was the site for the majority of the erythema (redness) and epithelial disruption.

The meaning of these studies is unclear with respect to the actual risk of epithelial damage under normal use conditions. The effects of intercourse on the observed interaction of spermicide with vaginal epithelium, including mechanical effects as well as the diluting effects of semen and increased vaginal secretions, are difficult if not impossible to predict. The studies cited above raised the concern that spermicidal products now in use, under the conditions of frequent insertion, may raise risk of HIV infection, but this has not been demonstrated in any study.

Studies conducted on women actually using spermicidal products during intercourse, such as suppositories and soluble films with less N9 than sponges, have failed to document any increased risk of epithelial damage. On the other hand, it appears that N9 products now existing may not be suitable for regularly scheduled insertions (i.e., whether sex occurs or not)—a strategy that has never been employed but that theoretically removes the actual act of protection from the sexual act, thereby reducing the probability of partner knowledge and increasing the probability of a higher use-effectiveness.

One important lesson of the series of irritation studies described above is that further study of epithelial damage should not rely on self-reported irritation by users, but on direct visualization of the cervix. Individual sensitivities to N9 appear to vary. Moreover, epithelial disruption and symptoms of irritation may be unrelated. This question requires a good deal more research.

Evidence in Favor of a Role for Spermicides in HIV Risk Reduction

Two observational studies from Africa have demonstrated the potential for spermicides to confer protection—in one case, substantial protection—against HIV infection (see Table 1). One was conducted among Cameroonian sex workers, who reported an average of 3.2 partners per week during the course of the study (Zekeng, Feldblum, Oliver, & Kaptue, 1993). Women were counseled to use both condoms and soluble suppositories, the latter containing a much lower dose of spermicide (100 mg N9) than do contraceptive sponges. After adjustment for other risk factors, including concurrent condom use, a 90% reduction in new HIV infections was seen in more consistent compared with less consistent users of suppositories. Genital ulcers did not increase with greater spermicide exposure; in fact, the most frequent users had fewer genital ulcers than the least frequent users of suppositories (Weir, Roddy, Zekeng, & Feldblum, in press). Unlike the Nairobi study, this study was also able to take condom use and actual sexual behavior into account, owing to the use of self-completed coital logs collected from the study subjects.

One puzzling finding of this study was that consistent condom use was not found to confer any benefit overall to women in the study. The investigators hypothesized that this result was caused by women overreporting their partners' condom use to please the investigators. This is a plausible argument to explain the observed noneffect of condoms (as compared with spermicides), given the long history of educational efforts stressing condom use in the area where this study was undertaken. One finding in support of this explanation, pointed out by the investigators, is that condom use *did* protect women against HIV when the analysis was confined to women who stated at intake that their partners used condoms. Reported partners' condom use at follow-up may have been more accurate among these women who had already succeeded in partner negotiation at the start of the study.

Another possible contributor to the observed low use-effectiveness of condoms is that condom breakage rates were very high. In this study, 73% of women reported at least one episode of breakage. Also, 39% of the women reported pain, irritation, or skin injuries from condoms, which may have led to condom removal before ejaculation. The investigators note in their discussion that safety issues of condom use among high-frequency users such as sex workers have received little attention.

One drawback to the study design used in Cameroon is the absence of a study group that used only spermicides. A "condoms vs. spermicides" research design is not feasible due to the dubious ethics withholding male condoms—currently considered the most effective AIDS prevention modality—among the spermicide users. In fact, the authors of the Cameroon study felt ethically compelled to provide condoms *and* spermicides to each subject, given the history of favorable research findings on spermicides and STD.

With a new analytical procedure that separates sexual episodes where condoms were used from those where they were not, it has been possible to estimate the effectiveness of spermicide use alone. These new analyses continue to show a strong dose-dependent protective effect of spermicides against gonorrhea and HIV comparable to that offered by male condoms (*RR* = 0.4), as well as an expected protective effect of condoms, which is slightly higher (*RR* = 0.3) (Feldblum & Weir, 1995; Weir *et al.,* 1994).

Care will need to be taken in all nonrandomized studies attempting to determine the efficacy of specific methods, since there is likely some association between inherent risk (or probability of exposure to HIV/STD) and use of a protective method. For example, it may be that women who choose to use spermicides correctly perceive themselves to be at higher risk, because their partners refuse to use condoms and are therefore more likely to carry an infection. If this is true, then unless the study is designed to allow for statistical adjustment for this unequal risk of exposure—often difficult and sometimes impossible—any true underlying reduction in risk with spermicide use will not be observed when comparing spermicide users to condom users.

A second study suggesting a possible benefit in the use of N9 in reducing risk of HIV infection was conducted among 110 Zambian couples discordant for HIV serostatus (Feldblum, Hira, Kamanga, Mukelabai, Weir, & Thomas, 1995) (see Table 1). Couples were counseled to use both spermicides and condoms and were then examined and interviewed at 3-month intervals for a mean follow-up of approximately 18 months. Coital logs were collected at each follow-up. Consistent condom use conferred strong protection for both male and female seronegative partners (*RR* = 0.2). However, in the case of consistent spermicide use, only a weak protective effect was seen overall (*RR* = 0.8), which was increased when considering only women (*RR* = 0.5, or a risk reduction of 50% as compared to inconsistent spermicide use). The investigators of this study hypothesize that the male partners of HIV+ women may have had outside unprotected sexual exposure to HIV, which might, in turn, have offset any risk reduction from N9 use with their main partners.

The most problematic aspect of this study was its small size, which severely limited the ability to draw any meaningful conclusions concerning protection. None of the results were statistically significant, likely due to the small number of couples followed. Also, because the condom intervention was so successful—78% of all coital episodes were protected by condoms—there was little chance to observe the effect of spermicide used alone on HIV risk. The investigators nevertheless undertook an analysis of acts where condoms were not used. The analysis failed to show a protective effect with use of N9 alone, likely due to the study's lack of statistical power.

In this study, as in the Cameroon study, visual examination of the vaginal and cervix with the aid of speculum revealed no increased epithelial damage to spermicide users, as compared to nonusers. In fact, there was evidence for a decreased incidence of infectious ulcers among spermicide users, due perhaps to a "treatment" effect of the spermicide or possibly to other behaviors of spermicide users not able to be adequately controlled.

It remains unclear whether the conflicting results among studies to date may be explained on the basis of different spermicidal products, different study methodologies, or different populations. N9, in very low doses, kills all STD organisms in the laboratory, but it does so by disrupting the cell membrane of bacteria and the viral envelope of viruses. Therefore, theoretically, it has the capacity to irritate and damage the mucous membranes of the vagina and cervix. Numerous studies among women that show protection from STDs such as gonorrhea with use of spermicides, however, imply that these theoretical effects do not necessarily occur under conditions of actual use during sexual intercourse. Because there appears to be no need to employ a very high dosage of spermicide to the vagina, which might in fact wear down the vaginal lining for some users, it appears prudent to restrict further research having to do with HIV infection to lower-dose methods (150 mg N9 or less). This is especially true in the case of women with frequent sexual encounters, such as sex workers. If, however, we discontinue research with these products, as some are advocating, we may be discarding one of the most useful, immediate prevention techniques available to women (Gollub & Stein, 1992).

RESEARCH AND REGULATORY CHALLENGES

Spermicides come in a variety of different forms listed in Table 2, which also gives the corresponding amount of N9 contained in the product. A central desirable characteristic of spermicides in the prevention of STD/HIV is that they may be used "clandestinely," without the partner's knowledge. Though this is probably true for diaphragms and cervical caps as well, current standards of care call for fitting of these latter methods, raising further obstacles to access and use (see below for a discussion of "fit-free" diaphragms).

Information is severely lacking on which forms of spermicides may be superior in coverage of the vagina and cervix, which may be more acceptable to women and their partners, and whether the protection obtained with spermicide is enhanced with use of another female barrier method, such as the cervical cap or diaphragm. Furthermore, while animal studies have demonstrated that spermicides may also be useful in the prevention of herpes and other viral infections (Whaley, Barratt, & Zeitlin, 1993), human studies to clarify the role of spermicide protection in non-HIV viral infections have not been conducted, with the exception of those conducted on

Table 2. Spermicidal Products for Women Listed in Ascending Order of Nonoxynol-9 Content[a]

Name	N9/application (mg)	Comments
Bioadhesive gel	52.5	1. Appeared in late 1994
Film	70–75	1. No applicator. 2. 0–5 min. waiting time. 3. Difficult to find on pharmacy shelves unless preordered.
Suppositories	100–150	1. No applicator. 2. Requires 15–20 min melting time.
Foams	100–125	1. Requires applicator. 2. No waiting time.
Jellies and creams	100–350[b]	1. Requires applicator. 2. No waiting time.
Sponge[c]	1000	1. 24-hour continuous wear. 2. Requires moistening.

[a]Sometimes the percentage of N9 is given on the product's packaging. The percentage depends on the weight of the product and may therefore be less useful in comparing the number of grams of N9 actually delivered to the vagina by different products.
[b]Very few jellies and creams contain as much as 350 mg N9/application. The vast majority contain approximately 100–125 mg/application, comparable to foams.
[c]The "Today" sponge was approved by the FDA as a drug-delivery system and does not necessarily stay in front of the cervix during intercourse, as do the diaphragm and cervical cap. It is therefore included on this table as a spermicide. The sponge was withdrawn from the market by the manufacturer in early 1995.

cervical cancer, for which a viral etiology (certain types of human papillomavirus) is most likely. In the United States, we have also not undertaken studies of the acceptability of spermicides that are used in other countries, including those based on the active ingredients menfegol, benzalkonium chloride, and chlorhexidine, even though these too kill STD microorganisms in the laboratory and in preliminary clinical studies (Lee, Utidjian, Singh, & Carpenter, 1972; Cutler *et al.*, 1977; Mendez, Castro, & Ortega, 1986; Siboulet, Bohbot, Catalan, & Siboulet, 1988). For some of these compounds, applications for FDA approval have been undertaken without success; with others, no attempt has been made. Liability issues loom large in a company's decision to undertake product development or engage in the FDA approval process. The sheer cost and length of this process—even for compounds with a substantial history of previous use—often dissuades private industry from going this route. Attempts on the part of the FDA to streamline the approval process for topical compounds and devices with the potential to reduce STD/HIV risk have so far been relatively unenergetic and fraught with bureaucratic and political delays.

The lack of priority-setting in the case of women and AIDS has thus posed further obstacles and disincentives to research and development efforts, crucial steps in achieving for women more choices in protection.

Currently, for example, a new protective method that combined a barrier with a spermicide would need clearance from two separate branches of the FDA, the one covering drugs and the other covering devices. Attempts to reform the agency and create a cross-divisional women's bureau appear to have been abandoned with little opportunity for public input.

Postcoital Application of Spermicides

Because spermicides inactivate HIV instantaneously in the laboratory, postcoital application might reduce the risk of HIV infection. Such a practice might be the only method possible for women in violent relationships or in others where negotiation is difficult and sex is not anticipated long enough in advance to apply a clandestine method with a limited duration of efficacy. Anecdotal evidence suggests that this approach may be utilized in some rape crisis centers in the United States. However, no research has yet been undertaken to determine whether risk of HIV is actually reduced with this approach. Such a study would require a very large number of women in most United States settings.

Diaphragms and Cervical Caps

The precise role of physical barriers such as diaphragms and cervical caps in AIDS prevention is unclear. Observational studies have demonstrated a range of protection associated with use of these devices against gonorrhea, chlamydia, and cervical cancer, similar to the case with spermicides used alone (Stone, Grimes, & Magdar, 1986; Cates & Stone, 1992; Rosenberg & Gollub, 1992). Although up to a 90% risk reduction has been found on occasion, a summary estimate of 50–75% was arrived at in a recent review (Rosenberg & Gollub, 1992). Controlled clinical trials of diaphragms and cervical caps for STD protection have not been conducted, nor are any currently under way.

The Role of the Cervix

Many questions surround the issue of use of physical barriers against STDs. For example, it is not known whether the protection observed is due to the mechanical coverage of the cervix, the fact that these barriers hold spermicide against the cervix, or both. Studies in which some women have used spermicides alone, and others in which women have used diaphragms *with* spermicides, have shown seemingly conflicting results—sometimes women using only the chemical methods show the lowest risk of infection (Peters, Thomas, Hagan, Mack, & Henderson, 1986; Celentano,

Klassen, Weisman, & Rosenhein, 1987; Slattery *et al.,* 1989). Part of the difficulty in interpreting these study data is that often no information is available concerning the consistency of use of either protective method; therefore, no information may be gleaned on method-effectiveness. Thus, a spermicide user may appear to be better protected from gonorrhea simply because she uses the spermicide more faithfully than a woman using both a diaphragm and spermicide. The extra effort associated with the diaphragm—in theory, a more efficacious method because it provides both physical and chemical protection—may paradoxically make it less use-effective in practice if it is used less.

Although sexual intercourse poses a substantially greater risk of HIV infection for women than for men, little is known at present about the preferred locus of entry of HIV in sexual transmission to women. Because of the early association found between risk of AIDS and genital ulcer disease for both men and women, the vagina came to be seen as the primary site of susceptibility for women. Animal evidence using extremely high doses of virus confirmed that infection could be contracted in the absence of a cervix (Miller, Alexander, Vogel, Anderson, & Marx, 1992). However, this may merely prove that, under the conditions of the experiment, the vagina is *sufficient* for infection; it says nothing about whether it is *necessary.* Nonulcerative diseases, such as chlamydia and gonorrhea, which infect the cervix and are often far more prevalent in a given population, also raise the risk of HIV (Wasserheit, 1992; Laga, 1992; also see Weir, Feldblum, Roddy, & Zekeng, 1994, for an alternative explanation of STD–HIV link). These findings imply a possible role for the cervix in HIV infection, especially if the cervix is rendered more vulnerable by preexisting STDs. Thus, rupture of the vaginal epithelium may not be the only, or even the main, mechanism of HIV infection for many women (Alexander, 1990).

There are several reasons to believe that the cervix could be especially susceptible to infection by HIV. The first reason is by analogy, because the cervix is often the preferred site of infection for other STDs, which invade and attach more easily to columnar epithelium (as compared to the squamous epithelium of the vagina) (Alexander, 1990; Schachter, 1990; Corey, 1990). Second, the cervix is far more prone to bleeding and irritation, thereby theoretically allowing for more contact with virus by circulating target cells.

Third, cervical changes occurring with menarche, pregnancy, and exposure to oral contraceptives may correlate with a changing risk of HIV infection (Bailey, 1993). For example, pregnancy increases the number of columnar cells exposed in the vagina (a condition known alternatively as "ectopy" or "ectropion") as well as the width of the transformation zone (zone of active metaplasia, or change in tissue type, lying between squamous and columnar cells) (Singer, 1975); pregnancy may also raise the observed risk of HIV infection (Chao *et al.*, 1991) and of cervical and vaginal shedding of virus (Henin *et al.*, 1993). Oral contraceptives, also associated with ectopy (Alexander, 1990; Stamm & Holmes, 1990; Moss *et al.*, 1991), have also been found, in some studies of HIV transmission (Simonsen *et al.*, 1990; Plummer *et al.*, 1991; Bulterys *et al.*, 1993), to raise risk of HIV. This, however, has not been the case for all studies of transmission (Lazzarin, Saracco, Musicco, Nicolosi, & the Italian Study Group, 1991; Allen *et al.*, 1991; European Study Group on Heterosexual Transmission of HIV, 1992; Hunter & Mati, 1992). Finally, in a study of genital shedding of in women, more cell-associated virus was present in the zones of ectopy as compared with other areas of the cervix (Clemetson *et al.*, 1993).

Taken together, this collection of observations seem to suggest a particular anatomical vulnerability that varies according to a woman's internal hormonal milieu, her stage of life, and her exposure to exogenous hormones. To date, no investigations have carefully followed a cohort of women through menarche, first pregnancy, and beyond that, into menopause, while also directly measuring cervical changes. Thus, while these observations are suggestive, they must be confirmed by more careful research.

It is also possible that the stage of the menstrual cycle influences risk of infection. To date, a sole study on the risk of gonorrhea infection and stage of the cycle has suggested an increased risk around the time of menstruation (McCormack, Reynolds, & the Cooperative Study Group, 1982). Studies on HIV, however, have suggested only an elevated risk of infection for the male partner when intercourse occurred during menstruation (European Study Group on Heterosexual Transmission of HIV, 1992). Thus, the effect of the cycle on infection risk is still poorly understood.

AIDS data from several African countries, based on reported cases of the disease, do suggest that young women may be at a particularly high risk of HIV transmission (Wawer *et al.*, 1991; United Nations Development Program, 1992; Bailey, 1993). Recent data reported by Centers for Disease Control and Prevention (CDC) also show that the median age of U.S. women diagnosed with AIDS acquired through heterosexual sex is 5 years younger than that of men with AIDS attributed to the same risk factor (CDC, 1994). In African countries with a high AIDS prevalence due to heterosexual sex, this apparent raised risk in young women has often been explained sociologically as due to a tendency for older men (who have a higher chance of being HIV-infected) to seek out younger women as sex partners (who are perceived to be "safe"). But biological forces may also be at work. In sexually active younger women with immature cervixes, there is a risk of increased direct exposure of columnar and metaplastic cells—those most vulnerable to invasion or penetration by pathogens—to ejaculate. Young women with an older age at first intercourse (sexual debut) appear to develop cervical and pelvic infection less frequently than do women who become sexually active at an early age (Moscicki, Winkler, Irwin, & Schachter, 1989; Duncan *et al.*, 1990).

Finally, recent evidence shows that genital shedding of HIV virus in HIV+ women occurs much more frequently from the cervix than from the vagina (Clemetson *et al.*, 1993). This may, however, denote a focus of established infection (and infectiousness), not necessarily a point of entry for the virus.

Thus, as regards transmission from and infection of the cervix, both during menses and in the absence of menstrual blood, there are compelling reasons to pursue studies of physical barriers for reducing risk of HIV. In particular, a long-wear physical barrier method for women may in practice be more acceptable in some international settings than will daily application of a chemical barrier.

Cervical Cap

No separate studies exist on the risk of STD with cervical cap use, although protection against STD infection is inferred from studies of the diaphragm (Cramer et al., 1987; Stone, 1990; Cates & Stone, 1992; Rosenberg & Gollub, 1992). Because the cap provides a tighter seal around the cervix than does the diaphragm, the cap could be more protective against organisms infecting the cervix. As with the diaphragm, it remains unclear whether spermicide offers more protection than the cap alone, against either pregnancy or disease. A single observational study collected information on women's use of spermicide and subsequent pregnancy rates; in this study, users of spermicide and cap did not enjoy more contraceptive protection than did those using the cap alone (Richwald, 1989). However, other factors, such as the women's sexual partners and practices, were uncontrolled, hence inference remains insecure.

Physical Barriers without Spermicide

The method-effectiveness of physical barriers such as diaphragms and caps used alone is a question of special importance to low-income population, since spermicides can be costly. A recent retrospective review of the pregnancy experience of women using diaphragms worn continuously without spermicidal gel suggested that the value of constant mechanical protection of the cervix may outweigh sporadic (and thus more error-prone) insertion of mechanical and chemical protection (Ferreira, Araujo, Regina, Diniz, & Faundes, 1993). This follows upon an older report of a new "fit-free" method of using diaphragms (Stim, 1980). Women using small-size diaphragms throughout the month showed a failure rate of only 2.8%, as compared with 9.8% for diaphragm/jelly users. However, a trial conducted in England among 110 women using Stims' suggested approach (nonspermicidal fit-free method) resulted in a substantially higher pregnancy rate than is usually associated with the diaphragm (no controls were available to compare pregnancy rates in that setting among a comparable group of women) (Smith, Farr, Feldblum, & Spence, 1995). The authors conclude that women should continue to be advised to use fitted diaphragms with spermicide. But the study did not answer the question of whether small-size (no-fit) diaphragms would be used more consistently. While the results tended to support the need for spermicide use, such use could also occur in conjunction with smaller diaphragms, which may be more comfortable and acceptable for long-term wear. A properly conducted prospective trial of both pregnancy and STD outcomes to investigate this hypothesis is urgently needed. Research should also focus on the effectiveness of cervical caps not available in this country (such as those constructed of hard plastic), which have already shown their capacity for month-long use as contraceptives (Grafenberg & Dickinson, 1944; Lehfeldt, Sobrero, & Inglis, 1961; Lehfeldt, 1970). Barriers that can be applied some time before coitus and that do not require daily insertion are of tremendous importance where privacy is impossible and where women are barred overtly by their partners from protecting themselves.

The Female Condom

The newly approved female condom (approved in the United States since May 1993), known in the United States by the trade name *Reality* (and in Europe as *Femidom*), was the first product to be approved under an FDA policy written in 1990, the intent of which was to fast-track the approval of anti-STD/HIV protective devices for women. The female condom is a 6-inch polyurethane sheath with one blind end containing a pliable movable ring that assists the user in insertion. The open end is framed by a second soft ring, sealed to the sheath, which rests against the users vulva (see Figures 1 and 2). The device was approved mainly on the basis of its performance as a contraceptive; clinical studies of pregnancy can be conducted more quickly than those on STDs, but admittedly the use-effectiveness of this device against STD will require further study. The range of contraceptive failure rates among women using the female condom, obtained from a carefully conducted FDA-overseen study, is comparable to that for other barrier methods for women and for men (Hatcher *et al.*, 1994): 5–21% annually (Trussell, Sturgen, Strickler, & Dominik, 1994). As

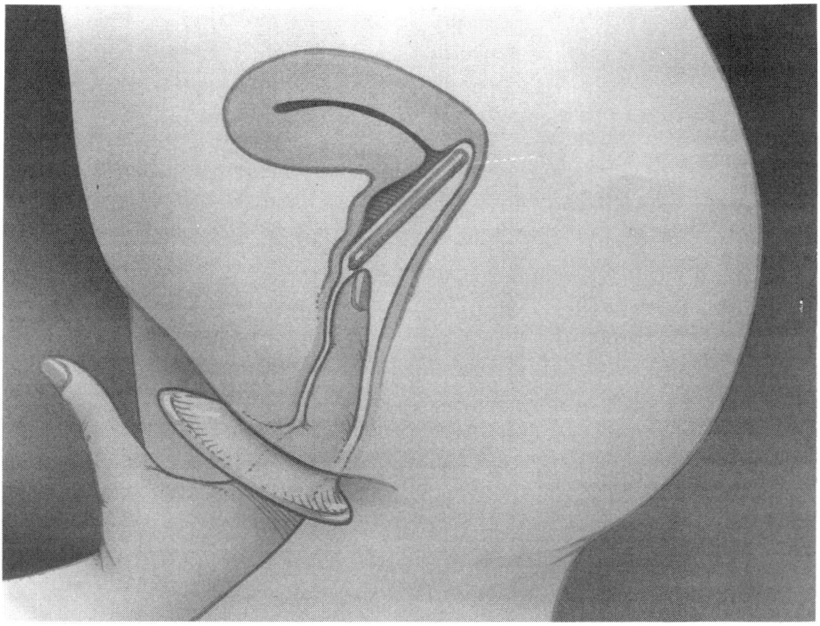

Figure 1. Final step in insertion of the Reality female condom.

with the male condom, improper or inconsistent use reduces the use-effectiveness.

Supplementary data also support the role of the female condom in STD prevention. In the lab, female condoms tear much less easily than do latex male condoms, and they prevent passage of virus particles as small as hepatitis B virus (smaller than HIV) (Drew, Blair, Miner, & Conant, 1990). In a study of women selected for their compliant use of the product, none experienced reinfection with *T. vaginalis,* as compared with women using the product only intermittently or not at all (Soper *et al.,* 1993).

Widespread use of the female condom will allow a better estimation of population effectiveness levels, both as a contraceptive and in disease prophylaxis. Acceptability studies of varying methodologies from the United States, Europe, Latin America, and Africa, conducted among small but diverse populations of women, have so far suggested that acceptability may be quite good among an important proportion (Bounds, Guillebaud, & Newman, 1992; Hernandez-Avila, 1992; Colimoro, 1993; Ford & Mathie, 1993; Liskin, 1993; Bassett, Ray, Nicolette, & Managazna, 1993; Gollub,

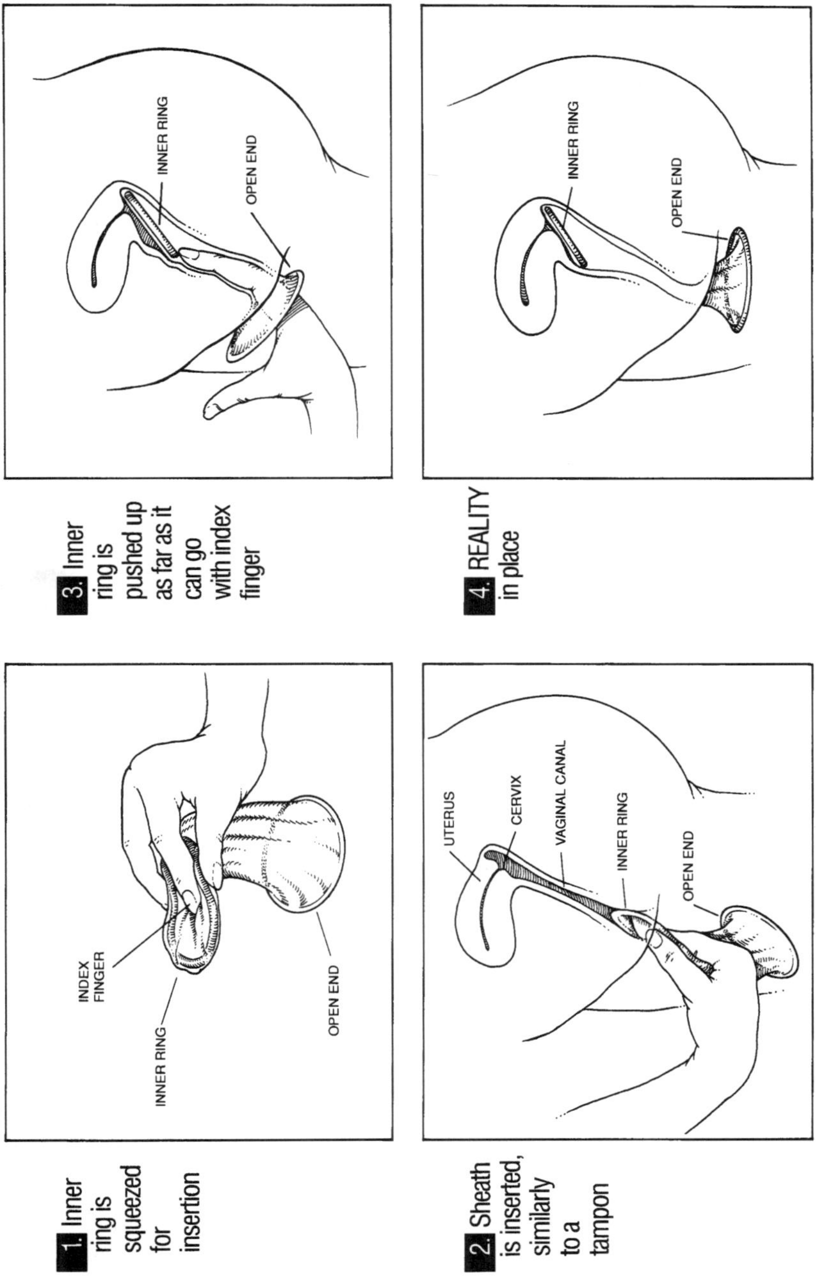

Figure 2. Procedure for inserting and positioning the Reality female condom.

Stein & El-Sadr, 1995). Features liked by women about this device included its soft feel, the sense of complete protection it conferred, and the experience of control over AIDS/STD protection. It appears that, in many cases, women's initial negative impressions of the large size of the device, the awkwardness of the two (inner and outer) rings, and the fear of internal damage or discomfort from the device did not persist after actual use experience. However, few of these studies have followed women for longer than a few months; therefore, long-term data on acceptability or continuation rates with the device are not yet available.

The female condom is visible to partners and is not liked by some for this reason. Surprisingly, however, focus group data have demonstrated that for many women whose partners are unwilling to don male condoms, the method will bring about a dramatic change in sexual dynamics (Gollub & Stein, 1993b; Shervington, 1993, 1994). "Once I have this inside me, what can he do?" one respondent summarized (Gollub & Stein, 1993a).

The female condom shows every promise of protecting as well as or better than a male condom. It tears less easily than latex and protects a woman's vulva, which is not possible with male condoms. Furthermore, it can be inserted long before any contact with pre-ejaculate, whereas use of the male condom depends on the man's erection. Despite these advantages, the female condom has encountered both political and professional resistance that did not meet the male condom, even though the latter was no better tested against AIDS at the time it was labeled for AIDS prevention. The female condom was assigned to a fast-track process of FDA approval but still required two FDA hearings to be passed. Its efficacy rates were compared to those for the male condom, even thought the latter were generated from inherently noncomparable studies that tend to spuriously elevate observed effectiveness. (Well-designed clinical trials on the male condom for contraception or disease prevention were never conducted.) Expert statistical comparisons of the female and male condom failure rates presented to the FDA showed no statistically significant differences, yet the agency ignored this evidence (Trussell, 1992; Trussell *et al.*, 1994). Although the material of the female condom is tougher and more resistant to tears than the male condom, the FDA has insisted that the label on the new device clearly state that it provides protection inferior to that of a male condom. The FDA also refused to allow the appearance of method-effectiveness rates on the label (the effectiveness with perfect use, 95%) and insisted that an invalid use-failure rate of 26% appear (obtained by rounding up a 12.2% 6-month failure rate, and doubling) instead of the rate that had been estimated according to sound statistical methods (21%). Finally, press releases from both the FDA and CDC following the female condom's approval have greatly undermined confidence in its use, and, although CDC's disposition toward the device has greatly improved, as of the publication date of this text, the female condom has never appeared in CDC-sponsored AIDS education television advertisements.

Part of the resistance to the female condom, indeed to all woman-controlled methods of STD prevention, lies in the misguided search for the *perfect* method. Some problems with this reasoning have already been mentioned: (1) Male condoms are not used by women and thus cannot possibly be the perfect method for women; (2) contraceptive research has shown that a variety of methods are needed in order to maximize the number of protected acts. To these two can be added the following observations: (3) Previous public health experiences has shown that imperfect methods often achieve great effectiveness on the population level and that important public health measures such as childhood vaccines have frequently been substantially less than 100% effective (Cates & Hinman, 1992). The goal of prevention efforts for women should therefore be to make available "different, mutually reinforcing techniques" to respond to the diversity of women seeking prevention (Cates & Hinman, p. 493). The utility of AIDS risk reduction messages (or "hierarchical messages") giving a *range* of protective options, as opposed to one sole, highly efficacious choice (such as the male condom), has been observed in other areas of the epidemic. In recognition that "Just say no" may be difficult if not impossible to achieve on a large scale, injection drug users have been offered clean needles as a risk-reduction approach. Anecdotal evidence and now preliminary research conducted on this approach have validated its role in reducing risky behaviors (Des Jarlais *et al.,* 1994).

In the case of women's risk of AIDS from sex, the New York State AIDS Institute has developed a hierarchy that begins with abstinence and mutual monogamy and methodically continues through male condom, female condom, diaphragm and spermicide, and finally spermicide use alone, stressing that this last option is not as efficacious as a male condom (see Table 2). Concern has been voiced by some, however, that increasing women's options by including anti-STD/AIDS strategies that are less method-effective that male condom (e.g., spermicides) may encourage women to abandon efforts to persuade their partners to use condoms. This raises the fundamental question of whether, under *any* circumstances whatsoever, it is ethical to withhold from women information that, given the realities of their lives, may help them care for themselves.

Expanding the information available to the public will always reduce the control over individuals' behaviors, because of the increase in personal choice. Those in favor of withholding information about possibly less-efficacious choices argue that the predicted success in inducing behavior change for the betterment of public health, *by means* of such proscription, justify the questionable ethics of this practice. The empirical evidence in this instance, however, suggests the opposite. Despite a longtime national

AIDS policy stressing only male condoms, no substantial increases in male condom use among the general public have been observed, and current use prevalence rates are low, as noted in the Introduction. Therefore, it may well be that heeding the ethical imperative to provide the public with full information, however imperfect, is completely consistent with the aim of public health, at least insofar as AIDS/STD prevention is concerned.

In fact, the promulgation of the male condom for AIDS prevention, as opposed to a more restricted message stressing abstinence and lifetime mutual monogamy, creates a de facto hierarchy and allows for human fallibility. Condoms are often not used correctly or consistently and can break, thereby exposing the individual to an increased risk of AIDS as compared to an absence of risk in the practice of abstinence or mutual monogamy. In view of this, some charge that condom promotion undermines AIDS prevention work. Yet the CDC appears not to be troubled by the risk of a "double message" in promoting male condoms. Then why the exceptionalism when it concerns women's methods of protection?

Women have experienced this kind of curtailment of choice before. One well-known example is that of the limitation of contraceptive options, both here and in many countries around the world. Often women are offered only, or a family planning service supplies only, nonbarrier methods of birth control (Depo-Provera, Norplant, oral contraceptives, or the IUD) because these methods are deemed to be "more effective." But these assessments tend to be made without substantial input by the users of such methods and frequently don't reflect their needs and concerns (giving rise to repeated attempts by grass-roots women's organizations in many of these countries to import and distribute or manufacture diaphragms) (Hardon, 1992). These examples reflect the obvious reality that women's choices will continue to be circumscribed where their economic status is low and their political power limited. (For an illustrative contrast, one might try to imagine the white gay male community tolerating a debate over whether its members should have access to alternative AIDS prevention or therapy modalities.)

Responding to the fears of many public policy makers, preliminary research by the New York State AIDS Institute concerned with actually measuring the impact (in terms of behavioral intent) of their hierarchical educational message to women has recently been undertaken in family planning clinics. Specifically, the research aims to determine whether women will understand the gradient of protection offered by the different methods presented, and if women successfully negotiating condom use with their partners will somehow arrest their efforts at this negotiation when confronted with other options not requiring negotiation ("condom migration"). Published results were not available at the time this chapter went to print; however, preliminary data, which are reassuring, have been presented

(Sorin, 1995). Other work aims to test the results of this message in an STD clinic setting (Gollub, French, Latka, O'Donnell, Stein, 1995).

In addition to the quest for perfection, another element to the resistance to women's methods such as the female condom may derive from dated and oppressive beliefs about women that maintain that women are unable to learn and practice consistent barrier use due to an inherent discomfort in touching their genitals. However, many would argue that discomfort in touching one's genitals is a learned behavior and neither gender-bound nor culturally bound. Since the advent of the pill, for example, women were not encouraged to use barrier methods of their own; such methods were seen as ineffective contraceptives. Prior to the pill, they were regularly used by many couples (Population Reports, 1984); yet many family planning clinics nowadays evince a lack of confidence in women as competent users. It is clear that promotion of barrier use to would-be users, by family planning professionals and other health educators, will determine in large part whether such methods will have a public health impact vis-à-vis AIDS. Many women may be willing to use such methods but will not initiate use unless they are given the opportunity, and the support of a provider.

Douching

The effect on AIDS risk of specific practices such as douching, of which a woman may be more in control than any methods so far discussed, and might choose to exercise, has not been studied. Douching, however, has been associated in some (Scholes *et al.,* 1993)—but not all (Rosenberg & Phillips, 1992)—studies with an increased risk of upper reproductive tract infections. It has been suggested that this may be due to a physical forcing of organisms into the endocervical canal and/or to a denudation of epithelium and natural lubrication, which acts to kill pathogens in the vagina, thus creating a more hospitable environment for infection. One central problem with studies that have been conducted is the difficulty of completely taking into account (controlling for) other behaviors of women who douche, which might actually be causing the infection (as opposed to the douching itself). Also, the definition of douching may vary among different populations of women (e.g., passive digital cleansing of the vagina without force vs. use of pressurized commercial douches).

To the extent that HIV "rides" with sperm in the ejaculate, douching will not be effective as a strategy to reduce risk of HIV infection, since sperm travel too quickly to be washed out of the vagina effectively by this practice. However, we do not know whether HIV infects in this manner (Anderson, 1992; Scofield, 1994).

Any application of caustic materials or drying agents to the vagina and/or vulva may increase the risk of HIV by promoting epithelial damage (Alexander, 1990). This risk would naturally be expected to increase dramatically if these practices were undertaken between partners and before intercourse occurred. This is currently the case in some African countries (Brown, Brown, & Ayowa, 1993).

Douching is practiced by a relatively large proportion of women, making public health recommendations regarding douching and STD/HIV both timely and important (Aral *et al.,* 1992). One as yet little-studied area is whether preparations to keep the vaginal pH low (acidic)—acidity being an important component of an STD/HIV defense system—would help prevent infection (Redondo-Lopez, Cook, & Sobel, 1990). One example of such a preparation is a lactobacillus douche, to replenish normal vaginal flora; another is a vinegar douche, which could be prepared at home. Immediate and expanded research here is warranted. If such preparations are effective, women who douched regularly might be steered toward such products, rather than counseled to stop douching altogether.

Withdrawal

A recent publication from an ongoing study of HIV-discordant couples provided the first actual evidence of a possible reduction in risk of HIV transmission to a woman associated with male partner withdrawal before ejaculation (De Vincenzi & the European Study Group, 1994). The rate of seroconversion among women whose partners withdrew about half the time was reduced by 80% as compared with women whose partners never or rarely practiced withdrawal. Among 12 couples who consistently practiced withdrawal, no seroconversions occurred. Corroboration of these important findings will be required in other settings. Information on withdrawal should be routinely collected in cohort studies measuring sexual HIV transmission.

Withdrawal has previously been shown to reduce the risk of cervical cancer (Peters *et al.,* 1986). There was a dose-dependent effect, by duration of this practice, with 10 or more years duration associated with a reduced risk of cervical cancer of 50%. A second study, however, showed the opposite effect (Rosenberg & Gollub, 1992).

Withdrawal, as compared to the partner's use of male condoms, may be more under a woman's control if partner nonuse stems from sexual insecurities and fear of loss of an erection. A woman may have a better chance of eliciting partner cooperation if she suggests withdrawal to avoid pregnancy, instead of to deter HIV infection.

Dental Dams

Latex dental dams are recommended for protection against HIV transmission between the mouth and the vulva and vagina. However, in recent years the use of plastic wrap has gained in popularity and is now often preferentially recommended by some AIDS groups, due to its larger size, its transparency, its lower cost, and its relative accessibility, as compared with dental dams. Actual data supporting protection against HIV are lacking, although plastic wrap has been found to block passage of herpesvirus, a virus of a size similar to that of HIV (Garland, Newnan, & de Crespigny, 1989). The oral–vaginal transmission route is thought to be considerably less risky than penile–vaginal intercourse. For women who have sex only with women, however, it increases in relative importance. The CDC has reported no cases of AIDS among women practicing woman-to-woman sex who have no other risk factors (such as heterosexual intercourse or intravenous drug use) (Chu, Buehler, Fleming, & Berkelman, 1990). However, this type of information is not routinely collected. Therefore, the number of women with AIDS who have engaged in woman-to-woman sex, in addition to heterosexual intercourse and/or IV drug use, is also not known. Case reports of possible HIV transmission between women exclusively having sex with women, with no other reported risk factors, have appeared in the literature (Marmor *et al.,* 1986; Monzon & Capellan, 1987).

FUTURE DIRECTIONS FOR RESEARCH AND ACTION

This chapter has sought to review current knowledge about HIV prevention methods. The gaps in knowledge reveal a formidable research agenda, ranging from the specific (do spermicidal foams coat the vagina better than suppositories?) to the more general, of which I will highlight four areas.

Rectal Intercourse

Virtually no research has been done on what protection a woman might use for rectal intercourse, even though this practice is considered to be substantially more risky than vaginal intercourse and is reported to be practiced by at least 10% of women from various national and international general population samples (Voeller, 1991; Ehrhardt *et al.,* in press). Clinic-based studies of women in the United States have sometimes reported a much higher frequency of this practice (greater than 50%) (Voeller, 1991). Voeller (1985) has pointed out that it is likely that in the United States, at least as many heterosexuals as gay men, if not more, practice rectal intercourse. In fact, in communities both in the United States and internationally, this practice is used as a method of contraception. Yet nearly all discussions of risk reduction among women focus exclusively on vaginal intercourse, while the issue of safe rectal intercourse is reserved exclusively for gay men.

Inquiries among pharmaceutical manufacturers have suggested that, among gay men, rectal lubricating preparations containing N9 in concentrations up to 1%, and in women, rectal use of Delfen foam, containing a far greater concentration (12%), have not been found to be irritating. However, no formal research appears to have been undertaken on this subject (Voeller, 1985). It is clear that this research is an urgent priority, especially since microbicide development has already commenced (see below). It is also conceivable that a modified female condom could be used for anal protection. Informal reports of gay men utilizing the device for this purpose have begun to suggest areas for improved acceptability of this practice.

Risk from Use of Nonbarrier Contraceptives

Reference has also been made to a potential risk from hormonal contraceptives and IUDs. A recent cross-sectional study based on Thai sex workers reported an HIV risk among Depo-Provera users of 2 1/2 times that of nonusers (Rehle *et al.*, 1992). These results are highly preliminary and require corroboration by better-designed studies. Previous small reports have not demonstrated such an association. Theoretically, however, Depo-Provera might raise the risk of HIV infection because of the vaginal bleeding it can induce (Hunter & Mati, 1992).

Use of IUDs has also recently been linked to a raised risk of HIV infection (2.5 times the risk of nonusers) (Kapiga, Shao, Lwihula, & Hunter, 1994). If menstrual blood is a vector for HIV, then IUDs, which can cause increased menstrual and intermenstrual bleeding, may be a mechanism explaining and observed increased risk of HIV infection (Alexander, 1990). On the other hand, IUDs likely cause a local inflammatory reaction in the endometrium, which could recruit HIV target cells to the endometrial surface. Because of previous associations between IUD use and other reproductive tract infections, avoidance of IUD use among women at "high" risk of AIDS and other STDs has been suggested, although the definition of "high" risk is problematic (Fathalla, 1990).

Hormonal contraceptive methods and IUDs are currently in widespread use around the world and are seen in some areas as especially suitable for young women. The health implications of even a small increased risk of AIDS with these methods would be dire. Further well-designed studies on risk of AIDS with use of these methods are both feasible and urgently needed. In the meantime, family planning programs would be well-advised to implement aggressive counseling on preventing STDs, and, at a minimum, to provide both male and female condoms as resources toward this end. As mentioned in the Introduction, counseling on "dual method" use—or, use of a nonbarrier contraceptive plus barrier STD protection—has generated a controversy in the family planning field. It has been observed among young people in communities at high risk that this practice has so far not been adopted (Healton, 1991). Others, however, have pointed out the great need for such counseling and our historic failure in this regard (Fathalla, 1990). The recent literature contains a number of appeals by those with an interest in women's reproductive health (including the avoidance of unwanted pregnancy) that recognize the multiple values represented by both women's and men's barrier methods, especially when used properly (Hatcher & Warner, 1992; Cates & Stone, 1992). These publications make the point, stated earlier, that consistent use of spermicides and barriers (male or female condoms as first choices, diaphragms or cervical caps as next best) together would result in excellent levels of both contraception and prevention of many STDs.

Finally, investigations of the potential effects of other exogenous hormone treatments, e.g. postmenopausal estrogens, should be undertaken immediately, since postmenopausal women may be at a heightened biological risk for HIV infection due to changes in the vaginal or cervical epithelium.

Microbicide

National and international outrage over the plight of women in the age of AIDS has lent tremendous force to the once faint and disparate calls for viricide research and development and has galvanized a social movement (Stein, 1990, 1993; Elias & Heise, 1993). Because of the immense toll in morbidity and mortality associated with conventional STDs as well as the link between STDs and HIV, the term "microbicide" has come to be preferred to "viricide." The attributes of the "ideal" microbicide may vary from woman to woman; however, important overall reliable features include that it be controlled by a woman without the knowledge of a man; be applicable both vaginally and rectally; be able to kill all STD pathogens, including HIV; and allow a choice between conception and contraception. It would be safe for repeated and long-term use, over a wide range of populations, including sex workers. Finally, the compound would be able to be applied long in advance of intercourse and would remain effective for long periods of time in the vagina (Stein, 1990, 1993; Elias & Heise, 1993; Elias, 1993).

Very recently, direct research on a microbicide has been undertaken in the United States by the Population Council, an international nonprofit agency (Lancet, 1993; WHO, 1993). With funds from the Swedish International Development Authority, the Rockefeller Foundation, and the U.S. Agency for International Development, basic research has led to the identification of potential compounds for testing, and phase I (safety) trials have begun. The most promising of these is a class of compounds called "polysulfated polysaccharides," which are highly effective at blocking transmission of HIV at concentrations well below those associated with any damage to epithelial cells (Elias, 1993; Pearce-Pratt & Phillips, 1993; Pearce-Pratt, 1995; Voelker, 1995). Among these, the compound carrageenan—found in ice cream, chewing gum, and over-the-counter cosmetics—shows the greatest potential as a future microbicidal formulation for women. Recently, the FDA approved the compound for Phase I clinical testing. In addition, preliminary acceptability research is under way to inform product development. To some extent, the lack of fundamental research into barrier methods for women has slowed progress toward a microbicide. For example, as mentioned above, whether a foam or a suppository provides more complete and long-lasting coverage of the vagina is still not known, although these products have been in use for decades as spermicides.

In addition to the basic research being undertaken by the Population Council, ongoing dialogue and consultation with domestic and international women's groups have been undertaken to address issues in development, testing, and introduction of this new technology.

Because the earliest appearance of a microbicide is still several years away, there is a persisting need for education about conventional methods of STD protection such as those discussed in the previous section. We cannot afford to be inactive over the testing phase of this new compound, which may still be threatened by any number of setbacks, from scientific to economic. In addition, high cost may limit accessibility to this product, especially in the first few years and beyond that in poorer communities in the United States and worldwide. Nevertheless, recent progress on the microbicide has been impressive and must continue.

SOCIOPOLITICAL IMPLICATIONS OF TECHNOLOGICAL ADVANCES FOR WOMEN

The specter of an invisible and imperceptible method of protection under the control of a woman, though still a distant prospect, brings with it a sense of uneasiness about future interest in improving the status of women and in encouraging active male participation and sharing of protection of genital/reproductive health. Will a microbicide leave women with even more responsibility, and men with less? Will no additional efforts be made to change norms in communication among couples once the "magic bullet" becomes available? Will the male condom once again become the poor relation to women's methods of contraception because it is no longer "necessary"?

These are all valid and troubling questions implying a need for a deeper search into the meaning of the movement to prevent STDs/HIV among women. This chapter opened with a reference to the AIDS epidemic in women as an expression of our oppression. This includes lack of equal access to economic resources, which would encourage women to leave relationships they consider to be bad for their health and well-being; and lack of an equal share of decision-making power in relationships, which often removes the decision to use protection from their control (Stein, 1990; Reid, 1991, 1992).

In addition to the advances to be made against women's historic oppression, activists and researchers alike have also recognized the crucial role to be played by improving basic sex education, by improving girls' knowledge and understanding of their own bodies, and by encouraging communication about sex and responsibility among boys and girls who are not yet sexually active. To these must be added a change in the arbitrary yet traditional separation of contraception and protection of genital and reproductive health for women, which is contrary to the goals of health promotion (Winikoff, 1991; Hunter & Mati, 1992; La Guardia, 1992). There is a growing appreciation of the ways in which mystery, fear, and embarrassment about the body have provided barriers to self-protection for women and communication between partners (Harlan, Bernstein, & Kessler, 1991; Ehrhardt, Yingling, Zawadzki, & Martinez-Ramirez, 1992; Carrington *et al.,* 1993; Gollub & Stein, 1993a). Therefore, initial small-scale successes have been demonstrated, in hospital settings and elsewhere, with programs that stress education about the body, participatory health care, and an unrushed and supportive provider-client relationship (Carrington *et al.,* 1993; Gollub & Stein, 1993a; Gupta & Weiss, 1993).

COLLECTIVE POLITICAL ACTION AND DIALOGUE

The extensive current lack of knowledge in regard to AIDS prevention in women is startling, especially considering that for some of these questions, the research opportunities have long existed and do not require sophisticated new technologies. It is therefore important to close this chapter with a call for activism and lobbying of our federal government to commit more resources to the issue of women and AIDS. Advances made to date have occurred more often as a result of such lobbying than not. Agencies of the Public Health Service must dedicate funds toward basic research related to women's risk from sex as well as investigations of all possible woman-controlled methodologies. Old beliefs in women's fragility and ineptitude are apparent in the paternalistic attitudes of regulatory agencies and among health care institutions. We must strive to enlighten those influencing policy at these agencies and institutions and call for an explicit recognition that male condoms have not sufficed as the only answer to the AIDS epidemic. New and experimental prevention techniques must be made available for women who, for whatever reason, cannot and are not being protected by existing technologies, in the same way as we have allowed access to experimental AIDS therapies for men (and, in theory, women) already infected with the virus. As long as products are inherently safe (without significant short-term and long-term adverse health effects), which vaginal barriers generally are, effectiveness against HIV infection may vary over a wide range and still be useful for women with no other options. After all, a male condom may be 90% effective for consistent users, but for a woman with a partner who says no, they are 0% effective. A recent meta-analysis of 18 studies on male condom effectiveness estimates a use-effectiveness from published studies of 69% (Weller, 1993). This finding strengthens the argument for additional and alternate prevention methods.

Most of all, as advocates, we must insist on interdisciplinary approaches, including community involvement, and must work against chasms between women from different advocacy communities. The issue of woman-controlled prevention techniques has become a contentious one, with accusations in some circles that such an approach works against women's empowerment in society by placing the burden of protection upon the woman. This assertion refuses to acknowledge a common dream among activists and scientists working in this area—that of an end to the oppressive policies and practices that place women at great risk of HIV infection. A lack of dialogue among ourselves at this crucial juncture will splinter and weaken the advocacy movement for women's protection against AIDS/STD. The variety of women's needs and situations must be respected. It would be a sad moment if, in the attempt to provide women with options for both the short and long term, any potential power to effect change were undermined by a disintegration of a cohesive women's community. Many have observed that the substantial strides forward in AIDS research and treatment realized in the United States during the 1980s were a function of the well-developed lobbying efforts of an articulate and powerful, mainly white, gay male community. In contrast, our traditional lack of power as women (our most fundamental risk factor for AIDS), as well as our diversity in social class and race, present a formidable challenge to creating a global women's advocacy group. Yet it is in our common experience as women that we must find our strength.

To this end, a critical eye must be turned toward research, its implications, and the justifications given for abandoning research on women's methods generally or specifically. Certain technologies may need to be tailored for use with some populations of women and may not be appropriate for others. Such technologies may be considered "limited" or "imperfect," yet, when considered for worldwide use, they may have the potential to save hundreds of thousands, even millions, of lives.

ACKNOWLEDGMENTS. I am grateful for the insightful comments provided by Dr. Zena Stein and Dr. Paul Feldblum on earlier versions of this manuscript.

REFERENCES

Alexander, N. J. (1990). Sexual transmission of human immunodeficiency virus: Virus entry into the male and female genital tract. *Fertility and Sterility, 54,* 1–18.

Allen, S., Lindan, C., Serufilira, A., Van de Perre, P., Rundle, A. C., Nsengumuremyi, F., Carael, M., Schwalbe, J., & Hulley, S. (1991). Human immunodeficiency virus infection in urban Rwanda. *Journal of the American Medical Association, 266,* 1657–1663.

Anderson, D. J. (1992). Mechanisms of HIV-1 transmission via somen. *Journal of NIH Research, 4,* 104–108.

Aral, S. O., Mosher, W. D., & Cates, W., Jr. (1992). Vaginal douching among women of reproductive age in the United States: 1988. *American Journal of Public Health, 82,* 210–214.

Bailey, M. (1993). The passage of adolescence. Paper delivered at the New York State Psychiatric Institute meeting on "Young women: Increased vulnerability for HIV/STD infection." New York, July 14, 1993.

Bassett, M., Ray, C. S., Nicolette, J., & Managazna, P. (1993). Acceptability of the female condom among CSWs. Eighth International Conference on AIDS in Africa (abstract TOP29). Marrakesh, Morocco, December 12–16, 1993.

Bounds, W. Guillebaud, J., & Newman, G. B. (1992). Female condom (Femidom): A clinical study of its use-effectiveness and patient acceptability. *British Journal of Family Planning, 18,* 36–41.

Bruce, J. (1987). Users' perspectives on contraceptive technology and delivery systems: Highlighting some feminist issues. *Technology in Society, 9,* 359–383.

Bulterys, M., Chao, A., Dushimimana, A., Habimana P., Nawrocki, P., Kurawige, J. B., Musanganire, F., & Saah, A. (1993). Multiple sexual partners and mother-to-child transmission of HIV-1. *AIDS, 117,* 1639–1645.

Campbell, A. A., & Baldwin, W. (1991). The response of American women to the threat of AIDS and other sexually transmitted diseases. *Journal of Acquired Immune Deficiency Syndromes, 4,* 1133–1140.

Carrington, B. W., Thompson, R. L., Mitchell, J. L., Namero, P. B., Gordon, T., Loftman, P. O., & Williams, S. B. (1993). The need for family planning services for women delivering with little or no prenatal care. *Women and Health, 20,* 1–9.

Catania, J. A., Coates, T. J., Stall, R., Turner, H., Peterson, J., Hearst, N., Dolcini, M. M., Hudes, E., Gagnon, J., & Wiley, J. (1992). Prevalence of AIDS-related risk factors and condom use in the United States. *Science, 258,* 1101–1106.

Cates, W., & Hinman, A. R. (1992). AIDS and absolutism—the demand for perfection in prevention. *New England Journal of Medicine, 327,* 492–494.

Cates, W., Jr., Stewart, F., & Trussell, J. (1992). Commentary: The quest for women's prophylactic methods—hopes vs. science. *American Journal of Public Health, 82,* 1479–1482.

Cates, W., & Stone, K. M. (1992). Family planning, sexually transmitted diseases and contraceptive choice: A literature update—part 1. *Studies in Family Planning, 24,* 75–84.

Celentano, D. D., Klassen, A. C., Weisman, C. S., & Rosenhein, N. B. (1987). The role of contraceptive use in cervical cancer: The Maryland cervical cancer case-control study. *American Journal of Epidemiology, 126,* 592–604.

Centers for Disease Control and Prevention (1994). Heterosexually acquired AIDS—United States, 1993. *Journal of the American Medical Association, 271,* 975–976.

Chalker, R. (1987). *The complete cervical cap guide* (pp. 175–176). New York: Harper & Row.

Chao, A., Bulterys, M., Musanganire, F., Mukafaranswa, B., Nawrocki, P., Dushimimana, A., Hoover, D., & Saah, A. (1991). Risk factors for HIV-1 among pregnant women in Rwanda. Poster No. MC 3097. Seventh International Conference on AIDS, Florence.

Chu, S. Y., Buehler, J. W., Fleming, P. L., & Berkelmen, R. L. (1990). Epidemiology of reported cases of AIDS in lesbians, United States 1980–89. *American Journal of Public Health, 80,* 1380–1381.

Clemetson, D. B. A., Moss, G. B., Willerford, D. M., Hensel, M., Emonyi, W., Holmes, K. K., Plummer, F., Ndinya-Achola, J., Roberts, P., Hillier, S., & Kreiss, J. K. (1993). Detection of HIV DNA in cervical and vaginal secretions: Prevalence and correlates among women in Nairobi, Kenya. *Journal of the American Medical Association, 269,* 2860–2864.

Colimoro, C. (1993). El condon femenino. Presentation at the Fourth National Congress on AIDS, Mexico City, October, 13–15.

Corey, L. (1990). Genital herpes. In K. K. Holmes, P. Mardh, P. F. P. F. Sparling, P. J. Wiesner, W. Cates, S. M. Lemon, & W. E. Stamm (Eds.), *Sexually transmitted diseases,* 2nd ed. (pp. 391–413). New York: McGraw-Hill.

Cramer, D. W., Goldman, M. B., Schiff, I., Belisle, S., Albrecht, B., Stadel, B., Gibson, M., Wilson, E., Stillman, R., & Thompson, I. (1987). The relationship of tubal infertility to barrier method and oral contraceptive use. *Journal of the American Medical Association, 257,* 2446–2450.

Cutler, J. C., Singh, B., Carpenter, U., Nickens, O., Scarola, A., Sussman, N., Wade, M., Volkin, L., Marsico, A., & Balisky, H. (1977). Vaginal contraceptives as prophylaxis against gonorrhea and other sexually transmissible diseases. *Advances in Planned Parenthood, 12,* 45–55.

Des Jarlais, D. C., Freidman, S. R., Sotheran, J. L., Wenston, J., Marmor, M., Yancovitz, S. R., Frank, B., Beatrice, S., & Mildvan, D. (1994). Continuity and change within an HIV epidemic: Injecting drug users in New York City, 1984 through 1992. *Journal of the American Medical Association, 271,* 121–127.

De Vincenzi, I., and the European Study Group on Heterosexual Transmission of HIV. (1994). A longitudinal study of human immunodeficiency virus transmission by heterosexual partner. *New England Journal of Medicine 331,* 341–346.

Drew, W. L., Blair, M., Miner, R. C., & Conant, M. (1990). Evaluation of the virus permeability of a new condom for women. *Sexually Transmitted Diseases, 17,* 110–112.

Duncan, M. E., Tibaux, G., Pelzer, A., Reimann, K., Peutherer, J. F., Simmonds, P., Young, H., Jamil, H., & Daroughar, S. (1990). First coitus and risk of sexually transmitted disease. *Lancet, 335,* 338–340.

Ehrhardt, A. A., Yingling, S., Zawadzki, R., & Martinez-Ramirez, M. (1992). Prevention of heterosexual transmission of HIV: Barriers for women. *Journal of Psychology and Human Sexuality 5*:1 & *2*:37–67.

Ehrhardt, A. A., Nostlinger, C., Meyer-Bahlburg, H., Exner, T. M., Gruen, R. S., Yingling, S. L., Gorman, J. M., El-Sadr, W., & Sorrell, S. J. (1995). Sexual risk behavior among women with injected drug use histories. *Journal of Psychology and Human Sexuality,* in press.

Elias, C., & Heise, L. (1993). The development of microbicides: A new method of HIV prevention for women. Working papers, No. 6. New York: The Population Council.

Elias, C. (1993). Roundtable on women's methods. Ninth International Conference on AIDS, Berlin, June 7–11, 1993.

Elias, C. (1995). A puzzle of will: Responding to reproductive tract infections in the context of family planning programs. In *Population council. Critical issues in reproductive health and population* (pp. 5–23). Presentations from a panel held on Professional Development Day at the USAID Cooperating Agencies meeting, Washington, DC., February 25, 1994.

European Study Group on Heterosexual Transmission of HIV (1992). Comparison of female to male and male to female transmission of HIV in 563 stable couples. *British Medical Journal, 304,* 809–813.

Fathalla, M. F. (1990). Relationship between contraceptive technology and HIV transmission. *Heterosexual transmission of AIDS.* New York: Alan Liss.

Feldblum, P. J. (1994). Spermicide acceptability among women and men at risk of STD. *International Society of Sexually Transmitted Disease Research,* August 28–31, 1995.

Feldblum, P., Hira, S., Kamanga, J., Mukelabai, G., Weir, S., & Thomas, J. Condom and Nonoxynol-9 use and HIV incidence in serodiscordant couples in Zambia. Unpublished abstract.

Feldblum, P. J., & Weir, S. S. (1995). The protective effect of nonoxynol-9 against HIV infection (letter). *American Journal of Public Health, 84,* 1032–1033.

Ferreira, A. E., Araujo, M. J., Regina, C. H., Diniz, S. G., & Faundes, A. (1993). Effectiveness of the diaphragm, used continuously, without spermicide. *Contraception, 48,* 29–35.

Ford, N., & Mathie, E. (1993). The acceptability and experience of the female condom, Femidom, among family planning clinic attenders. *British Journal of Family Planning, 19,* 187–192.

Garland, S. M., Newman, D. M., & de Crespigny, L. C. (1989). Plastic wrap for ultrasound transducers: Herpes simplex virus transmission. *Journal of Ultrasound in Medicine, 8,* 661–663.

Germain, A. (1993). Are we speaking the same language? Women's health advocates and scientists talk about contraceptive technology. In *Four essays on birth control needs and risks,* R. Dixon-Mueller and A. Germain (Eds.). New York: International Women's Health Coalition.

Gollub, E. (1993). The female condom: STD protection in the hands of women. *American Journal of Gynecological Health, Jul/Aug,* 9–10.

Gollub, E. (1995). STD/HIV prevention in the hands of women. HIV in Women Conference, Washington, DC, February 22–24, 1995.

Gollub, E., & Stein, Z. (1992). Nonoxynol-9 and the reduction of HIV transmission in women (letter) *AIDS, 6,* 599–601.

Gollub, E., & Stein, Z. (1993a). Woman-controlled HIV prevention: Meeting women's needs in an inner-city hospital setting. In Abstract No. PO-CO4-2627. *Proceedings of the International Conference on AIDS* (Berlin, June 6–11), *2,* 655.

Gollub, E., & Stein, Z. (1993b). The new female condom—item one on a woman's AIDS prevention agenda. *American Journal of Public Health, 83,* 498–500.

Gollub, E., & Stein, Z. (1995). Short-term acceptability of the female condom among women living or working in Harlem. *Family Planning Perspectives,* in press.

Gollub, E., French, P., Latka, M., & O'Donnell, J. (1995). Philadelphia Women's Health Sister Studies: Novel Approaches to Reducing STD/HIV Risk among Attending an STD Clinic (poster). HIV Infection in Women Conference, Washington, DC, February 22–24, 1995.

Grafenberg, E., & Dickinson, R. L. (1944). Conception control by plastic cervix cap. *Western Journal of Surgery,* 335–340.

Gupta, G. R., & Weiss, E. (1993). Women and AIDS: Developing a new health strategy. ICRW Policy Series No. 1. October, Washington, DC.

Hardon, A. (1992). The needs of women versus the interests of family planning personnel, policy-makers and researchers: Conflicting news on safety and acceptability of contraceptives. *Social Science in Medicine, 6,* 753–766.

Harlan, L. C., Bernstein, A. B., & Kessler, L. G. (1991). Cervical cancer screening: Who is not screened and why? *American Journal of Public Health, 81,* 885–891.

Hatcher, R. A., & Warner, D. L. (1992). New condoms for men and women, diaphragms, cervical caps and spermicides: Overcoming barriers to barriers and spermicides. *Current Opinion in Obstetrics and Gynecology, 4,* 513–519.

Hatcher, R. A., Trussell, J., Stewart, F., Stewart, G. K., Kowal, D., Guest, F., Cates, W., & Policar, M. (1994). *Contraceptive Technology,* Sixteenth Revised Edition (Chapters 8, 9, 27). New York: Irvington Publishers.

Healton, C. (1991). In harm's way—Urban minority youth and the AIDS epidemic. Doctoral dissertation. New York: Columbia University School of Public Health.

Henin, Y., Mandelbrot, L., Henrion, R., Pradinaud, R., Coulaud, J. P., & Montagnier, L. (1993). Virus excretion in the cervicovaginal secretions of pregnant and nonpregnant HIV-infected women. *Journal of Acquired Immune Deficiency Syndromes, 6,* 72–75.

Hernandez-Avila, M. (1992). Acceptability of female condoms among female prostitutes in Mexico City: Preliminary findings. Report to the Wisconsin Pharmaceutical Company.

Hunter, D. J., & Mati, J. K. (1992). Contraception, family planning and HIV. In L. C. Chen, J. S. Amore, & S. J. Segal (Eds.), *AIDS and women's reproductive health: Reproductive biology series.* New York: Plenum Press.

Kapiga, S. H., Shao, J. F., Lwihula, G. K. & Hunter, D. J. (1994). Risk factors for HIV infection and sexually transmitted diseases (STD's) among women attending family planning clinics in Dar-es-Salaam, Tanzania. *Journal of Acquired Immune Deficiency Syndromes, 7,* 301–309.

Kreiss, J., Ngugi, E., Holmes, K., Ndinya-Achola, J., Waiyaki, P., Roberts, P. L., Ruminjo, I., Sajabi, R., Kimata, J., Fleming, T. R., Anazala, A., Holton, D., & Plummer, F. (1992). Efficacy of nonoxynol-9 contraceptive sponge use in preventing heterosexual acquisition of HIV in Nairobi prostitutes. *Journal of the American Medical Association, 268,* 477–482.

Laga, M., Manoka, A. T., Kivuvu, M., Malele, B., Tuliza, M., Nzila, N., Goeman, J., Behets, F., Batter, V., Alary, M., Heyward, W. L., Ryder, R. W., & Piot, P. (1993). Non-ulcerative sexually transmitted diseases as risk factors for HIV-1 transmission in women: Results from a cohort study. *AIDS 7,* 95–102.

Lazzarin, A., Saracco, A., Musicco, M., Nicolosi, A., & the Italian Study Group on HIV Heterosexual Transmission (1991). Man-to-woman sexual transmission of the human immunodeficiency virus. *Archives of Internal Medicine, 151,* 2411–2416.

Lee, T. Y., Utidjian, H. M. D., Singh, B., & Carpenter, U. (1972). Potential impact of chemical prophylaxis on the incidence of gonorrhea. *British Journal of Venereal Diseases, 48,* 376–380.

Lehfeldt, H. (1970). Cervical cap. In M. S. Calderone (Ed.), *Manual of family planning and contraceptive practice.* Baltimore: Williams & Wilkins.

Lehfeldt, H., Sobrero, A. J., & Inglis, W. (1961). Spermicidal effectiveness of chemical contraceptives used with the firm cervical cap. *American Journal of Obstetrics and Gynecology, 82,* 446–448.

Leigh, B. C., Temple, M. T., & Trocki, K. F. (1993). The sexual behavior of US adults: Results from a national survey. *American Journal of Public Health, 83,* 1400–1408.

Liskin, L. (1993). Using female condom for AIDS prevention: Promises and problems (abstract TOP28). December 14, 1993. Eighth International Conference on AIDS in Africa, Marrakesh, December 12–16, 1993.

Louv, W. C., Austin, H., Alexander, W. J., Stagno, S., & Cheeks, J. (1988). A clinical trial of nonoxynol-9 for preventing gonococcal and chlamydial infections. *Journal of Infections Diseases, 158,* 518–523.

Marmor, M., Weiss, L. R., Lyden, M., Weiss, S. H., Saxinger, W. C., Spira, T. J., & Feorino, P. M. (1986). Possible female-to-female transmission of human immunodeficiency virus. *Annals of Internal Medicine, 105,* 969.

McCormack, W. M., Reynolds, G. H., & the Cooperative Study Group. (1982). Effect of menstrual cycle and method of contraception on recovery of Neisseria gonorrhoeae. *Journal of the American Medical Association, 247,* 1292–1294.

Mendez, F., Castro, A., & Ortega, A. (1986). Use-effectiveness of a spermicidal suppository containing benzalkonium chloride. *Contraception, 34,* 353–363.

Miller, C., Alexander, N. J., Vogel, P., Anderson, J., & Marx, P. A. (1992). Mechanisms of genital transmission of SIV: A hypothesis based on transmission studies and the location of SIV in the genital tract of chronically infected females. *Journal of Medical Primatology, 21,* 64–68.

Moatti, J. P., Bajos, N., Durbec, J. P., Menard, C., & Serrand C. (1991). Determinants of condom use among French heterosexuals with multiple partners. *American Journal of Public Health, 81,* 106–109.

Monzon, O. T., & Capellan, J. M. B. (1987). Female-to-female transmission of HIV. *Lancet, 2,* 40–41.

Moscicki, A. B., Winkler, B., Irwin, C. E., & Schachter, J. (1989). Differences in biologic maturation, sexual behavior, and sexually transmitted disease between adolescents with and without cervical intraepithelial neoplasia. *Journal of Pediatrics, 115,* 487–493.

Moss, G. B., Clemetson, D., D'Costa L., Plummer, F. A., Ndinya-Achola, J. O., Reilly, M., Holmes, K. K., Piot, P., Maitha, G. M., Hillier, S. L., Kiviat, N. C., Cameron, C. W., Wamola, I. A., & Kreiss, J. K. (1991). Association of cervical ectopy with heterosexual transmission of human immunodeficiency virus: Results of a study of couples in Nairobi, Kenya. *Journal of Infectious Diseases, 164:*588–91.

Niruthisard, S., Roddy, R. E., & Chutivongse, S. (1991). The effects of frequent nonoxynol-9 use on the vaginal and cervical mucosa. *Sexually Transmitted Diseases, 18,* 176–179.

Niruthisard, S., Roddy, R. E., & Chutivongse, S. (1992). Use of nonoxynol-9 and reduction in rate of gonococcal and chlamydial cervical infections. *Lancet, 339,* 1371–1375.

Pearce-Pratt, R., & Phillips, D. M. (1993). Studies of adhesion of lymphocytic cells: Implication for sexual transmission of the human immunodeficiency virus. *Biology of Reproduction, 48,* 431–445.

Persson, E. (1991). Family planning and prevention strategies for sexually transmitted diseases. *Advances in Contraception, 7,* 181–186.

Peters, R. K., Thomas, C., Hagan, D. G., Mack, T. M., & Henderson, B. E. (1986). Risk factors for invasive cervical cancer among Latinas and non-Latinas in Los Angeles County. *Journal of the National Cancer Institute, 77,* 1063–1077.

Plummer, F. A., Simonsen, J. N., Cameron, D. W., Ndinya-Achola, J. O., Kreiss, J. K., Gakinya,

M. N., Waiyaki, P., Cheang, M., Piot, P., Ronald, A. R., & Ngugi, E. N. (1991). Cofactors in male–female sexual transmission of human immunodeficiency virus. *Journal of Infectious Diseases, 163,* 233–239.

Population Reports (1979). Spermicides—simplicity and safety are major assets. Series H, No. 5: H78–118. Baltimore: Population Information Program, Johns Hopkins University.

Population Reports (1984). New developments in vaginal contraception. Series H, No. 7 (Jan/Feb): H157–H190. Baltimore: Population Information Program, Johns Hopkins University.

Redondo-Lopez, V., Cook, R. L., & Sobel, J. D. (1990). Emerging role of laeto bacilli in the control and maintenance of the vaginal bacterial microflora. *Reviews of Infectious Diseases, 5,* 856–872.

Rehle, T., Brinkmann, U. K., Siraprapasiri, T., Coplan, P., Aiemsukawat, C., & Ungchusak, K. (1992). Risk factors of HIV-1 infection among female prostitutes in Khon Kaen, Northeast Thailand. *Infection 20, 6,* 26/328–29/331.

Reid, E. Gender, knowledge, and responsibility. (1992). In J. Mann, D. J. Tarantola, & T. W. Netter (Eds.). *AIDS in the world.* Cambridge: Harvard University Press.

Reid, E. Placing women at the centre of the analysis. (1991). In: *Women and AIDS: Strategies for the future.* Canadian International Development Agency.

Roddy, R. E., Cordero, M., Cordero, C., & Fortney, J. A. (1993). A dosing study of nonoxynol-9 and genital irritation. *International Journal of STD and AIDS, 4,* 165–170.

Rosenberg, M. J., Feldblum, P. J., Rojanpithayakorn, W., & Sawasdivorn, W. (1987). The contraceptive sponge's protection against Chlamydia trachomatis and Neisseria gonorrhoeae. (1987). *Sexually Transmitted Diseases, 14,* 147–152.

Rosenberg, M. J., & Phillips, R. S. (1992). Does douching promote ascending infection? *Journal of Reproductive Medicine, 37,* 930–938.

Rosenberg, M. J., & Gollub, E. L. (1992). Commentary: Methods women can use that may prevent sexually transmitted disease, including HIV. *American Journal of Public Health, 82,* 1473–1478.

Rosenberg, M. J., Holmes, K. K., & the World Health Organization Working Group on Virucides (1993). Virucides in prevention of HIV infection. *Sexually Transmitted Diseases, 20,* 41–44.

Saracco, A., et al. (1993). Man-to-woman sexual transmission of HIV: Longitudinal study of 343 steady partners of infected men. *Journal of Acquired Immune Deficiency Syndromes, 6,* 497–502.

Sen, G., & Snow, R. C. (1994). Power and decision: The social control of reproduction. In *Harvard series on population and international health. Harvard Center for population and Development Studies.* (pp. 233–253). Cambridge: Harvard University Press.

Schachter, J. (1990). Biology of *Chlamydia trachomatis.* In K. K. Holmes, P. Mardh, P. F. Sparling, P. J. Wiesner, W. Cates, S. M. Lemon, & W. E. Stamm (Eds.), *Sexually transmitted diseases,* 2nd ed. (pp. 167–180). New York: McGraw-Hill.

Scholes, D., Daling, J. R., Stergachis, A., Weiss, N., Wang, S., & Grayston, T. (1993). Vaginal douching as a risk factor for acute pelvic inflammatory disease. *Obstetrics Gynecology, 81,* 601–606.

Sciarra, J. J. (1979). Vaginal contraception: Historical perspective. In G. I. Zatuchni, A. J. Sobrero, J. J. Speidel, & J. J. Sciarra (Eds). *Vaginal contraception: New developments.* New York: Harper & Row.

Scofield, V. L., Rao, B., Broder, S., *et al.* (1994). HIV interaction with sperm. *AIDS, 12,* 1733–1736.

Shervington, D. (1993). Acceptance of the female condom among low income African American women. *Journal of the National Medical Association, 85,* 341–347.

Shervington, D. (1994). Experiences of African-American women with the use of the Reality female condom. Proceedings, International Conference on AIDS, Yokohama, Japan, August.

Siboulet, A., Bohbot, J. M., Catalan, F., & Siboulet, A. (1988). Prevention locale feminine des MST. Resultats obtenus avec le benzalkonium sous la forme comprimes pharmatex. *Contraception-fertilité-sexualité, 16,* 403–411.

Simonsen, J. N., Plummer, F. A., Ngugi, E. N., Black, C., Kreiss, J. K., Gakinya, M. N., Waiyaki, P., D'Costa, L. J., Ndinya-Achola, J. O., Piot, P., & Ronald, A. (1990). HIV infection among lower socioeconomic stratum prostitutes in Nairobi. *AIDS, 4,* 139–144.

Singer, A. (1975). The uterine cervix from adolescence to the menopause. *British Journal of Obstetrics and Gynecology, 82,* 81–99.

Slattery, M. L., Overall, J. C., Abbott, T. M., French, T. K., Robison, L. M., & Gardner, J. (1989). Sexual activity, contraception, genital infections and cervical cancer: Support for a sexually-transmitted disease hypothesis. *American Journal of Epidemiology, 130,* 248–258.

Smith, C., Farr, M. G., Feldblum, P. J., & Spence, A. (1995). Effectiveness of the non-spermicidal fit—free diaphragm *Contraception* (in press).

Soper, D. E., Shoupe, D., Shangold, G. A., Shangold, M. M., Gutmann, J., & Mercer, L. (1993). Prevention of vaginal trichomoniasis by compliant users of the female condom. *Sexually Transmitted Diseases, 20,* 137–139.

Sorin, M. D. (1995). The women's methods of sexual HIV self-protection hierarchy in family planning (abstract). HIV Infection in Women Conference, Washington, DC, February 22–24.

Spira, A., Bajos, N., & the ACSF (Analyse des Comportements Sexuels en France) Investigators. (1992). AIDS and sexual behavior in France. *Nature, 360,* 407–409.

Stamm, W. E., & Holmes, K. K. (1990). Chlamydia trachomatis infections of the adult. In K. K. Holmes, P. Mardh, P. F. Sparling, P. J. Wiesner, W. Cates, S. M. Lemon, & W. E. Stamm (Eds.). *Sexually transmitted diseases,* 2nd ed. (pp. 181–193). New York: McGraw-Hill.

Stein, Z. A. (1990). HIV prevention: The need for methods women can use. *American Journal of Public Health, 80,* 460–462.

Stein, Z. A. (1992). The double bind in science policy and the protection of women from HIV infection. *American Journal of Public Health, 82,* 1471–1472.

Stein, Z. A. (1993). HIV prevention: An update on the status of methods women can use. *American Journal of Public Health, 83,* 1379–1382.

Stim, E. M. (1980). The nonspermicide fit-free diaphragm: A new contraceptive method. *Advances in Planned Parenthood,* 88–98.

Stone, K. M., Grimes, D. A., & Magdar, L. S. (1986). Personal protection against sexually transmitted diseases. *American Journal of Obstetries and Gynecology, 155,* 180–188.

Stone, K. M. (1990). Avoiding sexually transmitted diseases. *Obstetrics and gynecology clinics of North America, 17,* 789–799.

Stone, K. M., & Peterson, H. B. (1992). Spermicides, HIV and the vaginal sponge. *Journal of the American Medical Association, 268,* 521–523.

Strebel, A. (1993). Good intentions, contradictory outcomes? AIDS prevention and care for South African women. *Community Health Association of South Africa Journal, 4,* 22–25.

Trussell, J., Hatcher, R. A., Cates, W., Stewart F. H., & Kost, K. (1990). Contraceptive failure in the United States: An update. *Studies in Family Planning, 21,* 51–54.

Trussell, J. (1992). Testimony before the OBGYN Devices Committee of the Office of Device Evaluation, Center for Devices and Radiological Health, U.S. Food and Drug Administration, on the Reality female condom. Washington, DC, December 10.

Trussell, J., Sturgen, K., Strickler, J., & Dominik, R. (1994). Comparative contraceptive efficacy of the female condom and other barrier methods. *Family Planning Perspectives, 26,* 66–72.

United Nations Development Program: HIV and Development Programme (1992). Young women: Silence, susceptibility, and the HIV epidemic.

USDHHS. (1980). Vaginal contraceptive drug products for over-the-counter human use; establishment of a monograph; proposed rule-making. *Federal Register, 45 (421),* Friday, Dec. 12.

Vernon, R., & Ojeda, G. (1990). Incorporating AIDS prevention activities into a family planning organization in Columbia. *Studies in Family Planning, 21,* 335–343.

Voelker, R. (1995). Scientists zero in on new HIV microbicides. *Journal of the American Medical Association 13,* 979–980.

Voeller, B. (1991). AIDS and heterosexual anal intercourse. *Archives of Sexual Behavior,* 20, 233–276.

Voeller, B. (1985). Spermicides: An additional potential barrier to the sexual spread of the AIDS virus, LAV-HTLV-III. In Mariposa Occasional Paper #4B (pp. 1–8). New York: Mariposa Education and Research Foundation.

Wasserheit, J. N. (1992). Epidemiological synergy: Interrelationships between human immunodeficiency virus infection and other sexually transmitted diseases. *Sexually Transmitted Diseases, 19,* 61–77.

Watters, J. K., Estilo, J. J. Clark, G. L., & Lorvick, J. (1994). Syringe exchange and needle exchange as HIV/AIDS prevention for injection drug users. *Journal of the American Medical Association, 271,* 115–120.

Wawer, M. J., Serwadda, D., Musgrave, S. D., Konde-Lule, J. K., Musagara, M., & Sewankambo, N. K. (1991). Dynamics of the spread of HIV-1 infection in a rural district of Uganda. *British Medical Journal, 303,* 1303–1306.

Weir, S. S., Feldblum, P. J., Roddy, R. E., & Zekeng, L. (1994). Gonorrhea as a risk factor for HIV acquisition. *AIDS, 8,* 1605–1608.

Weir, S. S., Feldblum, P. J., Zekeng, L., & Roddy, R. E. (1994). The use of nonoxynol-9 for protection against cervical gonorrhea *American Journal of Public Health, 84,* 910–914.

Weir, S. S., Roddy, R. E., Zekeng, L., & Feldblum, F. (1995). Nonoxynol-9 use, genital ulcers and HIV infection in a cohort of sex workers. *Genitourinary Medicine* (in press).

Weisman, C. S., Plichta, S., Nathanson, C. A., Ensninger, M., & Robinson, J. C. Consistency of condom use for disease prevention among adolescent users of oral contraceptives. *Family Planning Perspectives, 23,* 71–74.

Weller, S. C. (1993). A meta-analysis of condom effectiveness in reducing sexually transmitted HIV. *Social Science in Medicine, 36,* 1635–1644.

Whaley, K. J., Barratt, R. A., Zeitlin, L., Hoen, T. E., & Cone, R. A. (1993). Nonoxynol-9 protects mice against vaginal transmission of genital herpes infections. *Journal of Infectious Diseases, 168,* 1009–1011.

Zekeng, L., Feldblum, P. J., Oliver, R., & Kaptue, L. (1993). Barrier contraceptive use and HIV infection among high-risk women in Cameroon. *AIDS, 7,* 725–731.

Zewdie, D. (1994). Men, women and AIDS. Plenary session, Eighth Conference on AIDS in Africa. Marrakesh, December 12–16, 1993.

4

Childhood Sexual Abuse and AIDS

Issues and Interventions

BEATRIZ PEREZ, GAIL KENNEDY, and MINDY THOMPSON FULLILOVE

In the past 20 years, the mental health professions have made much progress in understanding the human mind. Studies of neurochemistry, brain anatomy, and neurophysiology have led to new knowledge and new treatments. One of the most important areas of new knowledge is a series of discoveries that came, in large part, from patients' self-help groups, rather than researchers' laboratories. These are the advances that have been made in understanding the role of traumatic events—i.e., catastrophes that threaten the survival of the self—in the development of mental disorders. This understanding represents a major breakthrough because the study of trauma had been stymied for many years by theoretical models of the human psyche that placed too little weight on actual events. It took great effort to reorient the professions.

This work was accomplished by suffering men and women who needed—and demanded—help. Many of the men and women who had been to war in Vietnam came back in great distress, but they were offered little help in coping with painful, recurrent memories or terrifying nightmares. They organized "rap groups" and "drop-in centers" where they could share with each other what it had been like. They also put pressure on the Veterans Administration to provide mental health services to meet their needs. At the same time, the women's liberation movement began to provide advocacy and services for women who had been raped or were victims of domestic violence. Many of the professionals who have reshaped

---

BEATRIZ PEREZ, GAIL KENNEDY, and MINDY THOMPSON FULLILOVE • The Community Research Group, New York State Psychiatric Institute, New York, NY 10032.
Women at Risk: Issues in the Primary Prevention of AIDS, edited by Ann O'Leary and Loretta Sweet Jemmott. Plenum Press, New York, 1995.

the mental health disciplines actually became interested, concerned, and informed through their participation in these grass-roots self-help movements.

Out of those efforts have come research and treatment efforts that have outlined what traumatic events do to the mind. Probably the fact that trauma threatens physical, mental, or spiritual survival accounts for the deep injury it can cause. Survivors are left doubting their ability to protect and maintain themselves. This doubt can lead to a loss of faith in other people, of hope for the future, and of a sense of security in day-to-day events. People who have sustained intense, acute trauma may develop the disorder known as posttraumatic stress disorder. Those subjected to years of torture or abuse may have developed severe personality disorders, of which the most extreme is multiple personality disorder.

Childhood sexual abuse is one of the most serious traumas studied to date. Childhood sexual abuse can leave profound scars on the physical and mental health of the survivor. As a result of childhood sexual abuse, the survivor may have trouble caring for herself. This lack of self-protection can contribute to serious, and perhaps lifelong, problems. For example, a study of 511 women seeking care at a clinic in the rural Midwest found that 22% of the women had been sexually abused (Springs & Friedrich, 1992). The authors found that compared to nonabused women, abused women had significantly more health problems, had had more operations, engaged in more risk behaviors, and reported more physical and mental symptoms. Those who had suffered the most severe abuse rated most negatively on all these measures.

Studies have found that a history of childhood sexual abuse is a risk factor for many illnesses and conditions, such as adolescent pregnancy (Boyer & Fine, 1992), running away from home (Stiffman, 1989), drug use (Dembo *et al.,* 1988), prostitution (Simons & Whitbeck, 1991), sexually transmitted disease (Vermund, Alexander-Rodriquez, MacLeod, & Kelley, 1990), and gynecological problems (Springs & Friedrich, 1992).

AIDS may well be added to the list of illnesses for which childhood sexual abuse is considered an important precursor (Zierler *et al.,* 1991). Zierler and her colleagues, in a study conducted in 1991 among high-risk adults seeking HIV testing, found that 28% of the women interviewed reported a history of childhood sexual abuse. Women abused as children were 3 times more likely to have reported a history of commercial sex work and $2^1/_2$ times more likely to have reported early pregnancy than women who reported no such abuse. Men with a history of childhood sexual abuse had an increased risk of HIV infection (Zierler *et al.,* 1991).

It is possible that the increased likelihood of engaging in prostitution or drug use is the link between childhood sexual abuse and risk for HIV infection. Reported rates of childhood sexual abuse appear to be higher among substance-abuse clients than in the general population. A survey of clients entering substance-abuse treatment in Maine revealed that approximately three quarters of women had histories of childhood sexual abuse (Rohsenow, Corbett, & Devine, 1988). This rate is significantly higher than the rate of 27% obtained in a national, random telephone survey of 1481 women (Finkelhor, 1990). In a study of 100 women undergoing laparoscopy, those with a history of childhood sexual abuse were 6 times more likely than those without to report substance-abuse problems (Walker *et al.,* 1992).

Furthermore, among substance-using women, those with a history of childhood sexual abuse appear to be at higher risk for participation in commercial sex work than are substance-using women with no abuse history. In a study of drug-using women in New York City, 74 (51%) reported forced sexual experiences, of whom 34 (46%) were 16 or under at the time of the attack. Forced sex was associated with increased risk for participation in sex-for-drugs exchanges: Women with a history of sexual abuse were 2.9 times more likely to have engaged in that behavior than those without such a history (Paone, Chavkin, Willets, Friedmann, & Des Jarlais, 1992).

Childhood sexual abuse may play an important role in increasing risk for HIV infection. However, in order to understand this problem more fully, it is essential to examine the larger life context of people most at risk for HIV infection.

THE GEOGRAPHY OF THE AIDS–TRAUMA CONNECTION

AIDS has not struck randomly at the United States population. Rather, it has disproportionately affected marginalized populations: gay men, intravenous drug users, crack users, the homeless, and the mentally ill. These marginalized groups live in what Zwi and Cabral (1992) call "high-risk situations." They offered that term to differentiate the problems of "individual" risk from those of "group" risk. In high-risk situations, the forces that structure individual behavior increase the likelihood that a person will be exposed to HIV infection. For example, forced migration in a war-torn country—Rwanda is a case in point—will break up families, leave many penniless, increase despair, and otherwise disrupt normal social behaviors. Drug use and prostitution erupt in settings so deeply torn from their normal patterns of social interaction. The increase in these behaviors may lead to the spread of AIDS, but the high-risk behavior of the individual is directly linked to the effect of the war on the entire social group.

A common feature of high-risk situations is that they are characterized by high rates of trauma of all kinds. In fact, in the United States, it is not simply childhood sexual abuse that is present in the lives of women at risk for HIV infection. Rather, it is the broad range of traumas that cause injury and can lead to increased risk-taking and poorer self-care. Though traumatic events are defined by the American Psychiatric Association as "unusual" events (APA, 1987), they are actually all too common in the lives of the poor and the dispossessed. About 1% of "middle Americans" surveyed in the 1980s reported that they had experienced trauma (Kulka, Fairbank, Jordan, & Weiss, 1990). But nearly every resident of central Harlem, surveyed in 1993 by our research group, reported a history of one catastrophe or another. In fact, three fourths of the respondents in central Harlem reported three or more traumatic events. Emerging studies have found a high prevalence of traumatic events among gay men living in major centers of gay life. It is not surprising, given their experiences of marginalization and displacement, that the rates are high. Not only childhood sexual abuse, but also physical abuse, bias crimes, and other traumas, are found in the life stories of these men.

Given the "traumatic context" of people at risk for AIDS, childhood sexual abuse will often appear in the individual woman's life story as part of a constellation of traumatic events, occurring in a high-stress setting that offers minimal social support. It becomes difficult, under such circumstances, to separate the effects of childhood sexual abuse from other noxious factors. Rather, we believe that it is important to gain as broad an understanding as possible of the woman's life context, taking into consideration any and all traumatic events, the possibly toxic nature of the surrounding environment, and the presence or absence of social and emotional support.

How, then, should we describe the AIDS–trauma geography? There are several relationships that we believe are important. The first is that the community context puts people at risk to experience traumatic events. Victims of trauma, in turn, are more likely to engage in risky behavior. Finally, trauma is generally disabling. It adds to the list of problems and conditions that the HIV-infected individual must confront in the course of seeking care. Unfortunately, many of the manifestations of trauma-related illness will impede, rather than promote, help-seeking and compliance. Just at a point in their lives where they need to negotiate intensively with care systems, trauma survivors may not be able to be "good" patients.

In the following sections of this chapter, we will relate the unfolding story of our "Women and Trauma Project" in order to explore the interrelationships of trauma and AIDS and to draw lessons about the kinds of interventions and actions that women need. We hope that the stories convey some of the pain of trauma, as well as the hope of recovery.

THE "WOMEN AND TRAUMA PROJECT"

Since 1990, our research group has been working with women in recovery from drug addiction. That year, we began to conduct individual interviews and focus groups designed to tell us about sex-for-drugs exchanges, a risky sexual behavior linked to the spread of HIV among crack users. What we learned was that trauma and violence were an important, but unappreciated, aspect of the risky behavior (Fullilove, Lown, & Fullilove, 1992). In those interviews, participants suggested a "vicious cycle" of drug use and revictimization. Those caught up in this cycle described using drugs to dull the pain of childhood sexual abuse. While using drugs, they were likely to experience trauma. Some also became involved in sex-for-drugs exchanges, which exposed them to further trauma—notably rape or physical assault—necessitating even greater dependence on drugs.

One woman's story helps to illustrate this cycle of trauma and violence. In a series of interviews, the first in the spring of 1991 and the last in the winter of 1993, this woman, whom we shall call Paulette, shared with our research team the story of what had happened to her:

> *Story 1: "He was my firstborn."*
>
> Paulette, a 43-year-old black woman in recovery from heroin addiction, had discovered in the spring of 1991 that she was HIV-positive. She was extremely distraught when she first learned the news, and was especially distressed that the man she lived with didn't seem to care about what was happening to her. She felt helpless and hopeless.
>
> She began using drugs at age 13 to ward off the pain of being raped each night by her older stepbrother. She said:
>
>> [The drugs] made me forget about a lot of things and I knew that when I was high it didn't matter. It mattered to me but he did the things to me that he was doing, but then you didn't think about it. Like if I will feel numb.
>
> The sexual abuse was accompanied by belittling and degrading comments that made her feel isolated and worthless. Her stepbrother told her that no one else would ever want her because she was fat and unattractive. She felt that no one would listen to her if she reported the abuse. In fact, she felt that the abuse was her fault and that she would be blamed for it. She said of this:
>
>> I never wanted to talk about it before, 'cause I always thought it was something that I did, you know. That boy made me grow up to think that I was homely and, you know, nobody is ever going to want you, you know. I was always big—fat as a child—he made me really dislike myself.
>
> Paulette had a lasting resentment toward her father, who had placed her in a dangerous situation and was not available to protect her. She felt that if she told him about the abuse, he would do nothing to help her. She was sad that he had died with the past unresolved. She said of him:
>
>> I loved him because he was my father . . . but I hated that man. I hated that man with passion. . . . I never talked to him, you know. My father died, and, you know, and I never really told him, out of my own mouth, you know. I do love you, you know. Then when he died, that was something else I had

> on me. . . . I never even told him why I was angry at him, you know. maybe it was something that he would have done, maybe he wouldn't have, but I never even told him.

Paulette became pregnant at age 15 and had a baby boy, fathered by her stepbrother. She pretended that she had a boyfriend who was the father of the baby. She was filled with rage about what had happened to her, but was unable to direct that anger at her stepbrother, whom she feared. Instead, she took it out on the child:

> I took [the baby] and I smothered him into the wall and busted all of his mouth open. He was an innocent little baby, you know. I did that, I know now, I did that out of anger because I wanted to do that to my stepbrother, but I couldn't, you know. I hide it. I would tell everyone that I had a boyfriend, and I didn't. I knew that was his baby, you know. Sometimes I hated that baby and sometimes I loved him. I'm still going to cry because I know that I did that to my baby, you know, he—that was my baby—that was my firstborn.

In the wake of the sexual abuse she suffered as a young teenager, Paulette was always frightened, and used drugs to numb the pain that she felt. She was isolated, and found it hard to feel loved. Every action from another person—her lover's reaction to her HIV status, for example—was experienced as another rejection. She had a lifelong difficulty achieving intimacy and sexual satisfaction, even with men she trusted. "I just lay there and you do what you got to do," she said of sexual relations with her lover. To her credit, she was a consistent condom user.

The first interview with our team marked a turning point of sorts, as it was the one of the few times that Paulette had told her story. She began to take charge of that area of her life. For Paulette, letting go of the secret allowed her to begin discussions with members of her family. She shared the story with her relatives, finally including her son, who was in jail in an another state. The constant state of mental anguish was alleviated by the constant repetition of the tale. Over time the story itself changed slightly, not in content, but in tone. She seemed to grow stronger, her voice more forceful, as the story came out. Though still struggling to feel loved and secure, she was infinitely more hopeful about her chances for happiness.

The rape of Paulette, isolated from her mother and ignored by her father, set her life course. The rape filled her with enduring revulsion that was dulled only by drugs. It took 30 years for her to develop talking as an alternative method for handling the pain she felt. She turned the pain inward, hiding the trauma from her father. She also turned against her helpless baby. She suffered no matter what. For Paulette, the healing process depended fundamentally on developing a way to talk. She had never forgotten what had happened to her; she had just tried to wall it off from consciousness. She had many metaphors for this process. The past was "a skeleton in the closet," a "can of worms," a "trunk with the lid on." The shift from hiding to openness, from secrecy to sharing, was accompanied by a shift from victim to protector. She repeated over and over again that she didn't want what had happened to her to happen to the children in her care. To that end, she talked to them often, and tried to serve as the confidante she had never had.

Injuries to the Self

Frank Putnam, a leading trauma researcher, has proposed that damage to the sense of "self" is one way of understanding the injury caused by traumas such as childhood sexual abuse (1989). Trauma may cause the following disturbances in self-representation to develop: fragmentation or loss of sense of self, concerns about control, identity disturbances, body-image disturbances, and low self-esteem.

Women in recovery, burdened by multiple past traumas, are likely to report many of these symptoms. They are most often aware of feelings of low self-esteem. Women drug users are constantly told that, by their drug use, they have degraded themselves as women and failed their children. Insults add to the intensity of the shame they report. Paulette's story illustrates these issues of shame and low self-esteem.

Less often are women able to put into words the fragmentation of self with which they contend. But this fragmentation is common, as well. The following story illustrates some of the issues in the disturbed sense of self:

> *Story 2: "I fight back."*
>
> Penelope, a 34-year-old black woman in recovery from crack addiction, described herself as someone who takes no shit. She was angry much of the time, and she used that anger to keep people at a distance. The anger stemmed from sexual abuse in childhood. Her stepfather abused her nightly. When she told her mother, her mother made no effort to stop the abuse. Later, when a friend of the family attempted to molest her, Penelope fought back. Unable to injure him directly, she went to the local laundromat and destroyed his clothes. This was a satisfying experience, and supported her sense that, through her anger, she could be in control of her life.
>
> But there was another side to Penelope—and, in fact, a second name, Theresa. This other side was not angry or protective. This other side was more often the victim than the advocate. Penelope/Theresa had a very unstable relationship with her lover, who often physically abused her. Those attacks, rather than rousing her anger and indignation, seemed to deflate Penelope/Theresa, leaving her feeling helpless and sad. After one beating, she impulsively began an affair that offered solace and bolstered her flagging self-esteem. But that only added to the tension and hostility with her primary partner.
>
> For Penelope/Theresa, the world was split into fragments. From the vantage point of one segment, she was unable to perceive the other pieces. Driven by pain and frustration, she raced between the parts of her life. The image left in the minds of observers was one of terrible instability. At one point, she said about her life:
>
>> I feel angry all the time, you know, like it's never over. So, like when something happens, I just say, so what? . . . . I don't believe in anything good. I keep my walls up and people out. At least that's what I think I do, cause when you say about the fight, when I got hit, what walls? I didn't have no walls for that. But it's almost like as soon as I see it, you know, the two, the anger and the beating, I can't see it. It comes and goes, like I turn here and see one thing, but then I turn here and that thing is gone and I see this thing, and it hurts to see them both.

Penelope's fragmentation made it difficult—though not impossible—for her to acknowledge the widely divergent responses she had to painful situations. She acted impulsively when uncomfortable. She was not consistently able to keep herself safe. For example, with neither her primary partner nor her lover did she practice safe sex. She was unhappy a great deal of the time.

"Posttraumatic Sexual Style"

Paulette and Penelope/Theresa survived childhood sexual abuse, but in adult life, their "styles" were completely different. Here, we are using the word "style" in the manner of David Shapiro, author of the book *Neurotic Styles* (Shapiro, 1965). In that excellent work, he groups the oddities of behavior that seem to be associated with quirks of the personality that, while they have some features of full-blown neuroses, are in reality more matters of "style" than illness. Grouping the elements of style has been helpful in guiding therapeutic work, as the presence of one element of a style will alert the astute observer to search for others. Styles are not meant to either indicate or exclude illness: An individual may have an illness *and* a style.

In the stories of Paulette and Penelope/Theresa, we note that both women struggled with a consuming, helpless rage. But everything about each one's manner, carriage, and expression marked the two as different. Paulette was often depressed and tearful. She seemed to struggle through each day. Penelope/Theresa, by contrast, was more likely to be angry than tearful. She moved quickly from event to event, from relationship to relationship, from day to day.

In listening to many different women's stores, we have become convinced that the many patterns of response to trauma may be usefully grouped into a small number of categories of style. We have proposed four categories in our work: angry, passive, reenactment, and chaotic. The angry style is characterized by the consistent use of anger to control the world.

The passive style is characterized by the sense of helplessness that the woman projects and the constant search to be acknowledged as an object of pity.

The reenactment style characterizes those who seem to test fate by engaging in the same relationship over and over again, perhaps hoping to undo the past and achieve a new resolution in the present. There is an action element to this style—an embracing of danger—that makes it different from other styles, which all too frequently may also lead to new trauma.

The chaotic style is particularly important for women who have suffered extreme degress of trauma, beginning at a very early age. In the lives of these severely injured women, events and thoughts are often incoherent, flowing into and out of one another, propelled, as often as not, by a crisis or a new trauma. Crisis and chaos are so important that the woman's self is subsumed by them. In such cases, it often appears that there is an actual addiction to chaos as a form of life.

Following our system, Paulette's style would be described as passive, Penelope/Theresa's as chaotic. Each style carries with it particular patterns of sexual interaction. We have coined the phrase "posttraumatic sexual style" to link the posttraumatic style of thinking and acting to sexual thoughts and acts. In the stories of Paulette and Penelope/Theresa, it is clear that the need to negotiate the traumatic past becomes an important part of current sexual relationships. The traumatic past may shape the woman's style in choice of safe partners, adoption of safe sexual behaviors, and recognition and prompt treatment of sexually transmitted diseases (STDs). On the basis of this model of posttraumatic sexual styles, we have made the assumption that changing HIV sexual risk behaviors is closely linked to helping women understand and change their sexual styles.

Developing "Stress and Sex: A Course for Women"

On that assumption, we developed a psychoeducational intervention, directed at women in recovery from substance abuse. Psychoeducation is an intervention that can improve women's assessment of their need to use condoms and barrier protection. Psychoeducation was originally developed by psychiatrists to decrease hospitalizations among people with schizophrenia by increasing family knowledge of the signs and symptoms of the illness. Clinical researchers observed an association between family behavior, specifically acts of hostility, and the patient's risk for rehospitalization. They also observed that some "hostile" families had little understanding of the illness of schizophrenia: They had unrealistic expectations and became angry when their schizophrenic relative was unable to function at "normal" levels. The investigators presumed that inappropriate family functioning might be understood, not as primary family dysfunction, but rather as a failure to adapt to a "chronic disaster" (McFarlane, 1983). Providing skills and information relevant to the management of schizophrenia has proven to be a powerful intervention that has decreased risk for rehospitalization (Leff, Kuipers, & Berkowitz, 1983; Hogarty *et al.,* 1986, 1991).

Several elements of psychoeducation appear to play a key role in its effectiveness: providing accurate information on complex processes that are not part of ordinary life, incorporating into the educational process the emotional reactions to information about illness, and allowing participants to interact with each other and with group leaders. Utilizing these core elements, psychoeducational techniques have been adapted for treatment of many illnesses, including depression (Lewinsohn, Antonuccio, & Steinmetz, 1984), bulimia (Davis, Olmsted, & Rockert, 1990), drug addiction (Wallace, 1989), and HIV risk reduction (Sorensen, London, & Morales, 1991; Davis *et al.*, 1990). Depending on the issues involved, psychoeducational interventions may be targeted for patients, as well as for their families.

Our psychoeducational curriculum was developed by a team that included women in recovery, who provided guidance in developing appropriate and culturally sensitive materials; students in the M.P.H. program at the Columbia University School of Public Health, who developed the lessons and conducted the evaluation; and researchers, who guided the analysis of observations and other findings. The curriculum was developed through a series of drafts that were field-tested for effectiveness and accuracy. As the work progressed, the team developed or adopted many ideas for enhancing the learning process, ensuring cultural sensitivity, and developing a nonjudgmental group process.

Description of the Basic Course

The basic course, entitled "Stress and Sex: A Course for Women," is designed to be offered in four weekly, 1 1/2-hour sessions, each with clear goals and objectives that can be evaluated for mastery. The "Stess and Sex" course is guided by a leader's manual that was developed during the extensive field tests of the material. The course was developed for women in recovery from addiction; it is designed to be led by a peer counselor. A detailed outline of the goals, objectives, and mastery items is shown in Table 1.

Session 1, "Where We Were, Where We Are," is designed to introduce the concept of trauma and to aid women in developing a personal inventory of traumatic events. For many of the participants, this session is the first time they have spoken of these events or heard others speak of them. Women are encouraged to share their experiences of trauma, but the decision to participate is entirely voluntary. It is recognized that these are painful, personal matters that should be shared with others at individual discretion. As with other lessons in the curriculum, the session revolves around two worksheets that participants complete. Each worksheet is carefully designed to meet the goals of a particular segment of the curriculum. At the end of the session, participants are "debriefed" about the possibility that remembering and discussing traumatic events may lead to symptoms. They are informed that the peer leader is available to help them, as are other members of the clinic staff. At the end of each of

Table 1. Outline of "Stress and Sex: A Course for Women"

Goals	Objectives	Mastery
Session 1: Introduce concept of trauma.	1. Identify past trauma. 2. Discuss traumatic experiences. 3. Identify ways trauma has had an impact on feelings.	Participant can identify the following qualities of traumatic events: 1. Happen to many people. 2. Cause pain. 3. Leave lasting memories and feelings.
Session 2: Examine the links between trauma and sexual decision-making.	1. Define kinds of trauma in others' lives. 2. Identify effects of trauma. 3. Identify strategies used to cope. 4. Evaluate efficacy of strategies.	Participant can compare and contrast the ways in which traumatized women enter sexual relationships.
Session 3: 1. Provide information about HIV and STDs. 2. Examine ways in which men and women initiate sexual relationships.	1. Describe features of common STDs. 2. Identify the differences between seduction and coercion.	Participant can identify STDs that are lethal, incurable, or silent. Participants can compare and contrast seduction and coercion.
Session 4: 1. Practice correct use of barrier protection (sheaths and sheets). 2. Examine connections between trauma recovery and substance-abuse recovery.	1. Practice correct use of condom. 2. Practice correct use of dental dam. 3. Practice correct use of female condom. 4. Learn technique of genital self-examination. 5. List ways in which life has changed during recovery.	Participant can demonstrate correct use of condoms or dental dams.

sessions 1–3, participants are given homework to prepare for the next session.

Session 2, "Trauma in Our Lives," explores the ways in which trauma may shape relationships. The exercises use visual images to help women "see" the connection between the past trauma and current styles of interaction with others. Session 3, "Sex and the Happy Woman," provides intensive education about STDs. It also utilizes an audiotape of men discussing seduction and coercion to address the topic of consent in sexual relationships. It goes without saying that it is impossible for women to hear men talk among themselves: The tape provides an insight into what men say when they're together with no women around. For the many participants who have had experiences with forced sex, it provides an opportunity for them to reevaluate their right to say "no" in sexual relationships.

Session 4, "No Glove, No Love," helps women practice the mechanical skills of using a condom and a rubber dam. Because many women in the course will be having sex with other women, this exercise, like others in the course, underscores that safe sex is important in both same- and opposite-sex encounters. The course ends with an exercise that links the recovery from trauma to the recovery from addiction that women have already undertaken.

One of the exercises from the course is entitled "The Cat and the Fox." This exercise is based on a traditional African American allegory, illustrated by noted African American artist Don Miller. The allegory (see Fig. 1), which depicts two animals trying to protect themselves in a life-threatening situation, offers another way to look at the topic "No Glove,

Activity One:
The Cat and the Fox

Pass out copies of this story and read it out loud. Then allow the women to discuss any implications of the story for their own negotiations with their lovers.

Mr. Cat and Mr. Fox were talking one day and the cat said, "What you gonna do when the dogs come, Mr. Fox?"

"Oh, that's no problem, no problem at all," said Mr. Fox. "I got me a boatload of tricks. I'll just do my tricks. One of 'em will work. What you gonna do?"

"Well," said the cat, "I only got one trick—up the tree. I just hide in the tree where the dogs can't get me."

Just then the dogs came running up, barking and yapping, tearing after the fox and the cat. The cat went up the tree and though the dogs leaped and strained, they couldn't get him. The fox, down at the bottom of tree, started doing his tricks. But that didn't save him. Dogs got him and ate him up. Mr. Cat shook his head and said, "It don't pay to know too many tricks."

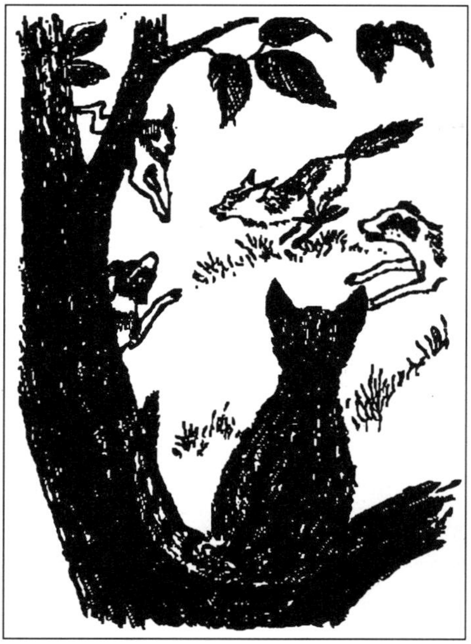

Figure 1. African American allegory as a teaching tool.

No Love." Metaphors are extremely important in the treatment of trauma, offering both distance and a way to "see" the problem (Terr, 1990).

Results in the Field

During the field tests, Sherri Uptegrow, the peer counselor working with the project, led the sessions. Each session was observed by two or more members of the team, who took notes. Each session was also audiotaped. The evaluation was designed to assess the extent to which the sessions met the stated goals of the curriculum. In examining the process, we paid careful attention to the problems that looked as though they might detract from the successful completion of the lessons, as well as examples of interchanges that worked.

"The Cat and the Fox" was an exercise that helped women make the connection between negotiating styles and outcomes. The exercise focuses on the concept that negotiating with a seducer is a bad idea. Seducers—whether male or female is of no importance—are on the offensive. They are determined to have sex, and given the slightest chance to succeed, they will. Any attempt to negotiate gives the seducer more opportunity to influence the outcome of the event. The exercise suggests that women will be safer if they refuse to negotiate. This is not to suggest that women refuse to have sex, but rather to emphasize that they can—and must—insist on the conditions under which sex will take place.

Story 3 relates a discussion on negotiation that took place during the field tests. In this story, Maribel actually took on the role of "seducer" with the telephone company—"promise them anything but give them what you have." Because the telephone company was clear, she was forced to live up to her promises:

> *Story 3: "I thought I didn't have to pay my phone bill."*
> During the discussion of the story, Sherri asks, "Who's negotiated something recently?"
>
> Maribel describes a negotiation with the phone company. She owed $225 for one month and $110 for another month. She negotiated a payment plan that involved paying all of the second month and a portion of the first month. She then paid only the fraction from the first month. "I had other bills," she explained. Her daughter was graduating, and she had other expenses. The phone company turned off her phone.
>
> Sherri: You tried to dope fiend your way out of paying, right?
> Maribel: I didn't think they would turn it off if I gave them some of the money. But they turned it off anyway. They didn't have the right to do that.
> Sherri: Wait, wait, wait. You didn't pay the bill, right?
> Maribel: Yeah.
> Sherri: So they cut off your phone. See, the point here is when we try to dope

> fiend, it doesn't work. The phone company was clear with you but you tried to evade your obligation to them. It just doesn't work.

In this story, a powerful agent—the telephone company—gets its way because it is clear, "No money, no phone." Maribel's efforts to circumvent ("dope fiend") the phone company are to no avail. By linking the allegory to real life, the discussion helps to ground the need for clear, real messages. This real-life application of the problems of negotiation helps to move the discussion to the problems of establishing safe sex relationships.

Some of the issues in teaching this material had to do as much with group process as with learning about safe sex. The lessons in the "Stress and Sex" course were developed to meet the needs of both homosexual and heterosexual women. One important incident arose during the second round of field tests that nearly derailed the group's work and emphasized the importance of the group's interactions for the course's success:

> *Story 4: "Homosexuality is disgusting!"*
>
> The two student observers noted that an intense discussion started after the group analyzed the story of a lesbian woman who kept reenacting past traumas.
>
> Lisa: When I was a child, I was disgusted by homosexuality. My mother is that way and it upset me. But now I talk to her and she tells me what it's like. I think it's wrong, it's in the Bible. But I know I know gay people and they're really nice.
>
> Sherri: Does that make a difference in terms of safe sex?
>
> Group: No!
>
> Tanisha: Homosexuality is disgusting! Gay women act like men. They turn me off when they start acting like men! That is so disgusting, it turns my stomach. Don't bring no homosexuals around me. [She says this in an intense, angry manner that is a blanket rejection of all homosexuals.]
>
> Tiny: [Reaches her hand toward Tanisha] I'm gay and I'm not like that. I'm not like a man.
>
> Sherri: Everyone is entitled to their opinion. Be true to yourself. [Turning toward Tanisha and Tiny] Be true to yourself. Remember, "Those that judge don't matter and those that matter don't judge" [a saying from 12-step fellowship].
>
> According to the observers, the meeting ended in a noisy exchange on homosexuality. Each participant was "debriefed" individually before she left. At the end of the session, the lesbian woman, Tiny, said that she thought it was a good group. However, later that evening, she began to be frightened and talked to Sherri about dropping out. Tanisha remarked that it was a good group and had made her remember many things from the past. The other participants were all upset that Tanisha had been so negative and rejecting in her style. At least one woman—Mary Louise—felt that she wanted to work with Tanisha in future sessions.

In the poor, inner-city community from which the participants came, there is a strong, complex tradition around homosexuality that is characterized by both overt rejection of homosexuality as an "abomination," following the Biblical admonition found in Leviticus 18:22–30 (*Original African American Study Bible,* 1993), as well as covert acceptance, especially if the homosexuality is appropriately "closeted." The use of a story that had a lesbian heroine touched off intense negative feelings in one participant. In trying to manage the situation, Sherri appealed to the opposite, nonjudgmental tradition. She had little success with Tanisha, although all the others supported Sherri's stance. Sherri did not condemn Tanisha's homophobia, which undoubtedly contributed to Tiny's pain, fear, and reluctance to return.

Tanisha's contentious homophobia threatened to derail the group. Sherri's strong personal connections with the group members were an essential factor that stabilized the situation. Other members of the clinic staff also intervened to help each of the women work through their feelings about the session. As the process continued, a clearer position emerged in support of the rights of homosexuals. The strong support provided by the clinic was, in our estimation, not only a solution for this problem, but also an important source of power for the intervention. Our team concluded, on the basis of this and other similar incidents, that this brief psychoeducational course is limited in what it can accomplish. Where it touches on deeply embedded prejudices and ignorance—as it must—it must be able to lean on the strong moral and social authority of the whole clinic. Only with the backing of the whole clinic can the brief course drive home its message. In that regard, the acceptance of homosexuality in the clinic was the foundation for working through homophobia in the group.

These observations helped us to place the curriculum in the context of the ongoing social life of the clinic. We realized that the curriculum could introduce important ideas and identify key problems. But this "Trauma 101" must be followed by other interventions. Our talks with many women confirmed that the residual effects of trauma were often pervasive disturbances that seemed to undermine major areas of women's functioning. Clearly, in order to address the long-term problems of recovery from trauma, we needed models of treatment that could be integrated into the clinical setting.

TREATMENT FOR TRAUMA-RELATED ILLNESS IN A DRUG CLINIC

In order to meet the long-term needs of women recovering from addiction and trauma, we began to develop models of individual and group treatment that could address the profound disturbances of self that affected not only sexual style, but also every area of a woman's functioning. In language consonant with the language of 12-step fellowship, we identified four areas of functioning that needed attention in the treatment milieu—the "4 *S*s": safety, sanity, serenity, and stability.

Safety, the first of the four *S*s, refers to keeping one's person free from harm. We include in this category practicing safe sex and avoiding violent relationships. This *S* comes first not only in the alphabet but also in clinical work. Theorists in the area of trauma treatment have proposed that safety should be the focus of the early stages of therapy, arguing that women must be safe before tackling other problems or exploring past traumas. We agree with this view in principle, but have learned that women living in high-risk situations may modify and control internally generated dangers, but are never safe from external threats.

Sanity, the second *S*, refers to a wide range of symptoms. In 12-step fellowship, there is a saying, "Insanity is repeating the same mistakes and expecting different results." We agree that a core problem among survivors of trauma is the tendency to re-create traumatic situations. Other disturbances of sanity that are important are the fragmentation of self and disorders of mood. Dissociative disorders are common among women we have interviewed and require careful assessment and treatment. Mood disorders—primarily depression—are also common problems deserving of care.

Serenity is the third *S*. The Serenity Prayer is another important saying in 12-step fellowship. In three short lines, it captures much of what modern theorists of coping attempt to teach. Basically, some problems can be solved. In those cases, active attention and self-assertion is required. Other problems are really out of one's personal control. In those instances, one must cope with the pressure and anxiety that often accompany feelings of helplessness. In these cases, too, there are specific actions that can be taken, but they have to do with stress and anxiety reduction or, in the language of 12-step fellowship, "turning the problem over to one's higher power." Paulette's search for comfort, in full awareness of the burdens she carried from the past, is an example of this.

Stability is the fourth *S*. Many people in the aftermath of trauma find it hard to maintain business as usual. Doing so becomes even more difficult when circumstances churn up painful memories. As in Penelope/Theresa's story, it is often easier to turn to a new relationship than it is to make the old one work. But such abrupt changes can cause great disturbances in personal and social networks. The inability to trust and the difficulty in redressing grievances that are such serious problems for many traumatized people make it difficult to keep friendships and love affairs going through the ups and downs of ordinary life.

The "4 *S*s" provide a convenient way to conceptualize trauma-related problems in the lives of women drug users. They provide a framework for planning interventions. This framework emphasizes safety as the foundation for therapeutic work. On that basis, women can begin to make connections between the traumatic experiences of the past and the dysfunctional behaviors of the present. This is a slow process that gradually allows an injured woman to heal old wounds.

CONCLUSION

Our work with women in recovery from substance abuse offers examples of the manner in which the problems of trauma and childhood sexual abuse are important for HIV prevention and treatment. Lessons can be extracted from these experiences that have relevance for women infected and affected by HIV/AIDS. The first lesson is that clinicians and other providers need to be prepared to ask women about their past traumas. Trauma is common in the lives of marginalized women living in high-risk situations. Knowledge of past trauma is essential for thorough treatment planning. In our experience, women appreciate being asked. It opens the door for more thorough evaluation and treatment.

The second lesson is that conversations about trauma will be far-ranging. They will open up deep emotions, ugly prejudices, and trivial daily problems. Such conversations expand the range and the depth of conversation, creating even more complexity. Treatment staff need a great deal of support to manage this complexity. Just as we needed the support of the whole clinic to handle one woman's homophobia, organizational support is critical to the effective management of these problems.

The third lesson is that there is much more to learn. Women's lives are complex: They have many responsibilities, across generations in time and space. Helping women heal the past and shape the future is a challenging task. We know all too little about how to help women recover from trauma; we know even less about helping poor women living in high-risk situations in their recovery work.

In sum, trauma and childhood sexual abuse in a woman's past are interwoven in her present. Helping women recover from trauma is an essential task in controlling the AIDS epidemic.

Acknowledgments. This work was supported in part by NIMH/NIDA Center Grant P50-43520. We wish to acknowledge our colleagues at the

Lincoln Medical and Mental Health Center Substance Abuse Division for their advice and guidance.

REFERENCES

Boyer, D., & Fine, D. (1992). Sexual abuse as a factor in adolescent pregnancy and child maltreatment. *Family Planning Perspectives, 24,* 4–11.

Davis, R., Olmsted, M. P., & Rockert, W. (1990). Brief group psychoeducation for bulimia nervosa: Assessing the clinical significance of change. *Journal of Counseling and Clinical Psychology, 58,* 882–885.

Dembo, R., Williams, L., Wish, E. D., Dertke, M., Berry, E., Getreu, A., Washburn, M., & Schmeidler, J. (1988). The relationship between physical and sexual abuse and illicit drug use: A replication among a new sample of youths entering a juvenile detention center. *International Journal of the Addictions, 23,* 1101–1123.

Finkelhor, D., Hotaling, G., Lewis, I. A., & Smith, C. (1990). Sexual abuse in a national survey of adult men and women: Prevalence, characteristics and risk factors. *Child Abuse and Neglect, 14,* 19–28.

Fullilove, M. T., Lown, E. A., & Fullilove, R. E. (1992). Crack 'hos and skeezers: Traumatic experiences of women crack users. *Journal of Sex Research, 29,* 275–287.

Hogarty, G. E., Anderson, C. M., Reiss, D. J., Kornblith, S. J., Greenwald, D. P., Javna, C. P., Madonia, M. J., & Group, T. E. R. (1986). Family psychoeducation, social skills training, and maintenance chemotherapy in the aftercare treatment of schizophrenia. I. One year effects of a controlled study on relapse and expressed emotion. *Archives of General Psychiatry, 48,* 340–347.

Hogarty, G. E., Anderson, C. M., Reiss, D. J., Kornblith, S. J., Greenwald, D. P., Ulrich, R. F., Javna, C. P., Carter, M., & Group, E. R. (1991). Family psychoeducation, social skills training, and maintenance chemotherapy in the aftercare treatment of schizophrenia. II. Two year effects of a controlled study on relapse and adjustment. *Archives of General Psychiatry, 48,* 340–347.

Kulka, R. A., Fairbank, J. A., Jordan, B. K., & Weiss, D. S. (1990). *Trauma and the Vietnam War generation.* New York: Brunner/Mazel.

Leff, J. P., Kuipers, L., & Berkowitz, R. (1983). Intervention in families of schizophrenics and its effect on relapse rate. In W. R. MacFarlane (Ed.), *Family therapy in schizophrenia* (pp. 173–187). New York: Guilford Press.

The Original African American Study Bible (King James version) (1993). Leviticus 18:22–33. Nashville: The James C. Winston Publishing Company.

Lewinsohn, P. M., Antonuccio, J. L., & Steinmetz, L. T. (1984). *The coping with depression course: A psychoeducation intervention for unipolar depression.* Eugene, OR: Castalia Publishing.

McFarlane, W. R. (1983). Multiple family therapy in schizophrenia. In W. R. McFarlane (Ed.), *Family therapy and schizophrenia* (pp. 141–172). New York: Guilford Press.

Paone, D., Chavkin, W., Willets, I., Friedman, P., & Des Jarlais, D. (1992). The impact of sexual abuse: Implications for drug treatment. *Journal of Women's Health, 1,* 149–153.

Putnam, Frank W. (1989) *Diagnosis and treatment of multiple personality disorders.* New York: Guilford Press.

Rohsenow, D., Corbett, R., Devine, D. (1988). Molested as children: A hidden contribution to substance abuse? *Journal of Substance Abuse Treatment, 5,* 13–18.

Shapiro, D. (1965). *Neurotic styles.* New York: Basic Books.

Simons, R. L., & Whitbeck, L. B. (1991). Sexual abuse as a precursor to prostitution and victimization among adolescent and adult homeless women. *Journal of Family Issues, 12,* 361–379.

Sorensen, J. L., London, J., & Morales, E. (1991). *Group counseling to prevent AIDS: Preventing AIDS in drug users and their sexual partners.* New York: Guilford Press.

Springs, F. E., & Friedrich, W. N. (1992). Health risk behaviors and medical sequelae of childhood sexual abuse. *Mayo Clinic Proceedings, 67,* 527–532.

Stiffman, A. R. (1989). Physical and sexual abuse in runaway youths. *Child Abuse and Neglect, 13,* 417–426.

Terr, L. (1990). *Too scared to cry: Psychic trauma in childhood.* New York: Harper & Row.

Vermund, S. H., Alexander-Rodriquez, T., MacLeod, S., & Kelley, K. F. (1990). History of sexual abuse in incarcerated adolescents with gonorrhea or syphilis. *Journal of Adolescent Health, 11,* 449–452.

Walker, E., Katon, W., Hansom, J., Harrup-Griffiths, J., Holm, L., Jones, M. L., Hickok, L., & Jemelka, R. P. (1992). Medical and psychiatric symptoms in women with childhood sexual abuse. *Psychosomatic Medicine, 54,* 658–664.

Wallace, B. C. (1989). Relapse prevention in psychoeducational groups for compulsive crack cocaine smokers. *Journal of Substance Abuse Treatment, 6,* 229–239.

Zierler, S., Feingold, L., Laufer, D., Velentgas, P., Kantrowitz-Gordon, I., & Mayer, K. (1991). Adult survivors of childhood sexual abuse and subsequent risk of HIV infection. *American Journal of Public Health, 81,* 572–575.

Zwi, A., & Cabral, A. (1992). Identifying "high risk situations" for preventing AIDS. *British Medical Journal, 303,* 1527.

5

Preventing AIDS in Female Adolescents

MARY JANE ROTHERAM-BORUS, LORETTA SWEET JEMMOTT, and JOHN B. JEMMOTT III

INTRODUCTION

The increasing incidence of HIV infection is having a pervasive cultural impact among adolescents in the United States. To be sure, adolescents currently represent fewer than 1% of all reported AIDS cases in the United States [Centers for Disease Control and Prevention (CDC), 1993b]. But this statistic underestimates the potential for HIV infection among adolescents. Young adults in their 20s constitute about 20% of all AIDS cases (1993b), and because several years typically elapse between the time a person is infected with HIV and the appearance of clinical signs sufficient to warrant a diagnosis of AIDS, many of these individuals were infected during adolescence.

AIDS prevention among adolescents is a national public health priority (Wilcox, 1990). However, the impact of AIDS goes far beyond the need for individuals to recognize and to implement strategies to protect themselves. Even though condom use is the most effective strategy available for preventing HIV among sexually active youths, it depends on the male's consent. Female adolescents are traditionally in a deferent role with their

---

MARY JANE ROTHERAM-BORUS • Division of Social and Community Psychiatry, Department of Psychiatry, University of California, Los Angeles, Los Angeles, CA 90024. *LORETTA SWEET JEMMOTT* • University of Pennsylvania School of Nursing, Philadelphia, PA 19104. *JOHN B. JEMMOTT III* • Department of Psychology, Princeton University, Princeton, NJ 08554.

Women at Risk: Issues in the Primary Prevention of AIDS, edited by Ann O'Leary and Loretta Sweet Jemmott. Plenum Press, New York, 1995.

male partners, which decreases the likelihood that they have the power to ensure condom use. This is especially the case for female adolescents who are involved with men several years older than themselves. In addition, parenthood is sometimes an explicit goal of sexual intercourse for adolescent women. Helping them decide how, when, and with whom to get pregnant, and how to protect themselves from HIV, is a central challenge for those designing programs for adolescent women. The female condom may be a solution. However, it has been introduced only recently, and there has not been substantial research evidence of its efficacy. To implement effective prevention programs, fundamental changes may be required in sex role relationships and in the strategies developed to safeguard female adolescents from HIV.

To address adequately the AIDS epidemic among female adolescents requires research that identifies (1) conceptual variables that influence HIV-risk-associated behaviors and (2) interventions that focus on these conceptual variables and use the most effective behavior-change strategies. There are three areas in which the need for effective HIV prevention programs is especially urgent: (1) prevention programs that consider stereotypic sex roles and recognize that girls cannot use condoms; (2) programs to assist in parenting decisions that have a developmentally tailored HIV testing component; and (3) intervention programs for youths who are HIV-seropositive. This chapter will review the challenges posed by HIV to young women and the pertinent developmental and cultural issues that are involved in implementing HIV prevention programs.

HIV INFECTION AMONG ADOLESCENTS

HIV infection among adolescents is a significant and growing problem. It has been estimated that half of the 14 million people with HIV worldwide were infected between the ages of 15 and 24 (Goldsmith, 1993). Although few of these HIV-positive youths are aware of their serostatus, increasing numbers will be identified as HIV testing is advocated as a prevention strategy to encourage access to prophylactic treatments (Knox & Clark, 1991). More than 1300 U.S. youths aged 13–19 years have developed AIDS. Given the long incubation period between HIV infection and diagnosis with AIDS (Goeddert *et al.*, 1990), it is likely that those with AIDS aged 20–30 years (about 20% of AIDS cases) became infected during their adolescence. Estimates of the prevalence of HIV-positive serostatus among adolescents vary depending on the population. For instance, it has been found that 0.03% of teenage military applicants (Burke *et al.*, 1990), 0.4% of Job Corps entrants (St. Louis *et al.*, 1991), 0.4% of those attending clinics in urban hospitals (D'Angelo, Getson, Luben, Stallings, & Gayle, 1989), and 0.7% of adolescents giving birth in New York City (Novick *et al.,* 1989) are HIV-seropositive. However, there are subgroups of youths at even higher risk. For example, 2.2% of youths attending sexually transmitted disease (STD) clinics are HIV-positive (Quinn *et al.,* 1988). Among runaways, HIV seropositivity has ranged from a low of 2.1% in Houston (Stricof, Novick, & Kennedy, 1990), to 5.3% in New York City (Stricof, Kennedy, Nattell, Weisfuse, & Novick, 1991), to 12% in San Francisco (Shalwitz, Goulart, Dunnigan, & Flanney, 1990). Gay male youths are likely to be at high risk as well, given that about one third of male adolescents with AIDS have had same-sex partners (CDC, 1993a). High seroprevalence rates among adolescents are concentrated geographically in AIDS epicenters, including Los Angeles, San Francisco, and New York City. Compared to adult women, female adolescents are at higher relative risk (CDC, 1993b). Their risk is about equal to that of males (D'Angelo *et al.,* 1989). Seroprevalence rates rise with age (Hayman *et al.,* 1990; Stricof *et al.,* 1991) and are associated with ethnicity. African American and Hispanic youths are at higher risk for HIV infection than are Anglo-Americans, and these minority youths are overrepresented among adolescent AIDS cases (CDC, 1994).

Substance use is also a key issue that must be directly addressed when considering the design of intervention programs for HIV-positive youths. While alcohol and drug use is high among high school seniors (Johnston, O'Malley, & Bachman, 1987) and American households (National Institute on Drug Abuse, 1991), it is even higher among HIV-positive youths (Fullilove, Fullilove, Bowser, & Gross, 1990). Among inner-city adolescents, use of drugs, particularly crack cocaine (Fullilove *et al.,* 1990; Minkoff *et al.,* 1990), is significantly related to HIV-risk-associated behavior. Adolescent samples with high seroprevalence rates (homeless, gay, and bisexual) report significantly higher rates of substance abuse compared with high school samples. For example, Rotheram-Borus *et al.* (1994) found that nearly one third of male minority gay/bisexual youths reported alcohol or drug use on a weekly basis. Similar findings have been observed in a study of white, middle-class gay youths by Remafedi (1987). Illicit drug use was 83%, with 58% of youths meeting DSM-III criteria for substance abuse (Remafedi, 1987). It is hypothesized that alcohol and drug use are part of a cluster of problem behaviors occurring during adolescence (Jessor & Jessor, 1977), and therefore substance use is likely to be related to sexual risk behaviors. Substance use is linked to HIV seropositivity for two reasons: (1) Sharing needles or syringes ("works") or other paraphernalia in injection-drug use is a direct transmission route for HIV infection; (2) substance use, like use of alcohol and other noninjectable drugs, can disinhibit sexual risk behavior, leading to HIV infection as a result of failing to use condoms during sexual intercourse (Fullilove *et al.,* 1990; Hingson, Strunin, Berlin, & Heeren, 1990), exchanging sex for drugs or money (Goldsmith, 1988; Fullilove *et al.,* 1990), and sexual activity with multiple partners (Koopman, Rosario, and Rotheram-Borus, 1994). Schilling *et al.* (1991) note that although injection-drug users are engaging in safer needle practices, there is less evidence that they are changing their sexual behavior. An intervention program specifically targeted to an adolescent population with high-frequency drug use is therefore essential to reduce risk behavior and limit the spread of HIV infection.

HIV-RISK-ASSOCIATED SEXUAL BEHAVIORS

Epidemiological studies have identified sexual behaviors that increase risk of sexually transmitted infection (Hatcher *et al.,* 1990; Kipke, Futterman, & Hein, 1990), and these behaviors are risky with respect to HIV infection. Thus, HIV-risk-associated sexual behaviors include having sex (vaginal or anal) that is unprotected (i.e., without a condom), having many sexual partners, and having sex with partners who engage in high-risk behaviors such as injection-drug use. The best way, of course, to avoid sexually transmitted infection, including HIV infection, is to practice abstinence. Avoiding these high-risk sexual behaviors, however, should substantially decrease the chances of HIV infection. Next, we review the literature on the extent to which the sexual practices of adolescents contribute to risk of HIV infection. Unprotected sexual behaviors, substance use that disinhibits sexual restraints, and intravenous-drug use place youths at risk for HIV [National Research Council (NRC), 1989].

Sexual Intercourse

About two thirds of adolescents studied report engaging in sexual intercourse by age 19 (Sonenstein, Pleck, & Ku, 1989; Strunin & Hingson, 1992). Sexual activity was initiated at earlier ages for each group of adolescents over the last 30 years (Hofferth, Kahn, & Baldwin, 1987; Sonenstein *et al.,* 1989). Sexual behaviors vary by gender, ethnicity, and cultural norms. More males engage in sexual intercourse than females (60% vs. 53%) (Forrest & Singh, 1990; Sonenstein *et al.,* 1989), and they do so at younger ages (Zelnik & Shah, 1983). Although white (57%) and Hispanic (60%) youths report similar rates of sexual intercourse (Sonenstein *et al.,* 1989), white females report more sexual activity than do Hispanic females (Aneshensel, Becerra, Fielder, & Schuler, 1990). African American adolescents, both males and females, report engaging in sexual intercourse more frequently than whites and at an earlier age (Zabin, Hardy, Smith, & Hirsch, 1986). In part, the greater reports of sexual experience among African American adolescents may be attributed to socioeconomic background. On average, rates of poverty and low socioeconomic background, which are associated with early sexual experience, are greater among African American adolescents than among white adolescents. However, some studies have found greater reports of sexual intercourse among African American adolescents even when socioeconomic background was controlled statistically (Hofferth *et al.,* 1987).

These ethnic differences for males and females suggest that interventions may have to be targeted differently for youths from different ethnic groups. It may well be that programs cannot be designed for "minority" youth, as the sexual patterns of African American and Hispanic youth are quite different. Furthermore, white youths initiate various sexual activities in a sequential pattern (kissing, petting, vaginal intercourse, oral sex), whereas African American youths do not (Smith & Udry, 1985). Petting and sexual intercourse are initiated at about the same age for African American youth. These differences in psychosexual milestones among white and African American youths are important in that they may suggest the need for different intervention approaches.

Unprotected Coitus

Consistent use of condoms is one of the ways adolescents can protect themselves from HIV infection. During the last decade, condom use among adolescents has risen substantially (Forrest & Singh, 1990; Hingson *et al.,* 1990). For example, 58% of male adolescents report using a condom during their last sexual encounter, an increase of 37% from 1979 figures (Sonenstein *et al.,* 1989). However, consistent condom use, a prerequisite for effective AIDS prevention, is not this high. Rates of consistent condom use have ranged from a low of 16% among youths in southern California (Rhodes, MacDonald, & Elder-Tarizy, 1990), to 25% in Newark (Keller *et al.,* 1991), to 30% in Philadelphia (J.B. Jemmott, L.S. Jemmott, & Fong, 1992a), to a high of 39% among males and 28% among females in a recent national survey (Anderson *et al.,* 1990).

Furthermore, there are apparent inconsistencies in the reports of condom behavior that raise questions regarding the extent of change. For example, Kimble, Hertzog, Fisher, and Fisher (1991) found that although 30% of high school youths in Massachusetts reported using condoms on every sexual occasion, only 24% of the sexually active students had actually purchased a condom in the past year, and only 12% reported keeping condoms nearby or carrying them consistently. Additionally, only 18% of the students surveyed reported that they always refused unprotected intercourse. Clearly, even youths who intend to reduce their HIV risk behavior were unlikely to do so effectively; only 10% of a sexually active sample who reported changing their behavior due to concern over AIDS had specifically noted increased condom use as their risk-prevention strategy (Strunin & Hingson, 1987).

Data on adolescent pregnancy and STDs provide additional evidence of failure to use condoms. About 1 in 10 United States women become pregnant during their high school years, and roughly 85% of these pregnancies are unintended (Jones *et al.*, 1986; Pratt *et al.*, 1984). Adolescents have higher rates of chlamydia, gonorrhea, syphilis, and hospitalization for pelvic inflammatory disease than any other age group (Bell & Hein, 1984; Kipke, Futterman, & Hein, 1990). Unprotected sexual intercourse is the primary HIV transmission route for adolescents (CDC, 1993a), particularly adolescent girls, who are far more likely to become infected as a result of heterosexual transmission. The risks of unprotected sexual activity are particularly problematic among inner-city African American adolescents. The adolescent pregnancy rate is nearly twice as high among African Americans as among whites. Moreover, the incidence of STDs is 2–3 times greater among African Americans than among whites, and low-income people in urban areas are more likely to contract an STD than are people of higher income or those who reside in suburban or rural areas (Cates, 1987; Hatcher *et al.*, 1990; Jones *et al.*, 1986; Pratt *et al.*, 1984; Zelnik, Kantner, & Ford, 1981).

Multiple Sex Partners

Risk for HIV/AIDS increases based on the number of sexual partners of unknown serostatus, and exposure varies based on the local community (NRC, 1989). In the United States, nearly 35% of high school students report engaging in sex with two or more partners in the past year (Miller, Turner, & Moses, 1990). There is little evidence that African Americans and whites differ in number of sexual partners. In a school with predominantly white, middle-class students, sexually active youth reported a lifetime mean of 2.7 partners (Brown, DiClemente, & Beausoleil, 1992), whereas in a largely African American and Hispanic school sample from a low-income inner-city community, a mean of 6.5 partners over the lifetime was reported (Keller *et al.*, 1991). However, it is well established that age of initial coitus is younger among African American adolescents (Zelnik & Shah, 1983).

Noncoital Sexual Behaviors

Research on sexual behavior, for the most part, has focused on coitus with the aim of understanding fertility. Consequently, little is known about the dynamics of noncoital sexual behaviors such as anal intercourse. This lack of knowledge is unfortunate because the behavior associated with the best-documented risk for sexual transmission of HIV is unprotected receptive anal intercourse. Although chiefly associated with homosexual men, there is growing recognition that it is a fairly common practice among heterosexuals (Reinisch, Sanders, & Ziemba-Davis, 1988). For example, drawing on data from seven studies, Reinisch *et al.* (1988) estimated that 39% (range 20–43%) of white middle-class women had ever participated in anal intercourse. There is some evidence that fewer African American women engage in anal intercourse. Wyatt *et al.* (1988a,b), studying women ages 18–36 in the Los Angeles area, found that 21% of African American women, as compared with 43% of a matched sample of white women, reported having ever experienced anal intercourse.

Gender Issues and Condom Use

There are a number of important issues related to gender that must be considered. Most important, it is not the female adolescent, but her male partner, who uses the condom. Thus, female adolescents cannot determine whether condoms are to be used in a sexual encounter; they can only negotiate condom use with their partners or influence their partners to use condoms. Thus, female adolescents' ability to ensure that condoms are used is limited. In this connection, a central issue is the power imbalance between female adolescents and their male partners. For a variety of reasons, female adolescents typically are perceived as having and exerting less interpersonal power in their relationships with men (Wells, 1980). The perception that it is difficult to find a steady, desirable male partner may contribute to the power inbalance. Another contributing factor is often an age differential. Thus, female adolescents typically date older males (Zelnik & Shah, 1983), who have greater power because of their maturity, life experience, and financial resources. Unfortunately, these older males frequently are more sexually experienced and more likely to be infected than are the adolescents' peers. The importance of a female adolescent's male partner has been demonstrated in both African Americans and whites. Studies of both African American and white adolescents have indicated that partner opposition to or reluctance to use birth control is associated with nonuse of contraception (Thompson & Spanier, 1978; Zabin & Clarke, 1981). Rebalancing power relationships would seem to be a reasonable goal for HIV prevention programs for female adolescents, particularly those programs that would enhance condom use.

Adolescents are affected by society's rules or scripts pertaining to appropriate role behavior, including sexual behavior (Erikson, 1950; Kohlberg, 1966; Mussen, 1969). In this connection, it has been suggested that adolescents are socialized to believe that the prescribed sex role behavior for women includes passivity, feigning sexual naiveté, disinterest (Frieze, Parsons, Johnson, Ruble, & Zellman, 1978), and denial of sexual activity, with concomitant reluctance to make requests about protected intercourse (Whitley & Schofield, 1986). In contrast, it has been suggested that adolescents are socialized to believe that the social norms for men dictate a role as sexual aggressor (Gross, 1978), in which conquests are more significant than relationships (Carroll, Volk, & Hyde, 1985) and communication is placed at a minimum. These stereotypical roles are repeatedly displayed by adolescents in focus groups, as female adolescents report that their role is to "say no" and male adolescents report that their role is to "get as much [sexual contact] as you can" (Rotheram-Borus, Koopman, & Bradley, 1989). A consequence of adolescents' strict adherence to prescribed sex role behavior is lack of communication about past sexual experiences or discussion of and cooperation around questions of abstaining from sexual intercourse or the use of condoms.

In addition to sex roles, youths also adhere to roles that are defined by and specific to their immediate peer group. These roles may be associated with a distinct set of social and behavioral norms (Walter, 1990), including norms for sexual behavior (DeLamater, 1987; Simon & Gagnon, 1986). Peers are one of the most important sources of adolescents' information about sexual behavior. Direct pressure from peers and the adolescents' perceptions of peer group norms influence youths' decisions about whether, when, how, and with whom to engage in sexual behavior. As adolescents attempt to define themselves as sexual beings, the degree to which they take on the prescribed roles of their gender or peer group may play a significant part in defining their risk acts and condom use. Prevention programs must be designed to address the different social roles of adolescents and the influence of peer norms on adolescent sexual behavior.

The Female Condom

Our discussion of condom use has focused on the male condom, which is currently the only widely available method for reducing risk of HIV infection during sexual intercourse. Recently, however, the female condom has been approved for use in the United States. In theory, then, one strategy for grappling with the power imbalance would be to encourage female adolescents to protect themselves and their partners by using the female condom. However, there are scant data on the efficacy of the female condom, and none are on adolescents. There is some evidence that rates of pregnancy (26%) are higher while using the female condom than while using the male condom (8%). Moreover, the female condom is not readily available to female adolescents, and the cost is prohibitive. Nevertheless, the female condom is a prevention method that women can control. High priority should be given to studies investigating its effectiveness as a strategy to reduce risk of sexually transmitted HIV infection.

HIV Risk and Stressful Life Situations

In addition to norms associated with gender and peer group roles, there are other constraints on adolescents' HIV risk behavior. Of particular importance for many adolescents is the stressful life situations that affect them. Adolescents who are incarcerated, homeless, or gay are all living under stressful life circumstances. Among youths in such life situations, HIV risk behaviors are likely to become more prevalent. For example, sexual intercourse is likely to be initiated earlier and with more partners. Consistent with this likelihood, studies indicate that over 90% of incarcerated youths, runaways, minority gay male youths, and psychiatrically hospitalized female youths are sexually active (D. G. Baker & Mossman, 1991; DiClemente, Lanier, Horan, & Lodico, 1991; Morris, Baker, Huscroft, Evans, & Zeljkovic, 1991; Pennbridge, Freese, & Mackenzie, 1992; Rotheram-Borus & Koopman, 1991b; Rotheram-Borus *et al.,* 1994), typically by 12.5 years of age (Rotheram-Borus & Koopman, 1991a).

APPLYING PSYCHOLOGICAL THEORIES TO HIV-RISK BEHAVIOR

At least four cognitive–behavioral models have been applied to adolescents' HIV risk behavior: the health belief (Becker, 1974), social cognitive theory (Bandura, 1989), the theory of reasoned action/planned behavior (Ajzen, 1991; Fishbein & Ajzen, 1975), and the peer influence models (Fisher, 1988). Each of these cognitive–behavioral models emphasizes different social–perceptual constructs.

The Health Belief Model

The health belief model asserts that HIV/AIDS risk acts are less likely if the adolescent has: (1) knowledge about the means of transmission and the consequences of contracting HIV, (2) knowledge about prevention strategies, (3) beliefs of susceptibility to HIV infection, and (4) beliefs that the benefits of performing preventive acts outweigh the costs. Supporting this model, reduction in HIV-risk-associated behaviors has been linked to knowledge of HIV, positive attitudes toward practicing safer sex, beliefs in high personal susceptibility, and perceiving AIDS as a serious threat in a variety of adolescent populations, including gay and bisexual male teenagers, runaways, adolescents in a random community sample, and adolescents in residential placements.

The Social Cognitive Theory

The social cognitive theory (Bandura, 1992, 1994) provides a comprehensive analysis of the determinants of behavior change. What makes the theory a particularly advantageous approach to health behavior is that it provides prescriptions for effective alteration of the presumed mechanisms that underlie health behavior. The theory has two key components, perceived self-efficacy and outcome expectancies. Perceived self-efficacy is defined as the conviction that one can successfully execute the behavior required to produce desired outcomes. Outcome expectancy is defined as a person's estimate that a given behavior will lead to negative or positive outcomes. Hence, within social cognitive theory, perceptions of self-efficacy and outcome expectancies are the key determinants of effective behavior change toward safer-sex practices. For example, strong perceptions of efficacy to negotiate condom use with a partner and to control sexual impulse, greater expectations of positive outcomes of condom use (e.g., preventing HIV infection), and lower expectations of negative outcomes of condom use (e.g., reduced pleasure, negative partner response) might all contribute to using condoms. Self-efficacy and outcome expectancies have been shown to be associated with sexual refusal and consistent condom use among adolescents. Similarly, perceptions of low self-control in sexual situations have been shown to predict a high-risk pattern of sexual behavior among runaway youths.

The Theory of Reasoned Action/Planned Behavior

The theory of reasoned action/planned behavior places emphasis on both the adolescents' own feelings about risk behavior and their perceptions of the opinions of their significant referents. According to the theory (Ajzen, 1991; Ajzen & Fishbein, 1980; Fishbein & Ajzen, 1975), specific behavioral intentions are the determinants of behaviors. Thus, for instance, people's use of a condom whenever they have coitus is a function of their intention to use a condom on all occasions of coitus. The theory further holds that a behavioral intention is determined by attitudes toward the specific behavior and subjective norms regarding the behavior. Thus, people intend to perform a behavior when they evaluate that behavior positively and when they believe significant others think they should perform it. The theory holds that the relative importance of the attitudes and subjective norms depends on the particular behavioral intention. For some intentions, attitudinal considerations may be more important than are normative considerations; for others, normative considerations may be the most important predictor. Considerable research has shown that attitudinal beliefs, particularly beliefs about the effects of safer sex practices on sexual enjoyment, predict HIV-risk-associated sexual behaviors. In addition, research has tied subjective norms to HIV-risk behaviors among adolescents.

The Peer Influence Model

Like the theory of reasoned action, the peer influence model places emphasis on normative considerations. More specifically, the peer influence model proposes that peers substantially influence each other's behavior, including intimate safer-sex acts (Catania, Kegeles, & Coates, 1990). Peer support has been related to consistent condom use among public high school students and incarcerated adolescents, to the frequency of sexual activity among private high school students, and to adolescent substance use.

In addition to personal beliefs and perceptions of norms, HIV-risk-associated behaviors may be related to a pattern of risk-taking or a failure to cope with distressing emotions and life stressors. Moreover, different risky activities cluster among adolescents. For example, alcohol consumption and marijuana use have been linked to inconsistent condom use among adolescents and sexual risk among high school students. Conduct problems have been associated with sexual risk acts and drug use among adolescents (Rotheram-Borus, Becker, Koopman, & Kaplan, 1991a). Psychological distress, including anxiety and depression, is expected to be related to sexual risk acts and substance use and may underlie risk-taking behaviors.

Models Specific to HIV Risk Behavior

In addition to general models of behavior, there are now two models of health behavior that have been generated specifically to account for HIV risk behavior: the AIDS Risk Reduction Model (ARRM) (Catania *et al.,* 1989) and the AIDS preventive behavior model (Fisher & Fisher,

1992). The models are similar. The ARRM was developed on the basis of research with adult gay men and identifies three sequential stages to change HIV risk acts: (1) the development of perceived risk for HIV, (2) the development of motivation to change personal risk behavior, and (3) the development of skills to implement behavior change.

HIV PREVENTION INTERVENTION APPROACHES

Prevention programs to reduce adolescents' risk of HIV infection have benefited from earlier research on interventions to reduce cigarette smoking (Schinke & Gilchrist, 1985), alcohol use (Dielman, Shope, Campanelli, & Butchart, 1987), substance abuse (Botvin, 1986; Pentz *et al.*, 1989; Polick, Ellickson, Reuter, & Kahan, 1984), and teenage pregnancy (Pittman & Govan, 1986; Schinke & Gilchrist, 1985). These programs demonstrated that prevention efforts can change adolescents' behavior (Dryfoos, 1990) and provided guidelines to identify critical program components. Successful programs have concentrated on providing access to accurate information, personalizing this information to motivate change, providing training in behavioral skills so that these decisions can be implemented in real-life situations, and reinforcing and rehearsing these skills to build competence and enhance self-esteem (Dryfoos, 1990). Recognizing the importance of the situational contexts and the necessity of structuring support for behavioral change, other program developers have utilized comprehensive community-based interventions that stress problem-solving, general health-related education, and access to services (Carrera, 1987; Sandova, 1988; Vincent, Clearie, & Schlucheter, 1987). In this section, we discuss studies that have tested interventions to reduce HIV-risk-associated behavior among female adolescents and highlight some of the issues raised in such research.

Number of Intervention Sessions

A prevention program implemented by Rotheram-Borus, Koopman, Haignere, and Davies (1991b) targeting change in high-risk sexual behavior has demonstrated effectiveness with a key adolescent population. The subjects were runaway youths from two shelters in New York City. The youths reported significant behavior change at 3 and 6 months following a small group intervention averaging 11 sessions (Rotheram-Borus, Koopman, Haignere, and Davies, 1991). Positive results appeared to persist among males and African American females for up to 2 years (Reid, Rotheram-Borus, Rosario, & Gwadz, 1993). The effectiveness of the program was positively correlated with the number of intervention sessions the adolescents attended. Those who participated in 15 or more training sessions showed the greatest behavior change. Among these adolescents, self-reported consistent condom use rose from 33% at baseline to 57% at the 3-month follow-up and 63% at the 6-month follow-up interview. Additionally, these adolescents showed a decrease from 20% at baseline to zero at the 3-month and 6-month follow-up points in a high-risk pattern of sexual behavior, characterized by infrequent condom use combined with either multiple partners or encounters or both (Rotheram-Borus *et al.,* 1991b). By 1 year, about 8% of youths had begun to relapse (Reid *et al.,* 1993). At 2 years following the implementation, the program was not nearly as successful with Hispanic females as with African American females.

Rotheram-Borus *et al.* (1994) instituted a similar program with 150 African American and Latino adolescents at a large community-based agency in New York City. Reductions in the number of unprotected sexual risk acts and increases in the proportions of condom use were found over 3 months. Changes in sexual risk acts were associated with increased skills in negotiation, the generation of aggressive problem-solving alternatives, and the use of condoms. The program's efficacy was greater when delivered over seven 1.5-hour sessions as compared with three 3- to 4-hour sessions. Although the duration and content of the sessions were similar, condensing the program into fewer and longer sessions over a shorter time span decreased the program's impact.

Girls, Inc. (1991), recently evaluated a successful pregnancy prevention program entailing a comprehensive workshop-based approach to behavior change. The program targeted both the delay of first intercourse and the consistent use of reliable contraceptives. Outcomes at the 1-year follow-up indicated that female adolescents who participated in the program were more than half as likely as nonparticipants to have postponed first sexual intercourse. Participants who were already sexually active were about one third more likely than nonparticipants to use contraception. Girls, Inc., also stressed program intensity as an essential element in achieving the program aims. Similar to Rotheram-Borus *et al.* (1991b), Girls, Inc., found that the more intensive the program, the greater its impact.

Hedonistic Beliefs and Self-Efficacy

J. B. Jemmott, L. S. Jemmott, and colleagues have implemented HIV prevention programs for adolescents. Their initial study focused on 157 inner-city African American male adolescents. In that study (J. B. Jemmott *et al.,* 1992a), they successfully reduced HIV-risk-associated behaviors.

Their approach drew from the theory of reasoned action and social cognitive theory. The intervention consisted of 5 hours of culture-sensitive, developmentally appropriate activities, including small group discussions, videos, interactive exercises, and role playing. Adolescents who were randomly assigned to an HIV prevention program subsequently scored higher in AIDS and STD knowledge, expressed less positive attitudes toward HIV-risk-associated behavior, and reported reduced intentions for such behavior as compared with those assigned to a control intervention on career opportunities. The 3-month follow-up data collected on 96% of the original participants revealed significant effects on self-reported sexual behavior—reduced frequency of coitus, fewer sexual partners, reduced unprotected sex, and a reduced incidence of anal intercourse.

In designing their HIV-risk-reduction intervention, J. B. Jemmott *et al.* (1992a) attempted to have an impact on a variety of theory-derived variables that might affect HIV-risk-associated sexual behavior. These variables included AIDS knowledge, prevention beliefs, hedonistic beliefs, and perceived self-efficacy. A study by J. B. Jemmott, L. S. Jemmott, Spears, Hewitt, and Cruz-Collins (1992b) is one of the few studies to contrast the effectiveness of more than one HIV-risk-reduction intervention. The study compared the effects on intention to use condoms of three interventions: (1) a social cognitive intervention designed to increase perceived self-efficacy to use condoms and hedonistic beliefs favorable to condom use; (2) an information-alone intervention designed to increase general AIDS knowledge and specific prevention beliefs; and (3) a general health promotion intervention designed to provide information about health problems other than AIDS. The results revealed that adolescents in the social cognitive condition registered greater postintervention intentions to use condoms than did those in the two control conditions. Although participants who received the information-alone intervention scored higher in AIDS knowledge and in the specific beliefs that condoms prevent pregnancy, STDs, and AIDS than did those in the health promotion condition, they did not express greater intentions to use condoms. In addition, participants in the social cognitive condition scored higher in perceived self-efficacy and favorable hedonistic expectancies—the two hypothesized mediators of the intervention effect.

Translating Findings into Community-Based Programs

Often, the results of intervention research remain buried in the pages of scientific journals, where they are unlikely to come to the attention of the community people and educators who could make the best use of them.

The ideal of translating research results into practical programs is seldom realized. Recently, L. S. Jemmott and J. B. Jemmott (1992) attempted to address this issue by adapting their HIV-risk-reduction intervention for use in a program for African American female adolescents implemented by a community-based organization, the Urban League of Metropolitan Trenton. Taking into account the constraints within which the community-based organization had to work, the 5-hour program was implemented in three sessions. The first session focused on factual information about the cause, transmission, and prevention of AIDS and the risks faced by African American women of childbearing age in New Jersey. The second session focused on beliefs regarding partner reactions and hedonistic beliefs. The third session focused on skill-building and self-efficacy to use condoms.

L. S. Jemmott and J. B. Jemmott (1992) reported significant effects of the program on intentions among 109 sexually experienced African American female adolescents. Analyses revealed that the adolescents had greater AIDS knowledge, more positive hedonistic beliefs about the effects of condoms on sexual enjoyment, greater self-efficacy to use condoms, and greater intentions to use condoms after the intervention as compared with before the intervention. Further analyses revealed that changes in hedonistic beliefs and self-efficacy were the key mediators of changes in intentions: Increases in hedonistic beliefs and self-efficacy predicted increases in intentions, whereas increases in AIDS knowledge did not.

Parents as Intervenors with Adolescent Women

The theory of reasoned action/planned behavior suggests that in addition to beliefs about the consequences of engaging in behavior and perceptions of behavioral control or self-efficacy, there are normative influences on adolescents' sexual behavior. Although considerable work has focused on the peer group as a source of normative influence, one potentially important but underutilized normative influence is the adolescents' parents. Parents, particularly mothers, are key socializing agents in the lives of female adolescents. A recent study by J. B. Jemmott *et al.* (1993) tested the effects on intentions to influence daughters' HIV-risk-associated sexual behavior of a social cognitive intervention for parents of African American inner-city female adolescents. The subjects were 50 mothers of African American female adolescents recruited from an adolescent medicine clinic of a children's hospital serving a low-income, inner-city, ethnic minority community. The participants were randomly assigned to: (1) an AIDS social cognitive intervention designed to increase perceived self-efficacy to influence their daughter's sexual behavior or one of two control conditions,

(2) an AIDS information-alone intervention designed to increase AIDS knowledge, or (3) a general health promotion intervention that provided information about important health problems other than AIDS. All the interventions were designed to encourage the mothers to influence their daughters' health-related behaviors, but the behaviors that were targeted depended on the condition to which they were randomly assigned (AIDS conditions vs. general health promotion). As hypothesized, participants in the social/cognitive condition reported greater postintervention intentions to influence their daughters' sexual behavior than did those in the two control conditions. In addition, participants in the social/cognitive condition scored higher in perceived self-efficacy—the hypothesized mediator of the intervention effect. Although participants who received the information-alone intervention subsequently had greater AIDS knowledge than did those in the health promotion condition, they did not express greater intentions to use condoms. These results highlight the potential value of a social cognitive approach to helping parents influence their children's AIDS risk behavior.

HIV Testing as a Prevention Strategy

Health care professionals increasingly endorse HIV antibody testing for adolescents, particularly those engaging in high-risk acts (Hein, Blair, Ratzan, & Dyson, 1993), as a risk reduction strategy. Although HIV testing is encouraged, it is not clear that it causes reductions in HIV-risk acts or increased prophylactic treatments among adults (Higgins *et al.,* 1991). Some studies of the impact of HIV testing among adults indicate that many do not change their behavior after being informed of their serostatus (Fox, Odaka, Brookmeyer, & Polk, 1987; Ostrow *et al.,* 1989). There is evidence to support the claim that the combined effect of HIV testing with thorough pre- and posttest counseling can have positive effects via the reduction of anxiety for those who test HIV-seronegative, while those who test HIV-seropositive do not experience an increase in psychiatric symptomatology (Perry, Fishman, Jacobsberg, Young, & Frances, 1991). However, most studies of HIV testing centers and the self reports of those who have undergone testing for HIV suggest that pre- and posttest counseling is far from ideal. Such counseling is often too brief, omitted or not recalled, or poorly done. Many have argued for testing in order to provide therapeutic interventions. However, adolescents who test positive may not realize such benefits if they cannot reasonably expect access to the health care, experimental drugs, or vaccines that provide the rationale for early testing (Bayer, Levine, & Wolfe, 1986).

At this point, it is unclear whether a well-designed HIV testing program with sufficient counseling and follow-up would be an effective adjunct to behavioral change to safer sex and drug-use practices. There are few data specifically on adolescents who have been tested for HIV (C. J. Baker, Huscroft, Morris, Re, & Firpo, 1992), and the available evidence on adolescent behavior change in response to testing is inconclusive. There is evidence that adolescents are likely to continue risk acts after learning their serostatus. Futterman (1991) found that HIV-positive females did not increase condom use and continued to contract STDs after knowing their test results; among HIV-positive male youths, 33% continued high-risk acts and only 33% increased condom use. Continued crack or cocaine use was associated with ongoing high-risk sexual practices following HIV testing (Futterman, 1991). In studies of high-risk youths of unknown HIV serostatus, it was found that only 48% of runaways and 68% of gay males anticipated disclosing positive serostatus to their sexual partners (Koopman, Rotheram-Borus, Dobbs, Gwadz, & Brown, 1992; Rotheram-Borus, Gillis, Gwadz, Reid, & Fernandez, 1993). In addition to risk of spreading HIV infection to others, learning one's serostatus may be associated with negative outcomes. Among 24 youths testing HIV-positive, suicidal ideation was common, but no suicide attempts occurred (Futterman, 1991). However, 21% of New York City high school students spontaneously reported that they would commit suicide if they were HIV-positive (Goodman & Cohall, 1989). Rotheram-Borus *et al.* (1993) also found that many youths claimed that if they were HIV-positive, they would attempt suicide or have sex with as many as possible in order to infect them, or would do both.

Although HIV testing is an important public health strategy for early identification of infection, testing can also be seen as a prevention strategy. For female adolescents who want to become pregnant, emphasizing the importance of condom use is not likely to be an effective prevention strategy. Under these circumstances, HIV testing may be an effective component of a comprehensive prevention strategy. Furthermore, the recent announcements on the utility of AZT to reduce vertical transmission from mothers to newborns will dramatically increase the pressure for HIV testing of sexually active female adolescents, particularly those living in stressful life circumstances. Accordingly, there is an urgent need to design developmentally appropriate standards for the HIV testing of adolescents. Although there have been several attempts to design guidelines for adolescent testing (English, 1989; Rotheram-Borus, 1990), no consensus has been reached. Many community-based agencies have been hesitant to test adolescents for HIV because of the concern that if HIV-positive youths were identified, there would be no services for them. In contrast, many providers attempting to serve HIV-positive youths believe that community sites are overprotecting adolescents by not perceiving them as capable of making their own decisions regarding testing. These are debates that have continued over the last 5 years and have not been resolved by a consensus of opinion. Resolution of these debates is central, however, especially for female adolescents who want to become pregnant.

CONCLUSION

In conclusion, although female adolescents initiate sexual activity somewhat later than male adolescents, their partners are likely to be older, at higher risk for HIV, and more powerful within the relationship. These circumstances often translate into less control over condom use on the part of female adolescents. The female condom, unfortunately, is not currently a realistic alternative for female adolescents. With broader availability and the initiation of new training programs, the female condom may be an important part of enhancing female adolescents' interpersonal power to protect themselves from HIV. The desire to become mothers is often a central barrier to HIV prevention among female adolescents. To maintain protection while wanting a baby will demand far greater utilization of HIV testing as a strategy of HIV prevention. To this point, HIV pre- and posttest counseling has not been effectively implemented (based on clinicians' reports) or evaluated. This is an important research priority.

The theoretical and empirical literature reviewed in this chapter suggests several conclusions about behavior change. Enhancing motivation for safe acts is an implicit agenda in the design of the context of the interventions. Motivation can be increased by structuring the delivery of the intervention within a group of peers rewarding each other for reporting safe acts and role-playing coping skills in high-risk situations. In addition, motivation can be increased by interventions that address key conceptual variables. For example, adolescents can be motivated by fear of HIV (Rhodes *et al.*, 1990). Individuals will be more likely to change their health behaviors if they perceive themselves to be at risk (Rosenstock, 1974; Maimen & Becker, 1974). Prerequisites to perceiving HIV as a problem include having accurate knowledge about HIV transmission and risk behaviors, recognizing that one's own behaviors may be risky, and acknowledging the limits of one's ability to implement safe acts and to cope effectively under conditions of high emotional arousal (Rotheram-Borus, Koopman, & Rosario, 1992). A successful intervention program must integrate the need for factual information with the importance of personalizing this knowledge for youth. The task of personalizing knowledge involves clarifying the manner in which emotional arousal and youths' limited behavioral skills place them at risk in the situations they encounter.

Although some level of perceived risk of HIV may be necessary, an overemphasis on fear arousal may be ineffective. In fact, Rotheram-Borus and her research team, on the basis of their clinical experience, recommend enhancing the advantages of safe acts, rather than attempting to motivate youth through fear. For example, adolescents might be shown pictures of adults with AIDS in the terminal stages of illness, which is likely to heighten fear of HIV transmission. The trouble with this tactic is that adolescents are likely to distance themselves emotionally, especially given the dissimilarity between the sick person and themselves. In contrast, taking youths to homes of babies infected with HIV is likely to elicit youths' protective feelings toward offspring. Protectiveness is a more comfortable emotional state than fear and is not as likely to engender avoidant behaviors and feelings. If death is discussed in the context of HIV, it would be important for youths to recognize the negative consequences, such as "who will have your boyfriend if you die" or "who will get your bedroom." Although recognizing the relationship between unsafe sex and HIV infection, and between HIV infection and death, is an implicit goal of the intervention, equating sex with death is undesirable. To this end, strategies that emphasize life fulfillment and realizing individual potential, rather than links between sex and death, may be most effective.

Motivation can also be increased by interventions that address the hedonistic beliefs regarding the consequences of safer sex practices for sexual enjoyment. Interventions that incorporated hedonistic beliefs have been found to be especially effective at changing intentions to use condoms (J. B. Jemmott *et al.,* 1992b; L. S. Jemmott & J. B. Jemmott, 1992). Quite apart from adolescents' beliefs about condoms, HIV-risk-reduction interventions need to address the reactions of adolescents' sexual partners, particularly the sexual partners' approval or disapproval of safer sex practices, including abstinence. Unlike many health behavior interventions, HIV-risk-reduction interventions have to take into account that the adolescent may not have complete control over the targeted behavior. Protected sexual intercourse is interpersonal behavior, and hence the sexual partner's beliefs are important. Trust is an issue that often arises during intervention-group discussions regarding convincing sexual partners to use condoms. Asking a partner to use condoms may suggest to the partner that the adolescent does not trust the partner. This is particularly likely if the partner has an established or long-term relationship with the adolescent. In contrast, it may be easier to establish condom use at the beginning of new relationships. Clearly, HIV-risk-reduction interventions have to take this barrier to condom use into account.

Several studies also suggested that interventions should address skills and perceived self-efficacy. Although skills and perceived self-efficacy are likely to be correlated—people who have the skills are also likely to feel efficacious—they are not identical, and it is unclear which of the two is more important to behavior change. A number of types of skills and efficacy have been highlighted in the literature. Perhaps the most widely recognized type of skill or perceived efficacy is negotiation or resistance skill—the ability of the adolescent to convince a sexual partner to practice protected sexual intercourse or to resist partner pressure to practice unprotected sexual intercourse. Much less attention has been paid to technical skill in condom use, particularly skill at using condoms without ruining the mood. However, this type of skill may be just as important as negotiation skill (J. B. Jemmott, L. S. Jemmott, & Hacker, 1992). HIV-risk-reduction interventions must teach adolescents how to use condoms. It is not enough to simply tell them they should use condoms. By increasing technical skill at using condoms, it may be possible to allay the adolescents' sexual partners' concerns about the adverse impact of condom use on sexual enjoyment. Clearly, if an adolescent successfully negotiates condom use, but then implements it in a clumsy manner, the experience may decrease the likelihood that the adolescent will attempt to use condoms in the future or may make it more difficult to negotiate future use with that sexual partner.

Adolescents must also be able to coordinate their thoughts, feelings, and actions to act safely in situations that place them at high risk for HIV. Adolescents often feel unable to control both excitement and anxiety. Physiologically, the emotions are similar. Deep breathing and relaxation techniques can help youths cope with both emotions. Effective verbal and nonverbal behaviors that help youths assert their goals in a culturally appropriate and gender-specific manner can be shaped by role playing, video workshops, dramatizations of soap operas, and practicing prepared scripts of handling difficult interpersonal problem situations.

In sum, risk of HIV is related to particular sexual behaviors. Gender roles and other role constraints can limit female adolescents' ability to reduce their risk. Attitudes, peer norms, perceived self-efficacy, and skills have been found to be important determinants of risk behavior. Several theories have been applied to HIV-risk-associated behavior, and a number of promising interventions have been implemented. Still, a great deal of work remains to be done. There have been relatively few intervention studies that examined effects on behavior using randomly assigned control groups. The effects of HIV testing on adolescents remain unclear. As research continues, a more complete understanding will emerge, which should help to curb the impact of HIV on young women.

ACKNOWLEDGMENTS. Preparation of this chapter was supported in part by National Institute of Nursing Research Grant R01-NR03123-01 and National Institute of Mental Health Grant R01-MH45668.

REFERENCES

Ajzen, I. (1991). The theory of planned behavior. *Organizational Behavior and Human Decision Processes, 50,* 179–211.

Ajzen, I., & Fishbein, M. (1980). *Understanding attitudes and predicting social behavior.* Englewood Cliffs, NJ: Prentice-Hall.

Anderson, J. E., Kann, L., Holtzman, D., Arday, S., Truman, B., & Kolbe, L. (1990). HIV/AIDS knowledge and sexual behavior among high school students. *Family Planning Perspectives, 22,* 252–255.

Aneshensel, C. S., Becerra, R. M., Fielder, E. P., & Schuler, R. H. (1990). Onset of fertility-related events during adolescence: A prospective comparison of Mexican American and non-Hispanic white females. *American Journal of Public Health, 80,* 959–963.

Baker, C. J., Huscroft, S., Morris, R., Re, O., & Firpo, R. (1992). Changes in sexual behavior in delinquent youth following risk reduction counseling (abstract). *Proceedings of the Eighth International Conference on AIDS, 8*(3), 201.

Baker, D. G., & Mossman, D. (1991). Potential HIV exposure in psychiatrically hospitalized adolescent girls. *American Journal of Psychiatry, 148,* 528–530.

Bandura, A. (1989). Perceived self-efficacy in the exercise of control over AIDS infection. In V. Mays, G. Albee, and S. Schneider (Eds.), *Primary prevention of AIDS* (pp. 128–141). Newbury Park, CA: Sage.

Bandura, A. (1992). A social cognitive approach to the exercise of control over AIDS infection. In R. DiClemente (Ed.), *Adolescents and AIDS: A generation in jeopardy* (pp. 89–116). Newbury Park, CA: Sage.

Bandura, A. (1994). Social cognitive theory and exercise of control over HIV infection. In R. DiClemente & J. Peterson (Eds.), *Preventing AIDS: Theories and methods of behavioral interventions. AIDS prevention and mental health* (pp. 25–59). New York: Plenum Press.

Bayer, R., Levine, C., & Wolf, S. M. (1986). HIV antibody screening: An ethical framework for evaluating proposed programs. *JAMA, 256,* 1768–1774.

Becker, M. H. (1974). The health belief model and personal health behavior. *Health Education Monographs, 2,* 324–508.

Bell, T. A., & Hein, K. (1984). Adolescents and sexually transmitted diseases. In K. Holmes *et al.* (Eds.), *Sexually transmitted diseases* (pp. 73–84). New York: McGraw-Hill.

Botvin, G. (1986). Substance abuse prevention efforts: Recent developments and future directions. *Journal of School Health, 56,* 369–374.

Brown, L. K., DiClemente, R. J., & Beausoleil, N. I. (1992). Comparison of human immunodeficiency virus–related knowledge, attitudes, intentions and behaviors among sexually active and abstinent young adolescents. *Journal of Adolescent Health, 13,* 140–145.

Burke, D. S., Brundage, J. F., Goldenbaum, M., Gardner, L. I., Peterson, M., Visintine, R., Redfield, R. R., & The Walter Reed Retrovirus Research Group. (1990). Human immunodeficiency virus infection in teenagers: Seroprevalence among applicants for US military service. *JAMA, 263,* 2074–2077.

Carrera, M. (1987). Multi-service family life and sex education program. Report from Children's AID Society, New York, 1987.

Carroll, J. C., Volk, K. A., & Hyde J. S. (1985). Differences between males and females in motives for engaging in sexual intercourse. *Archives of Sexual Behavior, 14,* 131–139.

Catania, J. A., Dolcini, M., Coates, T. J., Kegeles, S. M., Greenblatt, R., Puckett, S., Corman, M., & Miller, J. (1989). Predictors of condom use and multiple partnered sex among sexually-active adolescent women: Implications for AIDS-related health interventions. *Journal of Sex Research, 26,* 514–524.

Catania, J. A., Kegeles, S. M., & Coates, T.J. (1990). Towards an understanding of risk behavior: An AIDS Risk Reduction Model (ARRM). *Health Education Quarterly, 17,* 53–72.

Cates, W., Jr. (1987). Epidemiology and control of sexually transmitted diseases: Strategic evolution. *Infectious Disease Clinics of North America, 1,* 1–23.

Centers for Disease Control and Prevention. (1993a). HIV/AIDS surveillance report, July. Atlanta.

Centers for Disease Control and Prevention (1993b). HIV/AIDS surveillance report, No. 4. Year-end provisional report.

Centers for Disease Control and Prevention. (1994). *HIV/AIDS surveillance report, 6*(1), 13.

D'Angelo, L. P., Getson, P., Luben, N., Stallings, E., & Gayle, H. (1989). HIV infection in adolescents: Can we predict who is at risk? Paper presented at the Fifth International Conference on AIDS, Montreal.

DeLamater, J. (1987). Gender differences in sexual scenarios. In K. Kelley (Ed.), *Females, males, and sexuality* (pp. 127–139). Albany: State University of New York Press.

DiClemente, R. J., Lanier, M. M., Horan, P. F., & Lodico, M. (1991). Comparison of AIDS knowledge, attitudes, and behaviors among incarcerated adolescents and a public school sample in San Francisco. *American Journal of Public Health, 81,* 628–630.

Dielman, T., Shope, P., Campanelli, P., & Butchart, A. T. (1987). Elementary school–based prevention of adolescent alcohol misuse. *Pediatrician, 14,* 70–76.

Dryfoos, J. (1990). *Adolescents at risk: Prevalence and prevention.* New York: Oxford University Press.

English, A. (1989). AIDS testing and epidemiology for youth. *Journal of Adolescent Health Care, 10,* 52S–57S.

Erikson, E. (1950). *Childhood and society.* New York: Norton.

Fishbein, M., & Ajzen, I. (1975). *Belief, attitude, intention, and behavior: An introduction to theory and research.* Reading, MA: Addison-Wesley.

Fisher, J. (1988). Possible effects of reference group-based social influence on AIDS-risk behavior and AIDS prevention. *American Psychologist, 43,* 914–920.

Fisher, J. D., & Fisher, W. A. (1992). Changing AIDS-risk behavior. *Psychological Bulletin, 111*(3), 455–474.

Forrest, J., & Singh, S. (1990). The sexual and reproductive behavior of American women, 1982–1988. *Family Planning Perspectives, 22,* 206–214.

Fox, R., Odaka, N. J., Brookmeyer, R., & Polk, B. F. (1987). Effect of HIV antibody disclosure on subsequent sexual activity in homosexual men. *AIDS, 1,* 241–246.

Frieze, I. H., Parsons, J. E., Johnson, P. E., Ruble, D. N., & Zellman, G. L. (1978). *Women and sex roles.* New York: Norton.

Fullilove, R., Fullilove, M., Bowser, B., & Gross, S. (1990). Risk of sexually transmitted disease among African-American adolescent crack users in Oakland and San Francisco, Calif. *JAMA, 263,* 851–855.

Futterman, D. (1991). Medical issues with HIV-infected adolescents. National Pediatric Conference on AIDS. Washington, DC, January 1991.

Futterman, D., Hein, K., Kipke, M., Reulbach, W., Clare, G., Nelson, J., Orane, A., & Gayle, H.(1990). HIV+ adolescents: HIV testing experiences and changes in risk related sexual and drug use behavior (abstract). *Proceedings of the Sixth International Conference on AIDS, 6*(3), 254.

Girls, Inc. (1991). Truth, trust and technology: New research on preventing adolescent pregnancy. Summary report on the Girls VX program development and research project. New York: published by the author.

Goeddert, J. J., Kessler, C. M., & Aledort, L. M. (1990). A prospective study of human immunodeficiency virus type I infection and the development of AIDS in subjects with hemophilia. *New England Journal of Medicine, 321,* 1141–1148.

Goldsmith, M. (1988). Sex tied to drugs = STD spread. *JAMA, 260,* 2009.

Goldsmith, M. (1993). Invisible epidemic now becoming visible as HIV/AIDS pandemic reaches adolescents. *JAMA, 270,* 16–19.

Goodman, E., & Cohall, A. T. (1989). Acquired immunodeficiency syndrome and adolescents: Knowledge, attitudes, beliefs and behaviors in a New York City adolescent minority population. *Pediatrics, 84,* 36–42.

Gross, A. E. (1978). The male role and heterosexual behavior. *Journal of Social Issues, 34,* 87–107.

Hatcher, R. A., Stewart, F. H., Trussell, J., Kowal, D., Guest, F., Stewart, G. K., & Cates, W. (1990). *Contraceptive technology 1990–1992.* New York: Irvington.

Hayman, C., St. Louis, M., Petersen, L., Miller, C., Job Corps, & Centers for Disease Control. (1990). HIV infection in underprivileged teenagers: Update from the Job Corps. Paper presented at the Sixth International Conference on AIDS, San Francisco.

Hein, K., Blair, J., Ratzan, S., Dyson, D. (1993). Adolescents and HIV: Two decades of denial. In S. Ratzan (Ed.), *AIDS: Effective health communication for the 90s* (pp. 215–232). Philadelphia: Taylor & Francis.

Higgins, D. L., Galavotti, C., O'Reilly, K., Schnell, D. J., Moore, M., Rugg, D. L., & Johnson, R. (1991). Evidence for the effects of HIV antibody counseling and testing on risk behaviors. *JAMA, 226,* 2419–2429.

Hingson, R., Strunin, L., Berlin, B., & Heeren, T. (1990). Beliefs about AIDS, use of alcohol and drugs, and unprotected sex among Massachusetts adolescents. *American Journal of Public Health, 80,* 295–299.

Hofferth, S. L., Kahn, J. R., & Baldwin, W. (1987). Premarital sexual activity among U.S. teenage women over the past three decades. *Family Planning Perspectives, 19,* 46–53.

Jemmott, J. B., III, Jemmott, L. S., & Fong, G. T. (1992a). Reductions in HIV risk–associated sexual behaviors among African-American male adolescents: Effects of an AIDS prevention intervention. *American Journal of Public Health, 82,* 372–377.

Jemmott, J. B., III, Jemmott, L. S., Spears, H., Hewitt, N., & Cruz-Collins, M. (1992b). Self-efficacy, hedonistic expectancies, and condom-use intentions among inner-city black adolescent women: A social cognitive approach to AIDS risk behavior. *Journal of Adolescent Health, 13,* 512–519.

Jemmott, J. B., III, Jemmott, L. S., & Hacker, C. I. (1992c). Predicting intentions to use condoms among African American adolescents: The theory of planned behavior as a model of HIV risk associated behavior. *Journal of Ethnicity & Disease, 2,* 371–380.

Jemmott, J. B., III, Jemmott, L. S., Braverman, P., Boccher-Lattimore, D., Fong, G. T., Lerman, C., McCaffree, K., & Hacker, C. I. (1993, April). *Training mothers to reduce their daughters' HIV risk behavior: A social cognitive intervention.* Paper presented at the Annual Meeting of the Society of Behavioral Medicine, San Francisco.

Jemmott, L. S., & Jemmott, J. B., III. (1992). Increasing condom-use intentions among sexually active inner-city adolescent women: Effects of an AIDS prevention program. *Nursing Research, 41,* 273–279.

Jessor, S. L., & Jessor, R. (1977). *Problem behavior and psychosocial development.* New York: Academic Press.

Johnston, L., O'Malley, P., & Bachman, J. (1987). Psychotherapeutic, licit, and illicit use of drugs among adolescents: An epidemiological perspective. [Special issue]. *Journal of Adolescent Health Care, 8,* 36–51.

Jones, E. F., Forrest, J. D., Goldman, N., Henshaw, S., Lincoln, R., Rosoff, J. I., Westoff, C. F., & Wulf, D. (1986). *Teenage pregnancy in industrialized countries.* New Haven, CT: Yale University Press.

Keller, S. E., Bartlett, J. A., Schleifer S. J., Johnson, R. L., Pinner, E., & Delaney, B. (1991). HIV relevant sexual behavior among a healthy inner city heterosexual adolescent population in an endemic area of HIV. *Journal of Adolescent Health Care, 12,* 44–48.

Kimble, D., Hertzog, N., Fisher, J., & Fisher, W. (1991). AIDS education needs assessment for Worcester Massachusetts high schools. Unpublished manuscript.

Kipke, M., Futterman, D., & Hein, K. (1990). HIV infection and AIDS during adolescence. *Medical Clinics of North America, 74,* 1149–1166.

Knox, M., & Clark, C. (1991). Early HIV detection: A community mental health role. *Journal of Mental Health Administration, 18,* 21–26.

Kohlberg, L. (1966). A cognitive–developmental analysis of children's sex role concepts and attitudes. In E. Maccoby (Ed.), *The development of sex differences.* Stanford, CA: Stanford University Press.

Koopman, C., Rotheram-Borus, M. J., Dobbs, L., Gwadz, M., & Brown, J. (1992). Beliefs and behavioral intentions regarding virus testing among New York City runaways. *Journal of Adolescent Health Care, 13,* 576–581.

Koopman, C., Rosario, M., & Rotheram-Borus, M. J. (1994). Alcohol and drug use and sexual behaviors placing runaways at risk for HIV infection. *Addictive Behaviors, 19,* 95–103.

Maimen, L., & Becker, M. (1974). The health belief model: Origins and correlates in psychological theory. In M. H. Becker (Ed.), *The health belief model and personal health behavior.* Thorofare, NJ: Charles B. Slack.

Miller, H. G., Turner, C. F., & Moses, L. E. (Eds.) (1990). *AIDS: The second decade.* Washington, DC: National Academy Press.

Minkoff, H., McCalla, S., Delke, I., Stevens, R., Salwen, M., & Feldman, J. (1990). The relationship of cocaine use to syphilis and human immunodeficiency virus infections among inner city parturient women. *American Journal of Obstetrics and Gynecology, 163,* 521–526.

Morris, R., Baker, C., Huscroft, S., Evans, C. A., & Zeljkovic, S. (1991). Two year variation in HIV risk behaviors in detained minors. Paper presented at the Seventh International Conference on AIDS, Florence.

Mussen, P. H. (1969). Early sex role development. In D. A. Goslin (Ed.), *Handbook of socialization theory and research.* Chicago: Rand McNally.

National Institute on Drug Abuse (1990). *National household survey on drug abuse: Population estimates 1990.* Rockville, MD: U.S. Department of Health and Human Services, U.S. Public Health Service, Alcohol, Drug Abuse, and Mental Health Administration.

National Research Council (1989). *AIDS: Sexual behavior and intravenous drug use.* Washington, DC: National Academy Press.

Novick, L., Berns, D., Stricof, R., Stevens, R., Pass, K., & Wethers, J. (1989). HIV seroprevalence in newborns in New York state. *JAMA, 261,* 1745–1750.

Ostrow, D. G., Joseph, J. G., Kessler, R., & Soucy, J. (1989). Disclosure of HIV antibody status: Behavioral and mental health correlates. *AIDS Education and Prevention, 1*(1), 1–11.

Pennbridge, J., Freese, T., & Mackenzie, R. (1992). High risk behaviors among male street youth in Hollywood, California. *Aids Education Prevention, Supplement,* 24–33.

Pentz, M., Dwyer, D., Mackinnon, B., Flay, W., Hansen, E., Yang, E., & Johnson, C. (1989). A multicommunity trial for primary prevention of adolescent drug abuse: Effects on drug use prevalence. *JAMA, 261,* 3259–3266.

Perry, S., Fishman, B., Jacobsberg, L., Young, J., & Frances, A. (1991). Effectiveness of psychoeducational interventions in reducing emotional distress after human immunodeficiency virus antibody testing. *Archives of General Psychiatry, 48,* 143–147.

Pittman, K., & Govan, C. (1986). *Model programs: Preventing adolescent pregnancy and building youth self-sufficiency.* Washington, DC: Children's Defense Fund.

Polick, J., Ellickson, P., Reuter, P., & Kahan, J. (1984). *Strategies for controlling adolescent drug use.* Santa Monica: Rand Corporation.

Pratt, W., Mosher, W., Bachrach, C., & Horn, M. (1984). Understanding U.S. fertility: Findings from the National Survey of Family Growth, Cycle III. *Population Bulletin, 39,* 1–42.

Quinn, T. C., Glasser, D., Cannon, R. O., Matuszak, D. L., Dunning, R. W., Klein, R. L., Campbell, C. H., Israel, E., Fauci, A. S., & Hook, E. W. (1988). Human immunodeficiency virus infection among patients attending clinics for sexually transmitted diseases. *New England Journal of Medicine, 318,* 197–202.

Reid, H. M., Rotheram-Borus, M. J., Rosario M. R., & Gwadz, M. (1993). Effectiveness of HIV prevention with homeless youth over 2 years. Paper presented at the Ninth International Conference on AIDS, Berlin.

Reinisch, J., Sanders, S., & Ziemba-Davis, M. (1988). The study of sexual behavior in relation to the transmission of human immunodeficiency virus: Caveats and recommendations. [Special issue.] *American Psychologist, 43,* 921–927.

Remafedi, G. (1987). Male homosexuality: The adolescent's perspective. *Pediatrics, 79,* 326–330.

Rhodes, F., MacDonald, K., & Elder-Tarizy, K. (1990). Effects of AIDS education on knowledge, attitudes and risk behavior of adolescent youth. Paper presented at the meeting of the American Psychological Association, Boston.

Rosenstock, I. (1974). Historical origins of the health belief model. *Health Education Monographs, 2,* 328–335.

Rotheram-Borus, M. J. (1990). Prevention of HIV infection among adolescents. In S. Blumenthal, A. Eichler, & G. Weissman (Eds.), *Women and AIDS: Promoting healthy behaviors* (pp. 109–117). Washington, DC: Government Printing Office.

Rotheram-Borus, M. J., & Koopman, C. (1991a). Sexual risk behavior, AIDS knowledge and beliefs about AIDS among predominantly minority gay and bisexual male adolescents. *AIDS Education and Prevention, 3,* 305–312.

Rotheram-Borus, M. J., & Koopman, C. (1991b). Sexual risk behaviors, AIDS knowledge, and beliefs about AIDS among runaways. *American Journal of Public Health, 81,* 208–210.

Rotheram-Borus, M. J., Koopman, C., & Bradley, J. (1989). Barriers to successful AIDS prevention programs with runaway youth. In J. O. Woodruff, D. Doherty, & J. G. Athey (Eds.), *Troubled adolescents and HIV infection: Issues in prevention and treatment* (pp. 35–55). Washington DC: Georgetown University.

Rotheram-Borus, M. J., Becker, J., Koopman, C., & Kaplan, M. (1991a). AIDS knowledge, beliefs, and sexual behaviors of sexually delinquent and non-delinquent runaway adolescents. *Journal of Adolescence, 14,* 229–244.

Rotheram-Borus, M. J., Koopman C., Haignere, C., & Davies, M. (1991b). Reducing HIV sexual risk behaviors among runaway adolescents. *JAMA, 266,* 1237–1241.

Rotheram-Borus, M. J., Koopman, C., & Rosario, M. (1992). Developmentally tailoring prevention programs: Matching strategies to adolescents' serostatus. In R. J. DiClemente (Ed.), *Adolescents and AIDS: A generation in jeopardy* (pp. 212–229). Newbury Park, CA: Sage.

Rotheram-Borus, M. J., Gillis, J. R., Gwadz, M., Reid, H., & Fernandez M. I. (1993). *HIV testing of heterosexual, gay, and lesbian youth: Uses, abuses, and attitudes.* Poster presented at the IXth International Conference on AIDS/IVth STD World Congress, Berlin.

Rotheram-Borus, M. J., Rosario, M., Meyer-Bahlburg, H., Koopman, C., Dopkins, S. C., & Davies, M. (1994). Sexual and substance use acts of gay and bisexual male adolescents in New York City. *Journal of Sex Research, 31*(1), 47–57.

Sandova, J. (1988). Impact '88: Dallas' countywide plan for reducing teen pregnancy. *SIECUS Report, 16,* 1–5.

Schilling, R. F., El-Bassel, N., Schinke, S. P., Gordon, K., & Nichols, S. (1991). Sexual behavior, attitudes toward safer sex, and gender among a cohort of 244 recovering IV drug users. *International Journal of the Addictions, 26*(8), 859–877.

Schinke, S., & Gilchrist, L. (1985). Preventing substance abuse with children and adolescents. *Journal of Consulting and Clinical Psychology, 53,* 596–602.

Shalwitz, J., Goulart, M., Dunnigan, K., & Flannery, D. (1990). Prevalence of sexually transmitted diseases (STD) and HIV in a homeless youth medical clinic in San Francisco. Paper presented at the Sixth International Conference on AIDS, San Francisco.

Simon, W., & Gagnon, J. (1986). Sexual scripts: Permanence and change. *Archives of Sexual Behavior, 15,* 97–120.

Smith, E. A., & Udry, J. R. (1985). Coital and non-coital sexual behaviors of white and African-American Americans. *American Journal of Public Health, 75,* 1200–1203.

Sonenstein, F., Pleck, J., & Ku, L. (1989). Sexual activity, condom use and AIDS awareness among adolescent males. *Family Planning Perspectives, 21,* 152–158.

St. Louis, M. E., Conway, G. A., Hayman, C. R., Miller, C., Peterson, L. R., & Dondero, T. J. (1991). Human immunodeficiency virus infection in disadvantaged adolescents. Findings from the U.S. Job Corps. *JAMA, 266,* 2387–2391.

Stricof, R. L., Novick, L. F., & Kennedy, J. (1990). HIV-1 seroprevalence in facilities for runaway and homeless adolescents in four states: Florida, Texas, Louisiana, and New York. Paper presented at the Sixth Annual International Conference on AIDS, San Francisco.

Stricof, R. L., Kennedy, J. T., Natteu, T. C., Wersfuse, I. B., & Novick, L. F. (1991). HIV seroprevalence in a facility for runaway and homeless adolescents. *American Journal of Public Health, 81* (Suppl.), 50–53.

Strunin, L., & Hingson, R. (1987). Acquired immunodeficiency syndrome and adolescents: Knowledge, beliefs, attitudes, and behaviors. *Pediatrics, 5,* 825–827.

Strunin, L., & Hingson, R. (1992). Alcohol, drugs, and adolescent sexual behavior. [Special issue]. *International Journal of the Addictions, 27,* 129–146.

Thompson, L., & Spanier, G. (1978). Influence of parents, peers, and partners on the contraceptive use of college age men and women. *Journal of Marriage & the Family, 40,* 481–492.

Vincent, M., Clearie, A., & Schlucheter, M. (1987). Reducing adolescent pregnancy through school and community-based education. *JAMA, 257,* 3382–3386.

Walter, H. (1990). AIDS prevention for adolescents in school. Paper presented at Grand Rounds of the HIV Center for Clinical and Behavioral Studies, Columbia University, New York, October 1990.

Wells, K. (1980). Gender role identity and psychological adjustment in adolescence. *Journal of Youth and Adolescence, 9,* 59–73.

Whitley, B. E., & Schofield, J. W. (1986). A meta-analysis of research on adolescent contraceptive use. *Population and Environment, 8,* 173–203.

Wilcox, B. L. (1990). Federal policy and adolescent AIDS. In W. Gardner *et al.* (Eds.), *New directions in child development: Adolescents in the AIDS epidemic* (pp. 61–70). San Francisco: Jossey-Bass Inc.

Wyatt, G., Peters, S., Guthrie, D. (1988a). Kinsey revisited: I. Comparisons of the sexual socialization and sexual behavior of White women over 33 years. *Archives of Sexual Behavior, 17,* 201–239.

Wyatt, G., Peters, S., Guthrie, D. (1988b). Kinsey revisited: II. Comparisons of the sexual socialization and sexual behavior of Black women over 33 years. *Archives of Sexual Behavior, 17,* 289–332.

Zabin, L. S., & Clark, S. D., Jr. (1981). Why they delay: A study of teenage family planning clinic patients. *Family Planning Perspectives, 13,* 205–217.

Zabin, L. S., Hardy, J. B., Smith, E. A., & Hirsch, M. B. (1986). Substance use and its relation to sexual activity among inner-city adolescents. *Journal of Adolescent Health Care, 7,* 320–331.

Zelnik, M., Kantner, F., & Ford, K. (1981). Sex and pregnancy in adolescence. *Sage Library of Social Research, Vol. 133.* Beverly Hills, CA: Sage.

Zelnik, M., & Shah, F. K. (1983). First intercourse among young Americans. *Family Planning Perspectives, 15,* 64–70.

6

African American Women and HIV-Risk-Reduction Issues

LORETTA SWEET JEMMOTT, VERONICA CATAN, ADELINE NYAMATHI, and JOYCE ANASTASIA

INTRODUCTION

AIDS has become a major health problem in African American women between the ages of 18 and 44, making it one of the five leading causes of death among African American women in the United States [Centers for Disease Control and Prevention (CDC), 1992]. In New York and New Jersey, AIDS is already the number one cause of death among African American women ages 15–44 (Chu, Buehler, & Berkelman, 1990). Hence, African American women are disproportionately burdened by AIDS. Only 12% of the population in the United States is African American, yet 52% of women with AIDS are African American (CDC, 1991). For instance, through September 1993, there were 40,702 AIDS cases among women in the United States. Of these, 21,728 cases, or more than half, were African American women (CDC, 1993). It is estimated that over half of HIV-infected African American women (50%) are infected as a result of injection-drug use, and another 33% as a result of unprotected sex with HIV-infected partners (CDC, 1994). In addition, African American women are 9 times more likely to die from HIV infection than are white females (Department of Health and Human Services, 1992).

LORETTA SWEET JEMMOTT • University of Pennsylvania School of Nursing, Philadelphia, PA 19104. *VERONICA CATAN* • Columbia University School of Social Work, New York, NY 10032. *ADELINE NYAMATHI* • UCLA School of Nursing, Los Angeles, CA 90024. *JOYCE ANASTASIA* • Columbia University School of Nursing, New York, NY 10032.

Women at Risk: Issues in the Primary Prevention of AIDS, edited by Ann O'Leary and Loretta Sweet Jemmott. Plenum Press, New York, 1995.

The tragedy of HIV infection among African American women is compounded by the increasing rates among African American children. More than one half (52%) of the children under 13 years of age who have AIDS are African American. Compared with white pediatric AIDS cases, African American pediatric cases are more likely to have a mother who was exposed to HIV as a result of injection-drug use or heterosexual contact (CDC, 1991). For instance, 59% of their mothers were infected via injection-drug use and 41% were infected via sexual contact. It is projected that 72,000 to 125,000 children will be orphaned by AIDS by the end of the decade. Clearly, increased prevention efforts must be directed toward these women of childbearing age.

African American women with sexually transmitted diseases (STDs) are at increased risk for HIV infection (see Chapter 2). In general, inner-city African American women have disproportionately higher rates of chlamydia, syphilis, gonorrhea, and pelvic inflammatory disease than other women (Bell & Holmes, 1984; Hatcher *et al.*, 1990; Hayes, 1987; Hofferth & Hayes, 1987; Jones *et al.*, 1985; Pratt, Mosher, Bachrach, & Horn, 1984; Zelnik & Kantner, 1980). Like the risk of STDs, the risk of HIV infection is heightened by unprotected sexual activity. In addition, the presence of an STD and associated lesions may facilitate transmission of HIV. Since injection-drug users (IDUs) play an important role in the transmission of HIV infection to heterosexuals, the prevalence of IDUs in urban areas greatly heightens the risk of HIV infection for African American women who live in inner cities. Even if the women themselves do not inject drugs, they may have sexual relationships with men who are IDUs. The juxtaposition of elevated STD rates and the potential for perinatally transmitted HIV infection also suggests the urgency of intervening with African American women.

Fortunately, AIDS is preventable. In order to reduce the risk of AIDS among African American women, we need to know the key HIV-risk-associated behaviors in this population, the intervention-sensitive conceptual variables that determine those behaviors, and the most effective behavior-change intervention strategies. Unfortunately, despite the widely held view that the reduction of risk behavior is a critical component of any attempt to reduce the incidence of AIDS, efforts at behavioral prevention have been hampered because little is known about the reasons African American women engage in risk behaviors or about the most effective ways to change their behavior (Baum & Nesselhof, 1988; Becker & Joseph, 1988; Turner, Miller, & Moses, 1989). This chapter is an effort to fill that gap. First, this chapter will summarize and review the literature on African American women and AIDS-risk behaviors. Second, we will discuss conceptual variables that determine AIDS-risk behavior and culturally sensitive

HIV-risk-reduction intervention strategies. Third, we will discuss barriers and obstacles for HIV-prevention efforts for African American women.

AFRICAN AMERICAN WOMEN AND RISK OF SEXUALLY TRANSMITTED HIV INFECTION

The most effective way for an African American woman to avoid sexually transmitted HIV infection is to avoid having sex. Certain sexual activities are known to increase the chance of HIV infection (Hatcher *et al.,* 1990). The greater the number of times she has coitus without the protection of a condom, the greater her risk of HIV infection. Risk is heightened to the extent that she engages in unprotected vaginal, anal, or oral sex; has many sexual partners; has sex with people who have other sexual relationships; or has sex with a partner who is HIV-seropositive or who is at high risk because of his or her sexual activity or use of injection drugs with shared needles and syringes. Finally, to the extent that she engages in unprotected oral sexual activities, her risk is increased.

Nonuse of Condoms

Unfortunately, much of the sexual activity of African American women occurs without the protection of condoms. Studies have reported that sexually active African American women report not consistently using condoms (Belcastro, 1985; Mosher & Pratt, 1990; L. S. Jemmott & J. B. Jemmott, 1991). For instance, Belcastro (1985) found that about 42% of African American undergraduate women as compared with 27% of white undergraduate women reported never using condoms. Data from the 1982 and 1988 National Surveys of Family Growth have suggested that among women 15–44 years of age, African American women were less likely to use condoms than were white women in both 1982 and 1988 (Mosher & Pratt, 1990). In addition, L. S. Jemmott and J. B. Jemmott (1991) found that 60% of the 103 sexually active unmarried African American women undergraduates at an inner-city commuter university in northern New Jersey reported failing to use condoms 60% of the time they had coitus over a 3-month interval. Hence, failure to use condoms was their most common HIV-sexual-risk behavior.

Multiple Partners

Some evidence suggests that white women are more likely than African American women to have had only one nonmarital sexual partner. On the other hand, sexually experienced African American women undergraduates were less likely than their white counterparts to have had six or more partners (Belcastro, 1985). In a similar vein, Wyatt, Peters, and Guthrie (1988a,b) found that among white women aged 18–36, 52% reported having had 11 or more sexual partners since age 18 years, but among African American women, the figure was only 29%.

Noncoital Sexual Behaviors

Little is known about the dynamics of noncoital sexual behaviors such as anal intercourse and oral sex, especially among African American women. This lack of data is unfortunate because the behavior associated with the best-documented risk for sexual transmission of HIV is noncoital, namely, unprotected receptive anal intercourse. Although anal intercourse is chiefly associated with homosexual men, there is growing recognition that it is a fairly common practice among heterosexuals (Reinisch, Sanders, & Ziemba-Davis, 1988). When considering men who have engaged in anal intercourse, a greater percentage may have had such experience with women than with other men. Much better data are available on the noncoital sexual behaviors of white middle-class, well-educated individuals than on the noncoital sexual behaviors of other populations. However, the available data suggest that these behaviors may be somewhat less common among African Americans than among whites. Drawing on data from seven studies, Reinisch *et al.* (1988) estimated that 39% (range = 20–43%) of white middle-class women had ever participated in anal intercourse. In contrast, a study of African American college students at an East Coast university revealed that only 10% of African American women reported ever experiencing anal intercourse (Thomas, Gilliam, & Iwrey, 1989). In a similar vein, L. S. Jemmott and J. B. Jemmott (1991) found that only 16% of African American female undergraduates at a university in an inner-city area of New Jersey reported having ever experienced anal intercourse. One of the few studies to compare noncoital sexual behaviors in African Americans and whites was the study by Wyatt *et al.* (1988a,b) of women ages 18–36 years in the Los Angeles area. The study revealed that 21% of African American women, as compared with 43% of a matched sample of white women, reported having ever experienced anal intercourse.

As in the case of anal intercourse, evidence suggests tentatively that although oral sex is common among African Americans and whites, it may be less common among African Americans. For instance, studying college students, Belcastro (1985) found that reports of having ever engaged in heterosexual oral sex were lower among African American men and women than among their white counterparts. For instance, they found that 48%

of the African American college women and 81% of white women reported having engaged in fellatio. In addition, 34% of African American women and 50% of white women reported having engaged in cunnilingus with a man. Wyatt *et al.* (1988a,b) also found evidence of less oral sex among African Americans. For example, they found that 87% of white women and 70% of African American women reported having ever engaged in cunnilingus and that 93% of white women, but only 65% of African American women, reported having ever engaged in fellatio.

In summary, these data suggest that although African American women engage in a range of HIV-risk-associated sexual behaviors, the chief sexual risk behavior is the failure to use condoms during sexual intercourse. The key to risk of exposure to HIV and other STDs is not simply frequency of sexual intercourse or frequency of condom use, but the frequency of unprotected coitus. Thus, the higher rate of sexual intercourse among inner-city African American women must be viewed in light of their relatively low rates of condom use. A high rate of sexual intercourse would be less worrisome if condoms were used each time. A low rate of condom use would be less worrisome if the person had sexual intercourse only rarely. It is the combination—high rates of intercourse coupled with low rates of condom use—that is potentially deadly. It is this combination that heightens risk of exposure to HIV. However, sexual behavior is not the only HIV-risk-associated behavior among African American women. Injection-drug use plays a major role in HIV infection among African American women. Hence, the next section will focus on injection-drug use as an HIV-risk-associated behavior among African American women.

DRUG USE AS AN HIV RISK FACTOR

The primary HIV risk behavior for African American women is sharing contaminated drug-use paraphernalia (CDC, 1993). The next most frequent exposure category is being the sexual partner of an IDU. Among African American females, 50% of AIDS cases are the result of sharing needles for injection-drug use (CDC, 1994). Among African American males, a lesser percentage (36%) of AIDS cases are the result of needle-sharing (not because they use injection drugs less, but because many men were infected by having sex with other men). Of AIDS cases among African American women, 30% are the result of heterosexual contact, frequently with an IDU. Among women who contracted HIV infection heterosexually, 63% were sex partners of IDUs and had no history of injection themselves (Ickovics & Rodin, 1992). In New York City, almost 90% of the cases of heterosexual transmission have occurred from an IDU to a sexual partner who does not inject drugs (Des Jarlais & Friedman, 1988). There is evidence that this avenue of transmission may occur more frequently among African American couples. In a study of 12,000 multiethnic street-recruited IDUs in 19 cities, African American IDUs were more likely to report sex with a person who was not a drug user (Friedman, 1993).

Drug Use and Sexual Risk Behavior

Low-income African American women are at risk for HIV infection due to higher rates of drug use that involve both injection-drug use with contaminated needles and the association of crack cocaine use with prostitution and STDs (Chaisson *et al.,* 1989; Fullilove, Fullilove, Bowser, & Gross, 1990a). In addition, drug use, including use of alcohol and other noninjectable drugs, has been found to be associated with unprotected intercourse (Fullilove, Goldon, Bowsey, & Hulley, 1990b), which increases the risk for HIV infection. Cocaine, for example, lowers inhibition, and unprotected sex is frequently exchanged for cocaine or crack cocaine (Williams, 1990). Crack is also associated with having IDU sexual partners and with engaging in prostitution (Primm, 1991). As crack has become an easily accessible form of addiction, many female addicts prostitute themselves to pay for it. Since crack enhances libido and impairs judgment, the risk of unprotected sex is high for the addicted woman (Fullilove *et al.* 1990b). Risky sexual behavior also occurs among female IDUs. In many instances, women female IDUs will exchange sex for drugs.

Among IDUs, the great majority of males, approximately 75%, have their primary sexual relationship with women who do not inject drugs (Des Jarlais, Chamberland, Yancovitz, Weinberg & Friedman, 1984). In a survey of 5280 women who were sexual partners of IDUs, 62% reported that their partner never used a condom (Rosenshine, 1990). Among women, the cumulative incidence attributable to heterosexual contact per million population is over 11 times greater for African Americans and Hispanics than for whites (Holmes, Karon, & Kreise, 1990).

Social Conditions, Drug Use, and Sexual Behavior

It is clear that poverty is associated with the higher rates of HIV infection among African American women and that it affects the course of the disease once they are infected. With the serious risk for AIDS associated with drug use, especially in the African American community, the conditions that give rise to drug use cannot be ignored. There is evidence that drugs can be a symptom of urban poverty and oppression; both are major societal sources of stress (Blumberg, 1973; New York City Commission on Human Rights, 1987; Pearlin, 1989). For example, injection drug use in New York City is found primarily among lower-class minority groups (Stoneburner, 1988). In low-income urban areas around the country, 10–20% of newborn infants are exposed to cocaine *in utero,* again illustrating the association of drugs with poor urban areas. The report of the National Commission on AIDS also notes that drug trafficking is heaviest in inner-city areas, and injection drug use has been disproportionately associated with Northeastern urban life. African Americans most affected by HIV and AIDS are the ones who are poor and live in census-defined poverty areas of central cities (Bureau of the Census, 1992). In fact, it is fair to say that African Americans are disproportionately affected by HIV because they are disproportionately affected by poverty, a fact attributed by some to institutional racism (Marable, 1983).

Thus, this close connection between inner-city poverty and drug use is a major factor in the disparity between white and African American women in the number of AIDS cases. More than half of all African American and Hispanic children in this country live in cities as compared to 1 in 4 white children (Sabol, 1991). While 1 in 5 children in the United States are poor, almost 1 in 2 children living in female-headed households live below the poverty level. More than half of all African American children live in female-headed households, while only 1 in 6 white children do (Sabol, 1991). It is in these poor urban areas that one finds drugs, so important in the etiology of AIDS in the African American community. Hence, efforts to control AIDS must be aimed in part at eradicating the conditions that give rise to drug addiction (Gallo & Montagnier, 1988).

Being an impoverished African American woman adds to the problem of HIV and AIDS. It is particularly difficult for these women to change HIV-risk-related sexual behavior as they deal on a day-to-day basis with problems of poverty and are at increased risk for drug use, prostitution, and psychological dysfunction (Cochran, 1989; Gilliam, Scott, & Troup, 1989; Mays & Cochran, 1988). In addition, these women may be poorly educated, unemployed, lacking in medical knowledge and resources, and more likely to have higher rates of physical and mental illness, physical abuse, and low self-esteem compared to the general population (Wofsy, 1991). In addition, poor women who are homeless are at high risk for HIV infection due to the unavailability of socioculturally appropriate AIDS education, low rates of condom use, high rates of prostitution, and many other factors (Mays & Cochran, 1989; Cochran & Mays, 1989; Krueger, Wood, Diehr, & Maxwell, 1990; Nyamathi, Wayment, & Dunkel-Schetter, 1993b). Many of these impoverished women may perceive AIDS as having a low priority relative to their other problems (CDC, 1986; Mays & Cochran, 1989).

A study that used focus group interviews to assess the concerns of impoverished African American women who were homeless or drug-addicted and at risk for AIDS found that the women had serious concerns about basic necessities such as food, money, and a place to sleep (Nyamathi & Lewis, 1991). Many women discussed additional concerns that were a result of being homeless, such as physical violence, lack of love or affection, and extreme loneliness. Most women experienced worries about basic survival, about the dangers of unprotected sex with multiple partners, and about AIDS. To many women, the well-being of their children represented another major concern, particularly with regard to not being able to provide motherly love and having the children brought up by other family members.

Theoretical or empirical studies regarding concerns of impoverished women, who are at risk for AIDS, are quite limited. Such knowledge is critical, since these women have limited access to information related to risk reduction and have inadequate supports for the maintenance of risk-reduction strategies (Nyamathi & Flaskerud, 1992). It is unrealistic to believe that substantial progress can be made in eradicating HIV infection among African American women while ignoring the social conditions that foster the greater rates of infection in this population. Clearly, programs for impoverished African American women must address the most serious concerns of these women. These programs must also provide AIDS education, reinforce risk-reduction skills, supplement resources, and enhance self-esteem and control. Programs that include these characteristics may be most beneficial in reducing HIV-risk-associated behaviors (Wofsy, 1991; Stoneburner *et al.,* 1988; Nyamathi & Shin, 1990; Nyamathi, 1991b; Nyamathi, Leake, Faskerud, Lewis, & Bennett, 1993a).

COPING, SENSE OF COHERENCE, AND RISKY BEHAVIOR

African American women at risk for HIV infection tend to find ways to cope with their impoverished life situation. It is theorized that persons with a strong sense of coherence are likely to define an event as less stressful and be able to manage a problem more successfully than those with a weak sense of coherence (Antonovsky, 1979, 1987; Antonovsky & Sagy, 1986). There are a number of studies investigating the relationships among coherence and personal and environmental concerns, appraisal of threat, emotional distress, and high-risk behaviors in minority women who are homeless, IDUs, partners of IDUs, or prostitutes (Nyamathi, 1991a; Nyamathi *et al.,* 1993b). These studies reported a negative relationship between level of coherence and concerns. For instance, women strong in coherence reported less negative appraisals of threat, less emotional distress, and fewer high-risk behaviors than those with weak coherence. In studying self-esteem and coherence, these researchers reported that women who were high in self-esteem and stronger in sense of coherence reported significantly less emotional distress and significantly fewer high-risk behaviors, which included use of injection and noninjection drugs and unprotected sexual encounters. In addition, in studying coping, emotional distress, and HIV-risk behaviors, Nyamathi and her colleagues found that women who engaged in active coping were less likely to engage in risky behavior. Those who utilized avoidance coping were more likely to engage in risky behavior. Women who had higher self-esteem and more available support were less likely to appraise the condition of their lives as threatening and used more active coping. Results from focus groups of impoverished African American women who were homeless, IDUs, or prostitutes revealed that while the women were sexually active with multiple partners, few were sexually active on a personal level (Nyamathi & Lewis, 1991). These researchers report that for many women, prostitution represented a powerful problem-focused strategy. Given that many of these women experienced extreme environmental and personal concerns and had low self-esteem and minimal feelings of control, prostitution may have represented an easy outlet for supporting drug habits and, for some, the only available means of survival. Women most often used emotion-focused coping strategies. These strategies included using drugs and alcohol, using withdrawal or distancing strategies such as sleep or daydreaming, and using religion to seek comfort and strength. The spiritual inspiration and dedication of most women were also found to be a powerful strategy. However, when prayers were not answered, some women rejected religion. Often, women became frustrated when legal problem-focused strategies were unsuccessful in changing their situation. Consequently, it was common for them to fall back on the use of emotion-focused strategies (Nyamathi & Shuler, 1990).

These results suggest that continuing investigation of factors such as coherence that can lessen the seriousness of environmental stressors is imperative as it relates to women at risk for HIV infection. These results also suggest that personal resources such as social support and self-esteem are beneficial to well-being and health in part because they lead to less appraisal of threat, more adaptive coping, and less emotional distress. Evidence suggestive of the mechanisms whereby self-esteem and support have beneficial effects is valuable because it increases our understanding of stress and coping processes and suggests avenues of intervention. Coping behavior, for example, may be much easier to alter than social support or self-esteem. In fact, if more adaptive coping behavior can be promoted with beneficial effects on emotional well-being, a woman's basic sense of self-worth may be improved as a by-product. This approach may also lead in the long run to more abundant and effective social support. Thus, teaching adaptive coping behaviors may represent an important strategy in designing interventions for this population. Chesney and Folkman's preliminary findings on coping effectiveness training indicate that coping training may be a valuable HIV-prevention tool and does increase social support and lessen perceived stress (Chesney, 1994). However, continued investigation is essential to provide a clearer understanding of the psychosocial factors that influence risk behaviors among African American women.

In our effort to understand psychosocial factors related to HIV-risk-associated behaviors among African American women, we must begin to examine the role of theoretical frameworks for conceptualizing such factors and designing risk-reduction programs. The next section will describe the use of the social cognitive theory as a possible framework for conceptualizing and developing interventions to reduce HIV infection among African American women.

SOCIAL COGNITIVE THEORY AND HIV-RISK-REDUCTION RESEARCH

It may be possible to reduce HIV-risk-related behavior by encouraging people to modify their behaviors in ways that reduce their risk of HIV infection. The important question, then, is this: How might changes in risk-associated behavior be induced? In this connection, it might be useful to consider the social cognitive theory (Bandura, 1986, 1989), which provides a comprehensive analysis of the determinants of behavior change. What makes the theory a particularly advantageous approach to health behavior is that it provides prescriptions for effective alteration of the presumed mechanisms that underlie health behavior. The theory has two key components, perceived self-efficacy and outcome expectancies. Perceived self-efficacy is defined as the conviction that one can successfully execute the behavior required to produce desired outcomes. Outcome expectancy is defined as a person's estimate that a given behavior will lead to negative or positive outcomes. Hence, in social cognitive theory, perceptions of self-efficacy and outcome expectancies are the key determinants of effective behavior change toward safer-sex practices. For example, strong perceptions of efficacy to negotiate condom use with a partner and to control sexual impulse, greater expectations of positive outcomes of condom use (e.g., preventing HIV infection), and lower expectations of negative outcomes of condom use (e.g., reduced pleasure, negative partner response) might all contribute to using condoms. Skill-building interventions, based on social cognitive theory, can help women promote their health through a repertoire of cognitive and behavioral techniques, including problem-solving, personal coping, and interpersonal communication skills. Through these strategies, women can gain social and personal competence and reduce their risk for HIV infection.

Perceived Self-Efficacy

As described more fully in Chapter 1, a number of recent studies suggest that perceived self-efficacy is important for AIDS-risk-behavior change (O'Leary, Goodhart, Jemmott, & Boccher-Lattimore, 1992; Valdiserri *et al.,* 1980). Perceived self-efficacy to negotiate condom use with a partner has emerged as a strong predictor of sexual behavior change among gay men (McKusick, Coates, Morin, Pollack, & Hoff, 1990) and among adolescents (Hingson, Strunin, Berlin, & Heeren, 1990; L. S. Jemmott & J. B. Jemmott, 1992). In an additional study by L. S. Jemmott and J. B. Jemmott (1992), perceived self-efficacy was the best of several predictors of condom use among African American young women. A cognitive–behavioral risk-reduction intervention for African American young women that incorporated modeling, role playing, and other techniques known to enhance perceived self-efficacy was shown to be effective in increasing condom-use intentions, relative to a health promotion control condition and an AIDS information alone condition group (J. B. Jemmott, L. S. Jemmott, Spears, Hewitt, & Cruz-Collins, 1992b).

Outcome Expectancies Beliefs

In addition to perceived self-efficacy, outcome expectancies are likely to figure in HIV-risk-associated behavior. Negative outcome expectancies about condoms have been identified as important to condom use in a variety of populations (L. S. Jemmott & J. B. Jemmott, 1992; O'Leary *et al.,* 1992; Siegel & Gibson, 1988). For example, L. S. Jemmott and J. B. Jemmott (1992) reported that negative expected outcomes of condom use were associated with riskier sexual behavior among African American young women. The most obvious outcome expectancy is the belief that condoms can reduce the risk of sexually transmitted HIV infection, though several studies have suggested that knowledge of the cause, transmission, or prevention of AIDs is not sufficient to prompt safer behavior (Fisher & Fisher, 1994).

Another outcome expectancy is hedonistic expectancies or beliefs about the effects that the use of condoms will have on sexual enjoyment (L. S. Jemmott & J. B. Jemmott, 1991; Catania *et al.,* 1989; Manning, Balson,

Barenberg, & Moore, 1989a; Manning, Barenberg, Gallese, & Rice, 1989b; Valdiserri, Arena, Proctor, & Bonati, 1989a). For example, L. S. Jemmott and J. B. Jemmott (1991) reported that inner-city African American women students from an urban commuter university in northern New Jersey who believed more strongly that sex is still fun when a condom is used expressed more favorable attitudes toward using condoms. Such attitudes, in turn, were related to firmer intentions to use condoms in the next 3 months. Similarly, Valdiserri *et al.* (1989a) reported in their study of white women 19–25 years of age that those who believed that they would not enjoy intercourse if their partner used condoms were less likely to report past use of condoms than were their peers who did not hold this belief. Hence, it may be possible to change negative hedonistic expectancies through the use of intervention procedures that focus directly on beliefs about the adverse consequences of condom use for sexual enjoyment.

A third outcome expectancy is the partner's reaction to safer sex practices. Because risky sexual behavior takes place with another person, it is probable that women's risky sexual behavior is influenced by outcome expectancies regarding their romantic partners' approval of condom use or other safer-sex practices. That beliefs about how others would react are important is consistent with the theory of reasoned action, which has been demonstrated to be useful in facilitating behavior change among African American women (Ajzen & Fishbein, 1980; Fishbein & Ajzen, 1975; Fishbein & Middlestadt, 1987; L. S. Jemmott & J. B. Jemmott, 1991). The theory of reasoned action places emphasis on subjective norms as key determinants of behavioral intentions and behavior. For example, L. S. Jemmott and J. B. Jemmott (1991) reported that inner-city African American women undergraduates rated their sexual partners' opinions as more important to their use of condoms than the opinions of their mothers, fathers, friends, or church. Respondents also indicated they were more motivated to comply with the opinions of their sexual partners regarding condom use compared with the opinions of any other referent. Thompson and Spanier (1978) found that partner opposition to or reluctance to use birth control was a factor in respondents' nonuse of contraception. These results underscore the importance of sexual partners' opinions.

Partner reaction to condom use plays a critical role in the woman's making safer sex decisions if she is dependent on her relationship or perceives that there is a shortage of men. Low-income African American women may be particularly dependent on their romantic relationships. Moreover, there are more African American women who desire relationships than there are African American men for them to be involved with. Indeed, there is a widely perceived shortage of African American men (Guttentag & Secord, 1983; Semaj, 1982). Evidence indicates that when people of a given gender perceive that their gender is in short supply, they invest less in their romantic relationship and express less commitment to it (Guttentag & Secord, 1983; J. B. Jemmott, Ashby, & Lindenfeld, 1989). Thus, some African American women may perceive that their opportunities for other romantic relationships are limited or that they themselves are unattractive and consequently may be reluctant to risk alienating their romantic partner by pressing him to implement safer-sex practices.

In summary, the two theoretical components of the social cognitive theory, perceived self-efficacy and outcome expectancies, have utility in the reduction of HIV-transmission-related sexual behaviors among African American women. These studies suggest that it is important that HIV-risk-reduction programs address African American women's concerns about the adverse effects of condoms on sexual enjoyment and partner reaction to condom use and focus on increasing their perceived self-efficacy and skills at persuading their partner to use safer-sex practices. Such information might help remove not only hedonistic barriers, but also formidable normative barriers related to sexual partners' reactions. Since theory-based HIV-risk-reduction intervention research is needed to determine the effects of psychological variables on risky sexual behavior, the question that still remains is how to design theory-based interventions to reduce HIV-risk behaviors among African American women. The next section will discuss HIV-prevention strategies.

HIV-RISK-REDUCTION STRATEGIES

Recently, Loretta Jemmott and her colleagues implemented a study to examine the effects of a social cognitive intervention on condom use intentions among sexually active African American young women recruited from a family planning clinic (J. B. Jemmott *et al.,* 1992b). Participants were assigned to the social cognitive intervention designed to increase perceived self-efficacy and favorable outcome expectancies about the hedonistic consequences of using condoms or to one of two control interventions: an information-alone intervention designed to increase AIDS knowledge or a general health promotion intervention designed to provide information about important health problems other than AIDS. ANCOVAs revealed that women in the social cognitive condition subsequently had greater intentions to use condoms and scored higher in perceived self-efficacy to use condoms and favorable hedonistic expectancies as compared to those in the AIDS information-alone and general health promotion condition. Hence, outcome expectancies regarding the effects of precautionary practices on sexual enjoyment and perceived self-efficacy to implement such practices played an important role in decisions about condom use. These results highlighted the value of a social cognitive approach to AIDS-risk behavior.

There are five goals to consider when designing successful social cognitive interventions for African American women. The first goal is to increase African American women's knowledge about AIDS transmission and prevention. Since knowledge alone is not sufficient to promote safer sex practices, it is important to address attitudes and beliefs. A second goal is to bolster positive attitudes and outcome expectancies regarding condom use and increase personal perception of risk for sexually transmitted HIV infection. A third goal is to build self-efficacy with respect to avoiding situations and behaviors that place the woman at risk for HIV/AIDS. A fourth goal is to increase technical condom-use skills. Two types of technical skills are essential: negotiation skills and condom-use skills. For example, African American women who possess the technical skills for condom use may not know how to handle the communication necessary to negotiate safer sex practices with a partner or how to resist pressure regarding situations that place them at risk for AIDS. Finally, a fifth goal is to increase social support and resources for women to change their behavior and reduce their risk for HIV infection.

When teaching African American women about hedonistic beliefs, partner reaction beliefs, and condom-use skills, it is important to incorporate strategies to change their perception that condoms decrease sexual pleasure. One such strategy is to eroticize condoms (L. S. Jemmott & J. B. Jemmott, 1992; Whipple & Ogden, 1989). Women's believing that condoms do not ruin the mood or the pleasure of sex may increase their intentions to use condoms (L. S. Jemmott & J. B. Jemmott, 1991; J. B. Jemmott *et al.,* 1992b). In addition, if women know how to make the use of condoms fun and pleasurable, they can then teach their partner this new information as a way of encouraging condom use. Hence, this strategy may alter the outcome expectancy of partner reaction to condom use. In addition, women need to know where to get condoms and how to keep condoms available and to believe that it is perfectly appropriate for a woman to have condoms available.

When attempting to build self-efficacy and teach negotiation skills, it is important to remember that women who have low self-esteem or feel unempowered are more likely to engage in riskier sexual behaviors. They are less likely to encourage their partners to use condoms or even to question their partners' behavior. Merely introducing condom use to a partner may be difficult, causing problems to arise within a woman's relationship. Des Jarlais and his colleagues found that condoms are much easier to introduce into casual relationships than they are into committed relationships, since suggestions to use condoms can imply mistrust (Des Jarlais, Friedman, Goldsmith, & Hopkins, 1989). These issues should be addressed in the intervention.

Successful HIV-risk-reduction programs for African American women must also be culturally sensitive, use educational activities and videos with characters with whom participants can identify, have meaningful application to their personal lives, and be based on a sound theoretical framework. The intervention should include learning activities and exercises to build self-efficacy in the area of decision making, communication, negotiation, and condom use (J. B. Jemmott *et al.,* 1992b; Nyamathi *et al.,* 1993b). Most important, the intervention should incorporate strategies to build upon personal strengths of the African American woman. African American women need to learn how to talk with partners about how to protect themselves from AIDS and, if they are not able to convince their partners to use condoms, how to minimize their risk through other behaviors.

Mays and Cochran (1988) maintain that an approach based on a model of social responsibility rather than individualistic preservation may be more effective. Utilizing this approach, African American men are persuaded to practice safer sex so that they remain as fathers or supporters for their families. African American women are encouraged to be more assertive regarding condom use so that they will remain alive to take care of their parents and children. In short, the message is one of responsibility for the continued existence of the African American race. In particular, prevention approaches for ethnic minority individuals should focus on the individual as a responsible member of a family or social network. Ethnically based values of cooperation, unity, and collective responsibility may be particularly powerful motivators of behavior change among African Americans (Mays & Cochran, 1988).

Needle-Sharing-Prevention Strategies

With regard to sharing needles, there is considerable evidence that social norms among IDUs have changed, as a result of the AIDS epidemic, from sharing needles to not sharing needles (Des Jarlais & Friedman, 1988; Sorenson *et al.,* 1991; Deren, Tortu, & Davis, 1993). Deren *et al.* (1993), for example, made particular efforts to recruit African American women into their study of IDUs and their sexual partners by recruiting in the obstetrics and gynecological clinics of Harlem Hospital. A total of 653 women were recruited, 70% of whom were African American. These women received either an AIDS prevention information session or the information session plus two additional sessions in which they received skills training in needle-cleaning behavior and condom use. Of this group,

380 women were followed up 6 months later. Sharing of equipment to inject drugs decreased significantly, including renting works, using works given by others, and sharing cookers, cotton, and rinse water ($p<0.001$). As early as 1984, researchers found significant numbers of drug injectors increasing their use of sterile needles and reducing the number of people with whom they shared needles (Friedman *et al.,* 1987). In a similar study by Selwyn, Feiner, Cox, Lipshutz, and Cohen (1987), stopping or decreasing needle-sharing was the most common AIDS prevention method used in two groups studied, 136 methadone patients and 115 people in a prison detoxification unit.

Although the research evidence indicates an effort not to share, the fact that obtaining clean needles is proscribed by law in areas where the seroprevalence rate is highest makes this intention difficult to carry out (Des Jarlais & Friedman, 1994). There is no doubt that making clean needles available would decrease the incidence of HIV infection among African American women and other groups.

In our efforts to understand theoretical models and strategies to reduce the risk of HIV infection among African American women, we must also understand the barriers that preclude the provision of effective HIV-risk-reduction programs for this population. Therefore, the next sections focuses on the issues and barriers to HIV-risk-reduction programs for African American women.

BARRIERS TO THE PROVISION OF EFFECTIVE AIDS EDUCATION TO AFRICAN AMERICAN WOMEN

There are a number of barriers and obstacles that preclude the implementation of effective HIV-risk-reduction interventions for African American women. Some of these barriers are structural. Most, however, are not. This section will discuss those barriers.

One of the greatest barriers to effective implementation of AIDS programs for African American women is that the programs do not provide education in a culturally sensitive manner and do not reflect the distinct cultural and social realities of the African American population. Since the beginning of the AIDS epidemic, the scarce educational messages that have filtered down to minority communities have been interpreted by some as inappropriate, confusing, and offensive. In a society ravaged by poverty, homelessness, unemployment, drugs, and crime, the need to deliver messages that are culturally relevant and incorporate attempts to enhance lives and meet the needs of the people are our only hope of achieving health-promoting outcomes (Mays & Cochran, 1988). However, for many poverty-stricken minorities, involvement with drugs may provide not only a method of survival, but also a means of obtaining additional income. Driven by the desire to meet basic needs first, African American drug users or prostitutes who live with the risk of illegal activities may not be concerned with the additional risk of AIDS (Mays & Cochran, 1988). Therefore, regardless of what strategy is used in AIDS-prevention research, it needs to be sensitive to the cultural values of the participant and to be tailored to the cultural and political realities of the target community (Mays & Cochran, 1988). This approach is essential to the success of risk-reduction interventions aimed at ethnic minority women.

Since culturally determined values are crucial in designing and implementing AIDS-risk-reduction interventions for African American women, researchers and educators must understand the cultural values of African American people. These values are derived from African American history, gender relations, family structure, and economic and social survival (Tesh, 1988). Culturally determined values influence how perceptions of AIDS are created, how attitudes toward high-risk behavior are formed, and how habits that characterize high-risk behavior may be altered. The cultural values that inform sexuality among ethnic minority women cannot be understood apart from the context of racism, sexism, and economic oppression, which have shaped gender relations and family structure. Introducing behavioral concepts that propose to alter or go against cultural values or ignore structural variables can lead to social conflict. Proposed changes in the behavior may create guilt about acting against traditional cultural norms. Hence, HIV-risk-related behavioral change may not be promoted successfully without understanding the influence of cultural values on sexual behavior, drug use, and health behaviors or without understanding the relationship between individuals and their social world. Ignoring these relationships contributes to creating barriers to African American women's participating fully in AIDS prevention (Tesh, 1988).

Talking about sex is another barrier. It is difficult to convince women to discuss the benefits of condoms with their sexual partners, as many fear such discussion will either drive their men away or provoke physical abuse. Women who carry condoms with them may be perceived as loose women rather than as modest and innocent. Furthermore, while homosexuality and bisexuality are additional high-risk behaviors that are associated with AIDS, the view of these activities as perverted and obscene by African American communities accentuates the problem further by promoting denial, isolation, and segregation. Yet, despite these feelings, for some men, having affairs with men and a marriage may not be mutually exclusive. Often, the women are the last to know of these extramarital affairs. As a result, these women and their offspring are put at risk for HIV infection.

Another barrier to safer-sex programs for African American women is the "safer sex" message. AIDS education that promotes "safer sex" may threaten behavior patterns that African American women link with their survival. The suggestion that women should explore new forms of sexual behavior (e.g., nonpenetrative sexual techniques) as a means of preventing HIV transmission may be received ambivalently by women subject to victim-blaming because of stereotypes about their sexual behavior. Promoting "safer sex" may threaten behavior patterns that women link with their survival, which may lead to social conflicts, i.e., abandonment, guilt, and violence. In addition, the sex lives of many minority women are currently characterized by a lack of power and by multiple forms of otherness that are imposed on them from within and without their community. If they are to be supported to undertake behavior changes, their otherness has to be diminished, and behavior changes must be linked to the attitudes and beliefs that support their concepts of cultural and economic survival (Mays & Cochran, 1988).

A woman's sex partner can be her strongest barrier to implementing safer practices, especially since behavior change necessary for preventing sexual transmission of HIV requires the cooperation of another person, namely, the woman's sex partner. Unfortunately, many of the women most at risk depend on their male partners for economic security. Some women also fear that they may lose desired partners if they insist on condom use, since condoms may be taken to indicate unfaithfulness on the part of the woman, lack of trust concerning the man's own faithfulness, or infection with HIV or other STDs. Of particular concern is the plight of the woman experiencing domestic violence and coerced sex, for whom the recommendation of condom use may be impossible to execute. While the female condom will give women some control over the safety of their encounters, many of the problems that women experience in their attempts to be safe will persist because the presence of the female condom is quite obvious to their partners.

Use of condoms by prostitutes or drug-addicted women may be perceived as barriers. For prostitutes whose survival of self and family depends on income from prostitution, the use of condoms may seem a very restrictive proposal. Mays and Cochran (1989) contend that for the drug-addicted woman, motivation for a life-style change (i.e., drug abstinence and a change in social network) may require a change in perceived self-efficacy, self-esteem, perceived peer group norms, or beliefs about the controllability of the future. Exploring with a drug-addicted woman her ability to negotiate safer sex behaviors or safer drug paraphernalia use involves contending with issues of powerlessness, peer pressure, and need for personal intimacy. For the stricken ethnic woman, the prostitute, or the female drug abuser, it may be considerably easier to deny and underestimate personal vulnerability than to undertake significant behavior changes that accompany a major change in life-style.

Another barrier or potential obstacle for implementing successful HIV-risk-reduction interventions for African American women is related to their distrust of researchers and skepticism about behavior-change recommendations (Marin & Marin, 1991; R. L. Williams, 1980). Some examples of those obstacles are: (1) the belief that researchers are trying to exploit their community rather than to generate research that is useful to the community; (2) the belief that researchers will use the findings to support insidious stereotypes of ethnic minorities or to draw interpretations that disparage ethnic minority individuals; and (3) the distrust of AIDS-risk-reduction advice provided by government and health officials, which may be related to the often-cited infamous Tuskegee study (Thomas & Quinn, 1991). These issues present formidable challenges to those who seek to understand risk behavior among ethnic minority individuals. Research, education, and intervention strategies must consider the whole context of racism and distrust. Researchers must be aware of the issues and must be sensitive to the culture of ethnic minority individuals in the development of conceptual models and in the design and implementation of research and the interpretation of findings. In light of the enormity of the health problem that AIDS represents, it is hoped that sensitivity to the culture of the population, coupled with the involvement of members of the population in the research, may make these obstacles surmountable (Jemmott & Jones, 1993).

Another barrier could be the HIV-risk-reduction messenger, the person who brings the safer-sex message. The choice of who delivers the HIV-prevention message to the African American community is critical. The individual's or organization's political beliefs about the etiology of AIDS will determine how or whether that message is received and acted upon. Research on persuasion indicates that the effectiveness of a message is affected by the credibility that recipients attach to the source of the message (McGuire, 1985; Herek & Capitanio, 1994). Risk-reduction interventions may also be most effective if they are implemented by individuals with whom the participants can identify. For example, in the National AIDS Demonstration Research Project, indigenous outreach workers who were former drug users from the same community as the IDUs they worked with were highly effective in reducing risk behavior among IDUs (Singh *et al.*, 1993; Birkel, Golasezewski, Koman, Singh, & Catan, 1993). Peterson and Marin (1988) have also suggested that programs for ethnic minority IDUs should include ethnic minority staff, who may be more accepted by minority addicts because of their knowledge of minority cultural values.

Lack of familiarity with the people who make up the African American community is a barrier in implementing HIV-risk-reduction interventions for African American women. African American people are not a homogeneous group. Researchers and educators must be aware that a high degree of cultural variation exists between African American women in America who are African American, African, Haitian, Caribbean, and other cultural variations. Interventions need to consider how heterogeneity within ethnic minority groups might affect efforts to implement culturally sensitive interventions. It may well be that interventions that are designed to be culturally sensitive will be differentially effective depending on the individual's degree of acculturation or identification with the culture, region of the country, urban vs. rural living conditions, gender-by-race interaction effects, immigration status, and language capability. The implications for intervention strategies of these and other factors have not been well defined. Research programs have yet to grasp fully the behavioral implications of within-ethnic-group variation; therefore, change efforts may have missed key features of a subgroup's response to behavior-change messages.

Other barriers to HIV-risk-reduction research and education in this population include access to programs, lack of transportation and child care, and limited community resources to fund such programs. As we design our research projects or implement our HIV-risk-reduction programs, we must understand that before individuals take action, they must consider the negative consequences as well as the benefits. Barriers to action may occur when the action is considered inconvenient, expensive, unpleasant, painful, or upsetting. More research is needed to understand the barriers to reducing the risk of HIV infection among African American women. Yet, regardless of the numerous barriers and obstacles for implementing successful HIV-risk-reduction efforts for African American women, we must continue our HIV-prevention efforts. In the absence of a cure or preventive vaccination against HIV, behavior change remains the only available means for combatting the epidemic.

CONCLUSION

AIDS among African American women is a killer. To change the devastation caused by this disease, we must focus on prevention, for AIDS is preventable. We need to begin by assessing the determinants of risk behavior among African American women across socioeconomic backgrounds and by exploring the cultural values and structural determinants of attitudes and risk taking. If we understand the determinants of HIV-risk-associated behavior, we can design effective interventions to reduce those risks.

Culturally sensitive, empirically tested, and experimentally designed research interventions are needed to prevent AIDS among African American women. Most of the research has been from the standpoint of causal inference. Few of the studies were true experiments with random assignment to conditions. We also need more theory-based research. Particularly valuable would be experiments that test theory-based interventions. The use of theory should not be limited to the design of intervention procedures. Theory should also drive the selection of variables to be assessed. Measuring the putative social–psychological mediators of behavior change will provide a better conceptual understanding of risk behavior. Thus, statistical analyses might focus on whether the effects of an intervention are mediated by the conceptual variables it was designed to influence. In addition, if a theory-based intervention fails to change behavior, an examination of the putative mediators might shed light on why change did not occur or may suggest that the hypothesized variables are not important mediators. In this way, the key social–psychological variables that risk-reduction interventions should target might be identified (Jemmott & Jones, 1993).

More studies are needed evaluating the content, messages, skills resources, and length of interventions needed to reduce HIV infection. Studies are needed to investigate how many sessions are needed to achieve optimal behavior change. What about the content of the intervention? Most studies have used interventions that were highly focused on AIDS. An alternative approach that has not received much attention is to emphasize both specific AIDS content and more general life skills and resources. According to this view, people's concerns about the risk of AIDS may be secondary to more immediate economic and family problems. Under these circumstances, AIDS interventions may be more effective when they consider the broader context of people's lives. Further studies should test this hypothesis. We also need to examine which specific safer-sex messages are effective in changing behavior. For instance, should safer-sex messages be tailored to fit cultural values, relationship roles, and life-style characteristics? If so, how? We also need to examine which specific skills to include in interventions. For example, women might be taught ways to eroticize the use of condoms. Such an approach might also serve to reduce resistance to condom use among women's sexual partners and modify women's perception of adverse effects of condoms on sexual pleasure.

More studies are needed to increase our understanding of the issues that disenfranchised women face in confronting AIDS. Disenfranchised women suffer from problems often associated with poverty, such as unemployment, illicit drug use, physical and sexual abuse, discrimination, and homelessness. Although AIDS education and prevention campaigns have been launched by both public and private entities, these efforts have been slow to reach these women. Many programs are ineffective because they do not address demographic or cultural factors.

Researchers need to have a better understanding of the obstacles to HIV-risk-reduction intervention research. Studies have shown that there are potential obstacles having to do with ethnic minority individuals' distrust of researchers and skepticism about behavior-change recommendations (Marin & Marin, 1991; R. L. Williams, 1980). In light of the enormity of the health problem that AIDS represents, it is hoped that sensitivity to the culture of the population, coupled with the involvement of members of the population in the research, may make these obstacles surmountable.

In addition, research should focus on female-controlled prevention technology. The most critical feature of behavior change necessary for preventing sexual transmission of HIV for women is that it requires the cooperation of another person, namely, the women's sex partners. Unfortunately, many of the women most at risk depend on their male partners for economic security. Hence, female-controlled technology such as the female condom will give women some control over the safety of their encounters. However, many of the problems that women experience in their attempts to be safe will persist because the presence of the female condom is obvious to their partners. More research should address this issue.

Research on HIV-risk reduction among African American women is at an early stage of development. Few intervention studies have been conducted. Therefore, the inferences that can be drawn are limited. There is clearly a need for additional methodologically rigorous studies in this area, but there are also potential obstacles to such studies. We are optimistic that sensitivity to the values, beliefs, and concerns of the community will make it possible to implement the theory-based, culturally sensitive, methodologically sound, comprehensive studies that are needed to reduce HIV infection among African American women. These interventions should include not only information, but also coping effectiveness and skills training, supportive services, and resources for long-term behavior change. They should be implemented in a way that demonstrates that the change agent cares about the population.

As the number of infected African American women increases, more and more African American children will be affected. Implementing culturally sensitive, theoretically sound HIV-risk-reduction interventions that are perceived as helpful, that address the most serious needs, and that provide AIDS education, skills, and resources is our only hope of assisting African American women in reducing their risk of HIV infection.

REFERENCES

Antonovsky, A. (1979). *Health, stress and coping: New perspectives on mental and physical well-being.* San Francisco: Jossey-Bass.

Antonovsky, A. (1987). *Unraveling the mystery of health.* San Francisco: Jossey-Bass.

Antonovsky & Sagy, S. (1986). The development of a sense of coherence and its impact on responses to stress situations. *Journal of Social Psychology, 126,* 213–225.

Ajzen, I., & Fishbein, M. (1980). *Understanding attitudes and predicting social behavior.* Englewood Cliffs, NJ: Prentice-Hall.

Bandura, A. (1986). *Social foundations of thought and action: A social cognitive theory.* Eglewood Cliffs, NJ: Prentice-Hall.

Bandura, A. (1989). Perceived self-efficacy. In V. M. Mays, G. W. Albee, & S. F. Schneider (Eds.), *Primary prevention of AIDS: Psychological approaches* (pp. 128–141). Newbury Park, CA: Sage Publications.

Baum, A., & Nesselhof, S. (1988). Psychological research and the prevention, etiology, and treatment of AIDS. *American Psychologist, 43,* 900–906.

Becker, M., & Joseph, J. (1988). AIDS and behavioral change to reduce risk: A review. *American Journal of Public Health, 78,* 394–410.

Belcastro, P. A. (1985). Sexual behavior differences between black and white students. *Journal of Sex Research, 21,* 56–67.

Bell, T. A., & Holmes, K. K. (1984). Age-specific risks of syphilis, gonorrhea, and hospitalized pelvic inflammatory disease in sexually experienced U.S. women. *Sexually Transmitted Diseases, 7,* 291.

Birkel, R., Golasezewski, T., Koman, J. J., III, Singh, B. K., & Catan, V. (1993). Selected findings from the Horizontes AIDS Education Demonstration Project. *Health Education Quarterly, 20,* 523–538.

Blumberg, A. (1973). The politics of deviance: The case of drugs. *Journal of Drug Issues, Spring,* 105–113.

Bureau of the Census (1992). Washington, DC: U.S. Government Printing Office.

Catania, J. Coates, T., Kegeles, S., Estrand, M., Guydish, J., & Bye, L. (1989). Implication of the AIDS risk reduction model for the gay community: The importance of perceived sexual enjoyment and help-seeking behaviors. In V. Mays, G. Albee, & S. Schneider (Eds.), *Primary prevention of AIDS: Psychological approaches* (pp. 242–261). Newbury Park, CA: Sage Publications.

Centers for Disease Control and Prevention (1986). HIV/AIDS Surveillance Report. Atlanta: Centers for Infectious Diseases, Centers for Disease Control.

Centers for Disease Control and Prevention (1991). HIV/AIDS Surveillance Report, July 1–18. Atlanta: Centers for Infectious Diseases, Centers for Disease Control.

Centers for Disease Control and Prevention (1992). HIV/AIDS Surveillance Report. March 1–22. Atlanta: Centers for Infectious Diseases, Centers for Disease Control.

Centers for Disease Control and Prevention (1993). HIV/AIDS Surveillance Report. Atlanta: Centers for Infectious Diseases, Centers for Disease Control.

Centers for Disease Control and Prevention (1994). *HIV/AIDS Surveillance Report,* December 1–18. Atlanta: Center for Infectious Diseases, Centers for Disease Control.

Chaisson, R., Bacchetti, P., Osmond, D., Brodie, B., Sande, M., & Moss, A. (1989). Cocaine use and HIV infection in intravenous drug users in San Francisco. *JAMA, 261* 501–505.

Chesney, M. (1994). Coping effectiveness training for HIV positive gay men: Interim results from a clinical trial. Paper presented at the HIV Center for Clinical and Behavioral Studies, New York State Psychiatric Institute, September 22.

Chin, J., & Mann, J. (1990). HIV infections and AIDS in the 1990s. *American Journal of Public Health, 11,* 127–142.

Chu, S., Buehler, J., & Berkeiman, R. (1990). Impact of human immunodeficiency virus epidemic on mortality in women of reproductive age, United States. *JAMA, 264,* 225–229.

Cochran, S. D., & Mays, V. M. (1989). Women and AIDS related concerns: Roles for psychologist in helping the worried well. *American Psychologist, 44,* 529–535.

Cochran, S. D. (1989). Women and HIV infection: Issues in prevention and behavior change. In V. Mays, G. Albee, & S. Schneider (Eds.), *Primary prevention of AIDS.* Newbury Park, CA: Sage Publications.

Department of Health and Human Services (1992).

Deren, S., Tortu, S., & Davis, W. (1993). An AIDS risk reduction project with inner city women. In C. Squire (Ed.), *Women and AIDS* (pp. 73–89). Newbury Park, CA: Sage Publications.

Des Jarlais, D. C., Chamberland, M., Yancovitz, S., Weinberg, P., & Friedman, S. R. (1984). Heterosexual partners: A large risk group for AIDS. *Lancet, 2,* 1346–1347.

Des Jarlais, D. C., & Friedman, S. R. (1988). The psychology of preventing AIDS among injection drug users. *American Psychologist, 43,* 865–870.

Des Jarlais, D. C., Friedman, S. R., Goldsmith, D., & Hopkins, W. (1989). Heterosexual transmission of HIV from injection drug users: Regular partnerships and prostitution. In B. Voeller, J. Reinish, & M. Gottleib (Eds.), *AIDS and sex: An integrated biomedical and biobehavioral approach* (pp. 245–256). New York: Oxford University Press.

Des Jarlais, D. C., & Friedman, S. R. (1994). AIDS and the use of injected drugs. *Scientific American, 270*(2), 75–80.

Fishbein, M., & Ajzen, I. (1975). *Belief, attitude, intention, and behavior: An introduction to theory and research.* Reading, MA: Addison Wesley.

Fishbein, M., & Middlestadt, S. (1987). Using the theory of reasoned action to develop educational interventions: Applications to illicit drug use. *Health Education Research, 2,* 361–371.

Fisher J., & Fisher, W. (1992). Changing AIDS risk behavior. *Psychological Bulletin, 40,* 254–263.

Friedman, S. R. (1993). Racial differences in sexual behaviors related to AIDS in a 19-city sample of street recruited drug users. *AIDS Education and Prevention, 5,* 196–211.

Friedman, S. R., Des Jarlais, D. C., Sotheran, J., Garber, J., Cohen, H., & Smith, D. (1987). AIDS and self-organization among injection drug users. *International Journal of the Addictions, 22,* 201–220.

Fullilove, R., Fullilove, M., Bowser, B., & Goss, S. (1990). Risk of sexually transmitted disease among black adolescent crack users in Oakland and San Francisco, Calif. *JAMA, 263,* 851–855.

Gallo, R., & Montagnier, L. (1988). AIDS in 1988. *Scientific American, 259,* 40–48.

Gilliam, A., Scott, M., & Troup, J. (1989). Health education needs and social functioning of homeless women and their children (technical report). Hyattsville, MD: Institute of Minority Health and Human Development.

Guttentag, M., & Secord, P. (1983). *Too many women?* Beverly Hills: Sage Publications.

Hatcher, R. A., Stewart, F. H., Trussell, J., Kowal, D., Guest, F., Stewart, G. K., & Cates, W. (1990) *Contraceptive technology 1990–1992.* New York: Irvington Publishers.

Hayes, C. (1987). *Risking the future.* Washington, DC: National Academy Press.

Herek, G., & Capitanio, J. (1994). Conspiracies, contagion, and compassion: Trust and public reactions to AIDS. *AIDS Education and Prevention, 6,* 365–375.

Hingson, R. W., Strunin, L., Berlin, B., & Heeren, T. (1990). Beliefs about AIDS, use of alcohol and drugs, and unprotected sex among Massachusetts adolescents. *American Journal of Public Health, 80,* 295–299.

Hofferth S., & Hayes, C. (1987). *Risking the future,* Vol. 2. Washington, DC: National Academy Press.

Holmes, K., Karon, J., & Kreises, J. (1990). The increasing frequency of heterosexually acquired AIDS in the United States. *American Journal of Public Health, 80,* 858–863.

Ickovics, J., & Rodin, J. (1992). Women and AIDS in the United States: Epidemiology, natural history, and mediating mechanisms. *Health Psychology, 11,* 1–16.

Jemmott, J. B., III, Ashby, K. L. & Lindenfeld, K. (1989). Romantic commitment and the perceived availability of opposite sex persons: On loving the one you're with. *Journal of Applied Social Psychology, 19,* 1198–1216.

Jemmott, J. B., Jemmott, L. S., Spears, H., Hewitt, N., & Cruz-Collins, M. (1992). AIDS information, self-efficacy, hedonistic expectancies, and condom-use intentions: Testing the information alone hypothesis. *Journal of Adolescent Health, 13,* 512–519.

Jemmott, L. S., & Jemmott, J. B., III (1991). Applying the theory of reasoned action to AIDS risk behavior: Condom use among black women. *Nursing Research, 40,* 228–234.

Jemmott, L. S., & Jemmott, J. B., III (1992). Increasing condom-use intentions among sexually active inner-city adolescent women: Effects of an AIDS prevention program. *Nursing Research, 41,* 273–278.

Jemmott, J. & Jones, J. (1993). Social psychological and AIDS among ethnic minority individuals: Risk behaviors and strategies for changing them. In J. Pryor and G. Reeder (Eds.), *The social psychology of HIV infection* (pp. 183–224). Hillsdale, New Jersey: Lawrence Erlbaum.

Jones, E. F., Forrest, J. D., Goldman, N., Henshaw, S., Lincoln, R., Rosoff, J. I., Westoff, C. F., & Wulf, D. (1985). *Teenage pregnancy in industrialized countries.* New Haven: Yale University Press.

Krueger, L., Wood, R., Diehr, P., & Maxwell, C. (1990). Poverty and seropositivity: The poor are more likely to be infected. Seattle-King County Department of Public Health.

Manning, D., Balson, P., Barenberg, N., & Moore, T. (1989a). Susceptibility to AIDS: What college students do and don't believe. *Journal of American College Health, 38,* 70–73.

Manning, D., Barenberg, N., Gallese, L., & Rice, J. (1989b). College students' knowledge and health beliefs about AIDS: Implications for education and prevention. *Journal of American College Health, 37,* 254–259.

Marable, M. (1983). *How capitalism undeveloped black America.* Boston: South End Press.

Marin, G., & Marin, V. (1991). *Research with Hispanic populations: Applied social research methods series,* Vol. 23. Newbury Park, CA: Sage Publications.

Mays, V. M., & Cochran, S. D. (1989). Issues in the perception of AIDS risk and risk reduction activities by black and Hispanic/Latina women. *American Psychologist, 43,* 949–957.

McGuire, W. J. (1985). Attitudes and attitude change. In G. Lindzey & G. Aronson (Eds.), *Handbook of social psychology,* 3rd ed. (pp. 233–246). New York: Random House.

McKusick, L., Coates, T., Morin, S. F., Pollack, M. A., & Hoff, C. (1990). Longitudinal predictors of unprotected anal intercourse among gay men in San Francisco: The AIDS Behavioral Research Project. *American Journal of Public Health, 80,* 978–983.

Mosher, W. D., & Pratt, W. F. (1990). Contraceptive use in the United States, 1973–1988. *Advance data from vital and health statistics,* No. 182. Hyattsville, MD: National Center for Health Statistics.

New York City Commission on Human Rights (1987).

Nyamathi, A. (1991a). Sense of coherence in minority women at risk for HIV infection. *Public Health Nursing, 10,* 151–158.

Nyamathi, A. (1991b). Relationship of resources to emotional distress, somatic complaints, and high-risk behaviors in drug recovery and homeless minority women. *Research in Nursing and Health, 14,* 269–277.

Nyamathi, A., & Flaskerud, J. (1992). A community-based inventory of current concerns by impoverished homeless and drug addicted women. *Research in Nursing and Health, 15,* 121–129.

Nyamathi, A., Leake, Faskerud, J., Lewis, C., & Bennett, C. (1993a). Outcomes of specialized and traditional AIDS counseling programs for impoverished women of color. *Research in Nursing and Health, 16,* 11–21.

Nyamathi, A., & Lewis, C. (1991). Coping of African American women at risk for AIDS. *Women's Health Issues, 1,* 53–62.

Nyamathi, A., & Shuler, P. (1990). Focus group interview: A research technique for informed nursing practice. *Journal of Advanced Nursing, 15,* 1281–1288.

Nyamathi, A., & Shin, D. (1990). Designing a culturally sensitive AIDS education program for black and Hispanic women of childbearing age. *NAACOG's Clinical Issues in Perinatal and Women's Health Nursing, 1,* 86–98.

Nyamathi, A., Wayment, H., & Dunkel-Schetter, C. (1993b). Psychosocial correlates of emotional distress and risk behavior in black women at risk for HIV infection. *Anxiety Stress and Coping, 6,* 133–148.

O'Leary, A., Goodhart, F., Jemmott, L. S., & Boccher-Lattimore, D. (1992). Predictors of safer sex on the college campus: A social cognitive theory analysis. *Journal of American College Health, 40* 254–263.

Pearlin, L. (1989). The sociological study of stress. *Journal of Health and Social Behavior, 30,* 241–256.

Peterson, J. L., & Marin, G. (1988). Issues in the prevention of AIDS among black and Hispanic men. *American Psychologist, 11,* 871–877.

Pratt, W., Mosher, W., Backrach, C., & Horn, M. (1984). Understanding U.S. fertility: Findings from the National Survey of Family Growth, Cycle III. *Population Bulletin, 39,* 1–42.

Primm, B.J. (1991). AIDS: Today's and tomorrow's crisis. *Journal of Health Care for the Poor and Underserved, 1,* 73–85.

Reinisch, J. M., Sanders, S. A., & Ziemba-Davis, M. (1988). The study of sexual behavior in relation to the transmission of human immunodeficiency virus. *American Psychologist, 43,* 921–927.

Rosenshine, N. (1990). Preventing AIDS among female sexual partners of injection drug users: A unique training curriculum. *Network, 1,* 1–3.

Sabol, B. (1991). The urban child. *Journal of Health Care for the Poor and Underserved, 2,* 59–65.

Selwyn, P., Feiner, C., Cox, C., Lipshutz, C., & Cohen, R. (1987). Knowledge about AIDS and high risk behavior among injection drug users in New York City. *AIDS, 1,* 247–254.

Semaj, L. T. (1982). Polygamy reconsidered: Causes and consequences of declining sex ratios in African-American society. *Journal of Black Psychology, 9,* 29–43.

Siegel, K., & Gibson, W. C. (1988). Barriers to the modification of sexual behavior among heterosexuals at risk for acquired immunodeficiency syndrome. *New York State Journal of Medicine,* February, 25–36.

Singh, B. K., Koman, J. J., III, Catan, V. M., Soupley, K., Birkel, R. M., & Golasezewski, T. (1993). Sexual risk behaviors among injection drug using (IDU) human immunodeficiency virus (HIV) positive clients. *International Journal of the Addictions, 28*(8), 735–747.

Sorenson, J., Wermuth, L., Gibson, D., Choi, K., Guydish, J., & Batki, S. (1991). *Preventing AIDS in drug users and their sexual partners.* New York: Guilford Press.

Stoneburner, R., Des Jarlais, D. C., Benezra, D., Gorelkin, L., Sotheran, J., Friedman, S. R., Schultz, S., Marmor, M., Mildvan, D., & Maslansky, R. (1988). A larger spectrum of severe HIV-1-related disease in intravenous drug users in New York City. *Science, 242,*

Tesh, S. N. (1988). *Hidden arguments, political ideology and disease prevention policy.* New Brunswick, NJ: Rutgers University Press.

Thomas, S. B., Gilliam, A. G., & Iwrey, C. G. (1989). Knowledge about AIDS and reported risk behaviors among Black college students. *Journal of American College Health, 38,* 61–66.

Thomas, S., & Quinn, S. C. (1991). The Tuskegee Syphilis Study, 1932–1972: Implications for HIV education and AIDS risk reduction programs in the black community. *American Journal of Public Health, 11,* 1498–1505.

Thompson, L., & Spanier, G. (1978). Influence of parents, peers and partners on the contraceptive use of college men and women. *Journal of Marriage and the Family, 40,* 481–492.

Turner, C., Miller, H., & Moses, L. (1989). *AIDS, sexual behavior and intravenous drug use.* Washington, DC: National Academy Press.

Valdiserri, R. O., Arena, V. C., Proctor, D., & Bonati, F. A. (1989a). The relationship between women's attitudes about condoms and their use: Implications for condom promotion programs. *American Journal of Public Health, 79,* 499–503.

Valdiserri R. O., Lyter, D. W., Leviton, L. C., Callahan, C. M., Kingsley, L. A., & Rinaldo, C. R. (1989b). AIDS prevention in homosexual and bisexual men: Results of a randomized trial evaluating two risk reduction interventions. *AIDS, 3,* 21–26.

Whipple, B., & Ogden, G. (1989). *Safe encounters: How women can say yes to pleasure and no to unsafe sex.* New York: McGraw-Hill.

Williams, R. L. (1980). The death of white research in the black community. In R. L. Jones (Ed.), *Black psychology* (pp. 403–416). New York: Harper & Row.

Williams, T. (1990). *The cocaine kids.* New York: Wesley Press.

Wofsy, C. (1991). Clinical manifestations of HIV in women. *AIDS File, 5*(3), 3–5.

Wyatt, G. E., Peters, S., & Guthrie, D. (1988a). Kinsey revisited. I. Comparisons of sexual socialization and sexual behavior of white women over 33 years. *Archives of Sexual Behavior, 17,* 201–239.

Wyatt, G. E., Peters, S., & Guthrie, D. (1988b). Kinsey revisited. II. Comparisons of sexual socialization and sexual behavior of black women over 33 years. *Archives of Sexual Behavior, 17,* 289–332.

Zelnik, M., & Kantner, J. F. (1980). Sexual activity, contraceptive use and pregnancy among metropolitan-area teenagers: 1971–1979. *Family Planning Perspectives, 12,* 230–238.

7

Latinas and AIDS

Challenges to HIV Prevention Efforts

M. ISABEL FERNANDEZ

MAGNITUDE OF THE PROBLEM

AIDS is one of the most urgent and challenging health problems facing Hispanics living in the United States and its territories. Since 1989, Hispanics (approximately 9% of the population) have represented 15–16% of all male AIDS cases, 20–21% of all female cases, and almost 25% of all pediatric cases of AIDS. In the 3-year period from 1989 through 1992, 3626 Hispanic women were newly diagnosed with AIDS, representing a 171% increase from the cumulative cases among Hispanic women reported through December 31, 1989. The corresponding increase for non-Hispanic white women during the same time period was 139%. The AIDS case rate among Hispanics is $2^1/_2$ times higher than that among non-Hispanic whites (Diaz, Buehler, Castro, & Ward, 1993). Clearly, AIDS and HIV are disproportionately affecting Hispanic men and women.

What is not commonly recognized, but important to the development of effective prevention interventions, is that AIDS case rates and transmission patterns among Hispanics vary by birthplace, gender, and region of residence (Selik, Castro, & Pappaioanou, 1988, 1989; Diaz *et al.,* 1993). The northeastern states, in which Puerto Ricans are the largest subgroup of Hispanics, have consistently had the highest regional AIDS incidence among Hispanics. In fact, Puerto Ricans are 7 times more likely than non-Hispanic whites to be diagnosed with AIDS (Selik *et al.,* 1988, 1989). The lowest incidence of AIDS among Hispanics is found in the western states, particularly those that border Mexico, and 56–90% of Hispanics in these

---

M. ISABEL FERNANDEZ • Department of Psychiatry, University of Miami, Miami, FL 33136.
Women at Risk: Issues in the Primary Prevention of AIDS, edited by Ann O'Leary and Loretta Sweet Jemmott. Plenum Press, New York, 1995.

states are of Mexican origin (Diaz *et al.*, 1993; Selik *et al.*, 1989; Menendez *et al.*, 1990). Mexican-born Hispanics living in the South and West have consistently had the lowest rates of AIDS cases. Rates of AIDS cases among Hispanics in the Southwest are at levels similar to those in the non-Hispanic white population, and rates for Hispanics in Florida fall between the two (Sumaya, 1991; Castro, Valdiserri, & Curran, 1992). These trends and regional differences are supported by the results from HIV antibody testing among United States military service applicants, active duty military personnel, women attending family planning clinics, adolescents entering the Job Corps program, and blood donors [Centers for Disease Control and Prevention (CDC), 1987, 1988].

In a sense, the AIDS epidemic among Hispanics is a mosaic of epidemics, with different patterns and routes of transmission that vary by gender as well as geography and are influenced by life-style, sociocultural norms, and demographic characteristics. This chapter will briefly examine epidemiological trends in transmission of HIV infection among Hispanic women, propose several factors that have contributed to these trends, and discuss their implications for HIV-prevention efforts. Several recommendations for developing culturally competent and appropriate prevention interventions for Latinas will also be made.

WHICH HISPANIC WOMEN ARE MOST AFFECTED BY THE AIDS EPIDEMIC?

Before continuing, it is important to clarify that the term "Hispanic," although widely used to report health and economic data, is merely an umbrella term and label of convenience. This label is used to combine (many would say inappropriately) individuals with distinct historical, political, economic, and racial differences into a single category on the basis of one variable—a shared Spanish ancestry (Amaro, 1988). The use of this single label in reporting tends to obfuscate the distinct sociodemographic, cultural, and behavioral patterns that exist among Spanish-heritage subgroups in the United States—Mexicans, Puerto Ricans, Cubans, Central and South American countries, and Spain (U.S. Bureau of the Census, 1991a).

The HIV/AIDS Surveillance Report, published regularly by the Centers for Disease Control and Prevention, and the CDC AIDS Public Access Data Tape, utilize the single category "Hispanic" to report United States AIDS cases. This practice, often critiqued in the literature (Mays & Cochran, 1988; Amaro, 1988), masks the differential patterns of risk behaviors and transmission categories that emerge when the data are analyzed by country or territory of birth (Selik *et al.*, 1988, 1989; Diaz *et al.*, 1993). The practice therefore makes it difficult to identify which subgroup of Latinas are most at risk in a given area and hampers the development of effective and targeted HIV-prevention programs that incorporate the socioeconomic, cultural, and linguistic factors specific to the subpopulation of women being reached. It would be most useful for our national HIV-prevention efforts if data on Hispanic subgroup and gender were available by state or standard metropolitan statistical area, at a minimum, on an annual basis. If small cell size and confidentiality concerns make this difficult, combining data for two or three years would circumvent these issues while providing important information.

From the advent of the HIV epidemic, the majority of women with AIDS in the United States were either African American or Latinas (CDC, 1988), and this pattern has continued. Of the 40,702 cases of AIDS reported in adult and adolescent women as of October 31, 1993, almost 74% were in African American and Latina women. In the past few years, there has been a dramatic increase in the proportion of women among AIDS cases reported by the CDC (1988–1993). As of July 1988, women comprised 8.8% of the cumulative cases reported, while they comprised 15.3% of the cases reported in the 12-month period from October 1, 1992, to September 30, 1993. Latinas account for almost 20% of all cases among women reported in the 12-month period ending September 30, 1993, a far larger proportion than their representation in the United States population.

During the past decade, significant changes in the routes of HIV transmission in reported AIDS cases among Latinas have been observed. First, the proportion of reported cases attributed to intravenous-drug use has been steadily decreasing from 51.8% of the cumulative cases reported as of July 4, 1988, to 44% of the cases reported in the 12-month period ending September 30, 1993. Second, there has been a significant increase in the proportion of cases attributed to heterosexual contact, from 33.8% of the cases reported as of July 4, 1988, to 41% of the cases reported in the 12-month period ending September 30, 1993 (CDC, 1988–1993; Selik *et al.*, 1988).

In a recent article, Diaz *et al.* (1993) reported, for the first time, AIDS trends among Hispanics by gender, birthplace, and exposure category from 1988 through 1991. Among United States–born Latinas, intravenous-drug use was the predominant exposure category (55.8%). Heterosexual contact was the most prevalent route of exposure for Dominican (47.6%)-, Central American (46.9%)–, Cuban(39%)-, Mexican (35.8%)-, and South American (60%)–born Latinas. Although intravenous-drug use was the predominant exposure category for Puerto Rican–born Latinas (46.4%), heterosexual contact was a close second with 42% of the cases. This breakdown by birthplace provides some important information about foreign-born cases, but it masks subgroup differences among United States–born Latinas by combining them into a single category. The data on United States–born Latinas must be considered in conjunction with geographic differences in incidence and prevalence of HIV and AIDS and the regional distribution among the major Hispanic subgroups evident in the 1990 census. Unfortunately, specific data, which could be of great benefit for developing focused HIV-prevention efforts by gender, geography, and subgroup of United States–born Hispanics, are not available.

To date, these epidemiological trends suggest that of all Latinas with AIDS, Puerto Ricans living in the northeastern states and the island are most heavily affected. However, we should not look at these trends and determine that all our prevention resources should be targeted to United States–born or island-born Puerto Ricans—or, worse, conclude that only Latinas of Puerto Rican origin are at risk for HIV infection! No! These trends point to the pressing need for accurate information on the HIV risk behaviors and transmission patterns for men and women broken down by Hispanic subgroup and geography. This information is vital for developing specifically tailored prevention messages that address the real-life situations and actual HIV-risk patterns for each subgroup of Latinas. These risk patterns may involve the woman's own behavior or that of her partners.

It is also imperative that these data be put in their proper perspective. They tell a story that may be more than a decade old, given the long incubation period from initial HIV infection to presentation of an AIDS-defining condition, and may not accurately reflect present realities and patterns of transmission. Today, all women, Latinas included, are at increasing risk for HIV infection. The fastest-growing transmission category for women in general, and Latinas in particular, is heterosexual intercourse, not intravenous drug use. In 1992, heterosexual contact accounted for the largest proportionate increase in reported cases of AIDS in women (CDC, 1988–1993). For Latinas, the large gap between intravenous-drug use and heterosexual contact as primary exposure category is quickly diminishing. Epidemiological data on women who have recently seroconverted broken down by Hispanic subgroup, rather than data based on women diagnosed with full-blown AIDS, would be of tremendous assistance in directing focused prevention efforts.

WHY ARE LATINAS AT SUCH HIGH RISK?

There is precious little information currently available in the literature from which we can derive an empirically based answer to this complicated question. Very few behavioral or epidemiological studies have focused exclusively on Latinas, and even fewer studies that differentiate Latinas by Hispanic subgroup are available. Although researchers have identified several factors that may contribute to these disproportionately high rates of AIDS among Hispanic men and women, they did not often provide gender-specific effects. Among studies in which gender differences are reported, Latinas from all subgroups are combined into a single category, or Latinas are combined with African American women into the category of "minority women" and compared with non-Hispanic whites (Aruffo, Coverdale, & Vallbona, 1991; Biddlecom & Hardy, 1991; DiClemente, Boyer, & Morales, 1988; Mays & Cochran, 1988; G. Marin, 1988). Again, this lack of specific data is a barrier to the development of effective and targeted HIV-prevention messages.

First, data suggest that Hispanics, both adults and adolescents, have lower levels of knowledge and higher levels of misconceptions about HIV transmission than do non-Hispanic whites (Aruffo *et al.,* 1991; Biddlecom & Hardy, 1991; DiClemente *et al.,* 1988; G. Marin, 1988). Studies have shown that even when the proportion who correctly identify the major modes of HIV transmission is high, Hispanics continue to have misperceptions about transmission (Biddlecom & Hardy, 1991; Flaskerud & Ruiz Calvillo, 1991). For instance, Latinas consistently report believing the myths that people can become infected with HIV by donating blood and that one can discern a person's HIV serostatus by the way he or she looks (Nyamathi, Bennett, Leake, Lewis, & Flaskerud, 1993).

Second, Hispanic and African American women underestimate their personal risk for HIV infection to a greater extent than do nonminority women (Kalichman, Hunter, & Kelly, 1992; Williams, 1986; Mays & Cochran, 1988). These misperceptions about personal risk may in part be due to AIDS-prevention messages that lack cultural or personal relevance (Mays & Cochran, 1988; Prochaska, Albrecht, Levy, Sugrue, & Kim, 1990) or to Latinas' inability to perceive HIV as a real threat to themselves or their loved ones (Mays & Cochran, 1988; Prochaska *et al.,* 1990; Siegel & Gibson, 1988). Many Latinas and African American women continue to believe that only gay people or drug users are affected by HIV and AIDS.

Third, there are special socioeconomic, cultural, and psychological factors that affect Latinas' probability of adopting behavior patterns to reduce their risk for infection (Mays & Cochran, 1988; Kalichman *et al.,* 1992; De la Cancela, 1989), and these factors are mediated by Hispanic subgroup, geography, and local HIV seroprevalence rates. It is this third category that merits further discussion because of its importance for developing focused HIV-prevention programs. In fact, some claim that many prevention programs do not successfully reach Latinas because they do not address the specific economic and social contexts that shape their lives (Amaro, 1988). For instance, the life circumstances and relevant issues for Cuban American Latinas living in Miami could be radically different from those for Puerto Ricans living in New York City or Mexican American women living in Los Angeles. To be effective, prevention programs must be grounded in the individual realities and life contexts of the women they intend to reach. A program designed to reach Puerto Rican women living in the Northeast, where there is a higher prevalence of AIDS among Latinas, will need to address illicit drug use and migration patterns to and from the mainland United States. These issues are not relevant to Latinas in the Southwest.

FACTORS TO CONSIDER IN DEVELOPING HIV PREVENTION PROGRAMS FOR LATINAS

Socioeconomic Factors

There are dramatic and significant differences in the median age, economic status, and educational level among Latinas of Mexican, Puerto Rican, and Cuban origin. Women of Mexican origin constitute the largest subgroup of Hispanic women. As a group, they are the youngest and have the lowest education and income levels and the largest families. Women of Cuban origin are significantly older than the population as a whole, twice as likely as other Hispanic women to be college-educated, and much less likely to have incomes below the poverty level. Cubans have the smallest families and the lowest unemployment rates. Puerto Rican females have demographic profiles that resemble those of Mexican Americans, but are more likely than Mexican Americans to complete high school and have higher median incomes. However, a larger proportion of Puerto Ricans than Mexican Americans are living below the poverty line and have higher unemployment rates than Cubans. Females head 39% of Puerto Rican households as compared with 20% of Mexican American or 19% of Cuban households (U.S. Bureau of the Census, 1991a,b).

It is important to note that indicators of health status, which tend to correlate highly with socioeconomic variables, also vary across Hispanic subgroup. Puerto Ricans have the lowest health status, highest overall death rates, and highest infant mortality rates of any Hispanic subgroup, while Cubans have the highest health status and lowest death rates (U.S. Bureau of the Census, 1991a,b).

In short, with the exception of Cubans, Latinas are younger, poorer, and less educated than non-Hispanic women. They are overrepresented among women heads of households and among women in lower socioeconomic classes. They suffer from problems often associated with poverty, such as unemployment, illicit drug use, lower health status, physical and sexual abuse, discrimination, and homelessness (O'Leary, Jemmott, Suarez Al-Adam, Alroy, & Fernandez, 1991). Prevention researchers and service providers need to understand the sociodemographic situations of the Latinas they plan to serve and use this understanding to guide the development of focused prevention interventions.

Cultural and Religious Factors

The literature has characterized Latinas as having traditional cultural values, religious beliefs, and gender roles in which they are willing to sacrifice themselves for their children and as being passive and subordinate to men (Andrade, 1982; Canino, 1982; Giachello, 1985; Vasquez & Gonzales, 1981). Unfortunately, these characterizations, which typify only a small sector of the Latina population, are widely accepted and have come to stereotype Latinas in the United States. In addition to being dated, these generalizations were derived from clinical samples of primarily Mexican American women and do not take into account important mediators such as education, socioeconomic status, participation in the labor force, and residence in rural vs. urban settings (Amaro, 1988).

Unfortunately, the dearth of empirical data on these important differences among Latina subgroups has led many to use these gross generalizations and stereotypes to develop prevention programs. Of course, many of these efforts failed because they did not address the real-world circumstances and realities of their intended audiences. To be successful, prevention programs for Latinas who are educated, in the workforce, and economically independent should be very different than those for women who have low literacy, are economically dependent on their partners, and are homemakers.

Data indicate that Latinas from all subgroups have strong family orientations and that mothers play important and unique roles within the family structure (B. V. Marin & G. Marin, 1991). These characteristics appear to remain constant across sociodemographic variables. The role of Latina mothers in HIV-prevention efforts has not received adequate attention by researchers or service providers. Mothers could play important roles as credible sources of prevention messages or as opinion leaders (Rogers, 1982) to motivate individual or community-wide behavior change.

It is also widely believed that Latinas have a strong religious orientation and that Roman Catholic doctrine has tremendous influence on their life and reproductive decisions (O'Leary *et al.*, 1993). It is often assumed that

Latinas will follow papal decrees regarding birth control and condom use. However, studies have demonstrated that Mexican American, Puerto Rican, and Cuban women use contraceptives (Amaro, 1988; Marin *et al.*, 1981) and that Catholicism does not necessarily promote traditional reproductive behavior (B. V. Marin & G. Marin, 1991).

However, there are important differences between Latinas and non-Hispanic white women in contraceptive use that have implications for HIV-prevention efforts. Latinas are more likely to report never having used any contraceptive method, not currently using contraception, and not having used contraception at the time of first intercourse. Never-married Latinas were less likely than married Latinas and single non-Hispanic women to report using contraceptives (Moscher & Bachrach, 1986). Puerto Rican women have significantly higher rates of sterilizations than other Latinas or non-Hispanic women, and this may be a barrier to condom use among these women. Condom-promotion campaigns for these women and their partners may need to stress the disease-prevention aspect of condoms rather than focus on their contraceptive function.

To summarize, many HIV-prevention efforts to date have been guided by erroneous stereotypes that portray Latinas as having strong cultural values and as being passive and submissive to men and unwilling to use condoms because of strong religious beliefs. It is imperative that these stereotypes be abandoned and that more empirical data on variables that may mediate or moderate HIV-prevention efforts be available and used to develop appropriate programs for Latinas.

Acculturation

Acculturation, the process of adaptation in which immigrants may alter their attitudes and behaviors to more closely resemble those of the host society, is a variable that has traditionally been used in the social and health sciences as a predictor or determinant of a variety of behaviors (Padilla, 1979). Among Hispanics, "acculturation," measured in a variety of formats, has been found to predict health-related behaviors, including cigarette smoking, alcohol use, and early sexual initiation, and possibly to have different effects on each gender (Caetano, 1986; G. Marin, Perez-Stable, & Marin, 1989; Anashensel, Becerra, Fielder, & Weiss, 1990). For instance, highly acculturated Latinas smoke and drink more than less acculturated women, but highly acculturated Hispanic men may smoke and drink less than acculturated men.

Although there is little consensus in the literature about how best the construct of acculturation is to be measured and operationalized or even how it can best be utilized in research or service settings (Padilla, 1979), many continue to pursue this construct and determine its implications for

HIV-prevention efforts. Some researchers (B. V. Marin & G. Marin, 1992; B. V. Marin, 1995) found that in San Francisco, less acculturated Latinas were less likely to carry condoms than more acculturated Latinas, but acculturation did not appear to impact behaviors associated with condom accessibility among Hispanic men (B. V. Marin & G. Marin, 1992). Still others (Amaro, 1988; Magna *et al.,* under review) stipulated that machismo could lead less acculturated Hispanic men to engage in more risky and more frequent sexual activity, while traditional gender roles would serve to protect less acculturated Latinas because any sexual activity outside marriage would be considered taboo for any "honorable" woman. For instance, a Latina woman who has lived most of her life in the United States could be erroneously classified as highly acculturated as measured by English-language preference. In reality, she could hold very traditional values and attitudes. Thus a prevention intervention designed for acculturated Latinas may not be the most appropriate one for her.

While interesting, the implications of these data for HIV-prevention programs must be interpreted with caution. Of primary concern is that many of these findings were based on unidimensional (language-based) measurements of the variable that were psychometrically sound, but ignored the many other dimensions of the construct such as cultural awareness and ethnic loyalty (Padilla, 1979), the cultural context in which the process occurs (Cervantes & Castro, 1985; Szapocznik & Kurtines, 1979), and the existence of biculturality (Magana *et al.,* under review). In fact, the few articles found that focused on acculturation and gender differences in sexual attitudes and behaviors between Hispanic and non-Hispanic individuals (B. V. Marin, Tschann, Gomez, Kegeles, 1995c) did not measure acculturation directly, but used language of interview as a proxy measure! HIV-prevention interventions should take into account acculturation status, which implies a fuller understanding of the life context and reality of the individuals being reached, rather than acculturation level, which has stronger psychometric properties, but much less relevance.

Behavioral Factors

Intravenous-drug use and its associated pattern of sharing needles and syringes has long been identified as an HIV-related risk behavior for women, particularly Latinas and African Americans. Several new trends regarding gender differences among drug users have been reported (Brown & Weissman, 1993), but there is limited information for Hispanic subgroup differentiations. First, opiate use has been increasing among women at a higher rate than among men (Hoover, 1973). Second, the gender differences in patterns of illicit-drug use among adolescents and young adults have decreased (Clayton, Voss, Robbins, & Skinner, 1986).

Third, women are choosing crack cocaine, not heroin, as their preferred substance (Weissman, & The National AIDS Research Consortium, 1991).

Although there is a lack of data by Hispanic subgroup on the prevalence of intravenous-drug use, data from the Hispanic Health and Nutrition Evaluation Survey (Hispanic HANES) on use of nonintravenous drugs among Hispanics indicates that Puerto Rican women and men have higher rates of lifetime and current use of illicit drugs, including cocaine, than Mexican Americans or Cubans (Amaro, Whitaker, Coffman, & Hereen, 1988).

Data from the National AIDS Demonstration Research (NADR) projects with a total sample of 20,030 injection-drug users provide some information about subgroup differences and allow some comparison between United States mainland and island Puerto Ricans. Although Hispanics comprised 18% ($N = 3660$) of the total sample, only 7% were Puerto Ricans; the remaining 11% were from different Hispanic subgroups. Of the 1449 Puerto Ricans in the sample, 18.6% were women, while only 16.1% of the non–Puerto Rican group were women. Gender differences in HIV serostatus were not observed among the 9179 persons for whom these data were available. In this group, 43% of the Puerto Rican men and 44% of the Puerto Rican women in the sample were seropositive (Singer & Jia, 1993).

Interesting differences among mainland Puerto Ricans, island Puerto Ricans, and non-Hispanic whites in the NADR sample have been reported, but gender breakdown was not presented (Robles *et al.,* 1993). Mainland Puerto Ricans (40%) and island Puerto Ricans (41%) injected drugs much more frequently than non-Hispanic whites (27.6%). Non-Hispanic whites were more likely to inject drugs at friends' places, social gatherings, and in their own homes than were both groups of Puerto Ricans. Islanders were more likely to use shooting galleries (81%) than mainland Puerto Ricans (50.6%) or non-Hispanic whites (33%). Non-Hispanic whites were more likely to inject drugs with sex partners. Both Puerto Rican groups usually did not report injecting with sex partners, and island Puerto Ricans were least likely to report this behavior. A significantly higher number of whites reported injecting drugs with friends than did island Puerto Ricans. Islanders were less likely to share needles with more than one person (39.2%) than were mainland Puerto Ricans (49%) and non-Hispanic whites (55.5%). Both groups of Puerto Ricans were more likely to rent used needles than were non-Hispanic whites. Islanders were less likely to borrow used needles, but more likely to share the cotton and cooker, than the other two groups. A higher proportion of non-Hispanic whites reported sharing rinse water. This type of information, when collected locally and analyzed by gender, makes local prevention efforts more effective.

These differences have direct implications for prevention efforts for Latinas, particularly Puerto Ricans. Because a high proportion of Latinas with HIV/AIDS are infected due to their or their partners' injection-drug use, drug-abuse treatment and drug-abuse prevention messages should be integrated into HIV-prevention efforts for these women. HIV-prevention efforts should be linked in meaningful ways to drug treatment programs. HIV-prevention professionals and drug-abuse treatment providers should work collaboratively and develop holistic and integrated treatment/prevention programs that are women-focused and consider the social and economic realities of their lives. For many Latinas, the first step for HIV-related behavior change involves successfully completing a drug treatment program.

Unprotected sexual intercourse is the other relevant HIV-related risk behavior for Latinas. Addressing this risk behavior is complicated because prevention efforts need to address the woman's own behavior, the behavior of her partners, and the underlying seroprevalence of her community. The recent increases of heterosexual transmission previously cited indicate that Latinas are having sexual intercourse without using latex condoms. This inference is supported by high rates of primary and secondary syphilis, which are 5 times greater among Hispanic women (10.7%) and men (22.8%) compared to non-Hispanic whites (1.8% and 2.9%, respectively) (Vega & Amaro, submitted). This increase in syphilis in Hispanic women has been especially striking (24% increase) compared to that in Hispanic males (7%) and the minimal increase observed in non-Hispanic white women (Sumaya, 1991). Since increases in syphilis are an indicator of unprotected sex as well as a possible risk factor for enhanced transmission of HIV, prevention programs should focus on populations of Latinas in which syphilis is increasing.

What is not addressed by these data are the reasons Latinas engage in unprotected sex, who their partners are, and what can be done to help them and their partners change their risk behavior. In fact, there are few studies in the literature that focus primarily on Latinas and even fewer that focus on the behaviors of their partners. Several studies (B. V. Marin, Gomez, & Hearst, 1995a; B. V. Marin, Gomez, & Tschann, 1995b) identified the predictors and the prevalence of condom use among Hispanics. However, they focused primarily on men as opposed to women and did not provide data by Hispanic subgroup. The majority of the information on condom use among Latinas comes from studies of married women that focus on simple demographic predictors of condom use behavior rather than identifying the more complex psychological mechanisms that could better inform condom-promotion efforts (Mosher & Bachrach, 1986; Forrest and Singh, 1990).

One study (B. V. Marin, *et al.,* 1995c) examined gender and ethnic differences in condom use and its correlates among 435 Hispanics, primarily of Mexican American origin, and 736 non-Hispanic white unmarried heterosexual adults in San Francisco. Hispanic women reported fewer sexual partners than non-Hispanic whites of either gender or Hispanic men. Unmarried Spanish-speaking Latinas were less likely to be sexually active, and those who were sexually active used condoms at a lower rate than other groups. Less "acculturated" Latina adolescents delayed the initiation of sexual intercourse compared to non-Hispanic white adolescent females, but they were the most likely to become pregnant if sexually active. In general, condom use was low in all groups, but Spanish-speaking Hispanic women reported lower condom use than non-Hispanic white women.

It is imperative that these data be interpreted with caution and to understand that they represent only one particular subgroup of Latinas. To assume that Spanish-speaking Latinas are at low risk ignores the behaviors of their sex partners, which may be putting these women at risk of HIV infection. These few preliminary results and the current gap in the literature illustrate the pressing need for more behavioral research studies that target Latinas by subgroup. There is a desperate need for more empirical data on the determinants of risk behaviors, predictors of safe-sex alternatives (e.g., abstinence, monogamy, HIV testing, condom use), and the connection between local seroprevalence rates and risk of HIV infection for Latinas and their partners, to guide development of tailored prevention interventions for Latinas and their partners.

CHALLENGES OF HIV PREVENTION FOR LATINAS

After a decade of biomedical, epidemiological, and social research, there is no vaccine available, and HIV continues to spread. Behavior change was then and continues to be our primary weapon against HIV. Developing effective interventions that help prevent the initiation of risk behavior or assist individuals to change high-risk practices and adopt safer strategies continues to be the greatest challenge for HIV-prevention researchers and service providers.

One of the greatest barriers to developing effective prevention programs for women in general, and Latinas in particular, stems from lack of data at best, or inappropriately derived data, that were used to set national policy and make program decisions. For Latinas, this information gap is further widened by the paucity of gender- and subgroup-specific data from which to develop tailored prevention interventions. Instead of being grounded on the actual sociodemographic, cultural, and geographic factors of the women being served, development of many prevention programs was guided by commonly held beliefs or stereotypes. Even though the majority of women with AIDS have consistently been African Americans or Latinas, the overwhelming number of cases among homosexual men led to their being the primary focus of epidemiological studies and prevention and research efforts. Thus, in the first decade of the AIDS epidemic, development of the AIDS case definition, treatment guidelines, and prevention efforts was guided by data derived from gay men, with questionable relevance for women. Women-focused efforts suffered as a result.

This chapter has underscored the importance of revising the current surveillance report to include the standard information (exposure category and gender) by Hispanic subgroup for both foreign-born and United States–born Hispanics. With the proper assurances of confidentiality and anonymity, I have stressed the need for more locally derived surveillance data (e.g., by metropolitan statistical area) on both AIDS cases and newly diagnosed cases of HIV infection by exposure category, gender, and race/ethnicity using Hispanic subgroups. Availability of this information would be of great assistance to the development of effective prevention interventions by providing more accurate pictures of current local trends, rather than flashbacks of what occurred in the last decade.

However, these changes and the additional data on seroconversions will yield only a part of the information needed for advancing prevention efforts for Latinas. These data will provide little assistance in understanding why these women engage in risky practices or how to best motivate and assist them to adopt safer behaviors. The answers to these questions will be derived from behavioral science research efforts. Studies that focus on development and testing of behavior-change interventions for Latinas in each subgroup are desperately needed.

The scope of the HIV epidemic demands that these behavioral science studies follow the new research paradigm proposed by Kelly, Murphy, Sikkema, and Kalichman (1993). These studies must be put on a fast track that implies combining formative work and intervention testing in the context of a single study. We do not have the luxury of spending the next 5 years identifying determinants of risk behaviors without testing a behavior-change intervention. This urgency also implies abandoning traditional academic research models and entering into real partnerships with community-based service providers that work with the women we want to reach through our prevention efforts. It requires involving community members in all phases of the research process and making dissemination of successful interventions a top priority.

The urgency of the HIV epidemic also demands better integrating prevention and treatment services. Doing so requires broadening the current focus of many prevention efforts to include persons living with HIV or AIDS and the scope of traditional treatment services to include much more than medical care or case management. It necessitates that health care professionals and drug treatment staff incorporate prevention efforts into their daily activities, from routinely recommending HIV testing in high-seroprevalence areas to referring patients to more intensive behavior-change programs existing in their communities.

While these challenges are great, they are not insurmountable. There are numerous promising ideas and potential avenues previously discussed, such as Latina mothers, that need to be explored. But above all, we must stop and listen to the women themselves. It is they who can inspire and guide prevention efforts. With their wisdom and this new paradigm, we can curb the further spread of HIV.

REFERENCES

Amaro, H. (1988). Considerations for prevention of HIV infection among Hispanic women. *Psychology of Women Quarterly, 12,* 420–443.

Amaro, H., Whitaker, R., Coffman, G., & Heeren, T. (1990). Acculturation and marijuana and cocaine use: Findings from the Hispanic HANES. *American Journal of Public Health, 80,* 54–60.

Amaro, H. (1992). Reproductive choice in the age of AIDS: Policy and counselling issues. In C. Squire (Ed.), *Women and AIDS: Psychological perspectives* (pp. 20–41). New York: Sage Publications.

Anashensel, C. S., Becerra, R. M., Fielder, E. P., & Weiss, N.S. (1990). Onset of fertility related events during adolescence: A prospective comparison of Mexican American and non-Hispanic white females. *American Journal of Public Health, 80,* 959–964.

Andrade, S. J. (1982). Social science stereotypes of the Mexican American woman: Policy implications for research. *Hispanic Journal of Behavioral Sciences, 4,* 223–244.

Aruffo, J. F., Coverdale, J. H., & Vallbona, C. (1991). AIDS knowledge in low-income and minority populations. *Public Health Reports, 108*(2), 115–119.

Biddlecom A., & Hardy, A. (1991). AIDS knowledge and attitudes of Hispanic Americans: United States 1990. *Advanced Data Vital Statistics, 10,* 207.

Brown, V., & Weissman, G. (1993). Women and men injection drug users: An updated look at gender differences and risk factors. In B. S. Brown & G. M. Beschne (Eds.), *Handbook of risk of AIDS: Injection drug users and sexual partners* (pp. 173–193). Westport, CT: Greenwood Press.

Caetano, R. (1986). Patterns and problems of drinking among U.S. Hispanics. In Report of the Secretary's task force on black and minority health (pp. –). Washington, DC: U.S. Department of Health and Human Resources.

Canino, G. (1982). The Hispanic woman: Sociocultural influences on diagnosis and treatment. In R. Becerra, M. Karno, & J. Escobar (Eds.), *Mental health of Hispanic Americans* (pp. –). New York: Grune & Stratton.

Castro, K. G., Valiserri, R. O., & Curran, J. (1992). Perspectives on HIV/AIDS epidemiology and prevention from the Eighth International Conference on AIDS. *American Journal of Public Health, 82*(11), 1465–1470.

Centers for Disease Control and Prevention (1987). Trends in immunodeficiency virus infection among civilian applicants for military service—United States: October 1985–December 1986. *Morbidity and Mortality Weekly Report, 36,* 273–276.

Centers for Disease Control and Prevention (1988–1993). HIV/AIDS Surveillance report.

Cervantes, R., & Castro, F. (1985). Stress, coping and Mexican American mental health: A system review. *Hispanic Journal of Behavioral Sciences, 7*(1), 1–73.

Clayton, R. R., Voss, H. L., Robbins, C., & Skinner, W. G. (1986). Gender differences in drug use: An epidemiological perspective. In B. A. Ray & M. C. Braude (Eds.), *Women and drugs: A new era for research,* (pp. –). NIDA Monograph 65, DHHS Publication No. 86-1447. Rockville, MD: NIDA.

De la Cancela, V. (1989). Minority AIDS prevention: Moving beyond cultural perspectives towards sociopolitical empowerment. *AIDS Education and Prevention, 1,* 141–153.

Diaz, T., Buehler, J. W., Castro, K. G., & Ward, J. W. (1993). AIDS trends among Hispanics in the United States. *American Journal of Public Health, 83*(4), 504–509.

DiClemente, R. J., Boyer, C. B., & Morales, E. S. (1988). Minorities and AIDS: Knowledge, attitudes and misconceptions among black and Latino adolescents. 55–57.

Flaskerud, J. H., & Ruiz Calvillo, E. (1991). Beliefs about AIDS, health and illness among low-income Latina women. *Research in Nursing and Health, 14,* 431–438.

Forrest, J., & Singh, S. (1990). The sexual and reproductive behavior of American women, 1992–1988. *Family Planning Perspectives, 22,* 206–214.

Giachello, A. (1985). Hispanics and health care: Hispanics and the social service system. In P. S. J. Cafferty & W. C. McCready (Eds.), *Hispanics in the United States: A new social agenda* (p. 201). New Brunswick, NJ: Transaction Books.

Hoover, J. E., (1973). Crime in the U.S. *Uniform crime reports.* Washington, DC: U.S. Government Printing Office.

Kalichman, S. C., Hunter, T. L., & Kelly, J. A. (1992). Perceptions of AIDS susceptibility among minority and non-minority women at risk for HIV infection. *Journal of Consulting and Clinical Psychology, 60*(5), 725–732.

Kelly, J. A., Murphy, D. A., Sikkema, K. J., & Kalichman, S. (1993). Psychological interventions to prevent HIV infection are urgently needed: New priorities for behavioral research in the second decade of AIDS. *American Psychologist, 48,* 1–10.

Magana, J. R., de la Rocha, O., Fernandez, M. I., Amsel, J. L., Nava, P., & Moreno, R. (1995). Revisiting the dimensions of acculturation: Cultural theory and psychometric practice (under review).

Marin, B. V., Gomez, C. A., & Hearst, N. (1995a) Prevalence of multiple heterosexual partners and condom use among Hispanics and non-Hispanic whites. *Family Planning Perspectives* (in press).

Marin, B. V., Gomez, C. A., & Tschann, J. M. (1995b). Condom use among Hispanic men with multiple female partners: A nine-state study. *Public Health Reports* (in press).

Marin, B. V., & Marin G. (1990). Effects of acculturation on knowledge of AIDS and HIV among Hispanics. *Hispanic Journal of Behavioral Sciences, 12,* 110–121.

Marin, B. V., & Marin, G. (1992). Predictors of condom accessibility among Hispanics in San Francisco. *American Journal of Public Health, 82,* 592–595.

Marin, G. (1988). AIDS prevention among Hispanics: Needs, risk behaviors and cultural values. *Public Health Reports, 104,* 441–415.

Marin, G., Perez-Stable, E. J., & Marin, B. V. (1989). Cigarette smoking among San Francisco Hispanics: The role of acculturation and gender. *American Journal of Public Health, 79,* 196–199.

Mays, V., & Cochran, S. (1988). Issues in the perception of AIDS risk and risk education activities by black and Hispanic/Latina women. *American Psychologist, 43,* 949–957.

Menendez, B., Drucker, E., Vermund, S. H. (1990). AIDS mortality among Puerto Rican and other Hispanics in New York City. *Journal of Acquired Immune Deficiency Syndromes, 3,* 644–648.

Moscher, W. D., & Bachrach, C. A. (1986). Contraceptive use, United States, 1982. DHHS Publication No. (PHS) 86-1988. Hyattsville, MD: National Center for Health Statistics.

Nyamathi, A., Bennett, C., Leake B., Lewis, C., & Flaskerud, J. (1993). AIDS-related knowledge, perceptions, and behaviors among impoverished minority women. *American Journal of Public Health, 83*(1), 65–71.

O'Leary, A., Jemmott, L. S., Suarez-Al-Adam, M., Alroy, C., & Fernandez, M. I. (1993). Women and AIDS. In S. Mattero (Ed.), *American women in the nineties: Today's critical issues* (pp. 173–192). Boston: Northeastern University Press.

Padilla, A. M., Ed. (1979). *Psychological dimensions on the acculturation process: Theory, models and some new findings.* Boulder: CO. Westview Press.

Prochaska, T., Albrecht, G., Levy J., Sugrue, N., & Kim, J. (1990). Determinants of self-perceived risk for AIDS. *Journal of Health and Social Behavior, 31,* 384–394.

Robles, R. R., Colon, H. M., Matos, T. D., Reyes, J. C., Marrero, C. A., & Lopez, C. M. (1993). Risk factors and HIV infection among three different cultural groups of injection drug users. In B. S. Brown & G. M. Beschne (Eds.), *Handbook of risk of AIDS: Injection drug users and sexual partners* (pp. 256–274). Westport, CT: Greenwood Press.

Rogers, E. M. (1983). *The diffusion of innovation.* New York: Free Press of Glenco.

Seigle, K., & Gibson, W. (1988). Barriers to the modification of sexual behavior among heterosexuals at risk for acquired immunodeficiency syndrome. *New York State Journal of Medicine, 88,* 66–70.

Selik, R. M., Castro, K. G., & Pappaioanou, M. (1988). Distribution of AIDS cases by racial/ethnic group and exposure category. United States, June 1, 1981–July 4, 1988. *Morbidity and Mortality Weekly Report, 37,* 1–10.

Selik, R. M., Castro, K. G., & Pappaioanou, M. (1989). Birthplace and the risk of AIDS among Hispanics in the U.S. *American Journal of Public Health, 79* 836–839.

Singer, M., & Jia, Z. (1993). AIDS and Puerto Rican injection drug users in the United States. In B. S. Brown & G. M. Beschne (Eds.), *Handbook of risk of AIDS: Injection drug users and sexual partners* (pp. 227–255). Westport, CT: Greenwood Press.

Sumaya, L. von (1991). Major infectious diseases causing excess morbidity in the Hispanic population. *Archives of Internal Medicine, 151,* 1530–1520.

Szapocznik, J., & Kurtines, W. (1979). Acculturation, biculturalism and adjustment among Cuban-Americans. In A. M. Padilla (Ed.), *Psychological dimensions on the acculturation process: Theory, models and some new findings* (pp. 139–159). Washington, DC: American Association for the Advancement of Science.

U.S. Bureau of the Census (1991a). *Race and Hispanic origin, 1990.* Census Profile No. 2. Washington, DC: U.S. Department of Commerce.

U.S. Bureau of the Census (1991b). *The Hispanic population in the United States: March 1990.* Current population reports, population characteristics, Series P-20, No. 449. Washington, DC: U.S. Department of Commerce.

Vasquez, M. J. T., & Gonzalez, A. M. (1981). Sex roles among Chicanos: Stereotypes, challenges, and changes. In A. Baron, Jr. (Ed.), *Explorations in Chicano psychology* (pp. 50–70). New York: Praeger.

Vega, W. A., & Amaro, H. Health status of Latino populations. Annual Review of Public Health (submitted).

Weissman, G., & The National AIDS Research Consortium (1991). AIDS prevention for women at risk: Experience from a national demonstration research project. *The Journal of Primary Prevention, 12,* 49–63.

Williams, L. S. (1986). AIDS risk reduction: A community health education program for minority high risk group members. *Health Education Quarterly, 13,* 407–421.

8

Drug-Using Women and HIV
Risk-Reduction and Prevention Issues

GLORIA WEISSMAN and VIVIAN BROWN

INTRODUCTION

While drug-using women have been the group of women most at risk for HIV infection since the beginning of the AIDS epidemic, these women are also those for whom risk reduction to prevent acquisition of infection is most problematic. A number of recent studies strongly suggest that for drug-using women, there are significant educational, cultural, economic, psychological, physical, and social barriers that affect their ability to change risk behaviors and to participate in prevention programs (V. Brown & Weissman, 1993; G. Weissman & the NARC, 1991a,b). This chapter will discuss those barriers, some of the strategies that have been used to overcome them, and areas in which more work is needed. Our chapter in the next volume in this series will discuss issues that affect access to care for drug-using women with HIV disease.

The psychosocial realities faced by drug-using women, who are at very high risk to contract HIV, include:

- A significant likelihood of sexual, other physical, or psychological abuse (both current and past).
- Significant feelings of powerlessness, psychological distress, and depression.
- A lack of consistent social supports and related systems and resources.
- A lack of available, appropriate, and accessible drug treatment.

GLORIA WEISSMAN • Health Resources and Services Administration, Rockville, MD 20857. *VIVIAN BROWN* • PROTOTYPES, Culver City, CA 90230.

Women at Risk: Issues in the Primary Prevention of AIDS, edited by Ann O'Leary and Loretta Sweet Jemmott. Plenum Press, New York, 1995.

Many of these factors are well documented in the literature. Several investigators have found that women who abuse substances often come from families that provided little nurturance and had inadequate social support networks (Comfort *et al.,* 1990; Fiks, Johnson, & Rosen, 1985; Tucker, 1979) and from families with histories of substance abuse, mental problems, physical and sexual abuse, and foster care placement (Lex, Teoh, Lagomasino, Mello, & Mendelson, 1990; Pearlman, West, & Dalton, 1982). Often, chemically dependent women have been victims of violence and abuse, including rape, incest, child abuse, and domestic violence (Faulkner, Cogan, Nolder, & Shooter, 1991; Hurley, 1991; Mondanaro, 1981). Addiction among women is frequently associated with prostitution (Hser, Chou, & Anglin, 1990), and female prostitution is often accompanied by an abusive relationship between the female addict and a male pimp.

There have been data reported suggesting that women drug abusers are physically ill more often than their male counterparts (Roskies, Iida-Miranda, & Strobel, 1975; Uhlenhuth, Lipman, Balter, & Stern, 1974) and tend to have more medical problems (Andersen, 1977, 1980; B. S. Brown, Garvey, Meyers, & Stark, 1971; Flaherty, Bencivengo, & Olson, 1978; Mondanaro, 1981; Tucker, 1979). Female drug abusers are often troubled by gynecological complications, sexually transmitted diseases (STDs), urinary tract and bladder infections, and menstrual irregularities. Many of these medical problems have important implications for HIV risk and for HIV-related care.

A significant percentage of addicted women also have a co-occurring psychological disorder. Clarkin and Kendall (1992) reported that data from the Epidemiologic Catchment Area indicate that alcohol or drug abuse occurs in a significant percentage of individuals with diagnosed psychological disorders, including schizophrenia, affective disorders, and anxiety disorder. V. B. Brown, Ridgely, Pepper, Levine, and Ryglewicz (1989) suggest that the rate of substance abuse among the chronically mentally ill may be double that among the general population. Much of the research on dual diagnosis, however, has focused on samples of males. A recent study indicated a significant occurrence of comorbidity among incarcerated women (Ingram-Fogel, 1991).

RISK-REDUCTION ISSUES

New Studies

Recent data on drug-using women in the context of the AIDS epidemic come from two large community-based research studies. These studies have reached not only very large numbers of drug-using women, but also other groups of women not studied before. Whereas most earlier studies of drug-using women tended to be general household surveys, investigations of clients in treatment, or research on prison populations, these samples consist of women found in the community who may not have been in treatment or in prison and who are at known risk for HIV either through their own drug use or that of their sexual partners.

The first of these is the National AIDS Demonstration Research (NADR) program, which was launched by the National Institute on Drug Abuse (NIDA) in 1987. The program included 63 sites around the mainland United States, in Hawaii, along the United States–Mexico border, and in Puerto Rico. The purpose of the NADR program was to test the efficacy of strategies for reaching and intervening with two populations at significant risk for contracting and transmitting HIV—injection-drug users (IDUs) not currently in drug treatment programs and the sexual partners of IDUs.

Eligible individuals were interviewed using the AIDS Initial Assessment (AIA), a standard baseline instrument. The AIA elicited general demographic and health information, information on knowledge and attitudes about AIDS, and information on sexual and drug-use practices, including behaviors associated with the sharing and cleaning of drug injection paraphernalia. Individuals were then assigned to an AIDS-prevention intervention. Participants were reinterviewed at 6-month follow-up intervals with another standardized instrument, the AIDS Follow-Up Assessment. Large numbers of women were reached through the NADR program.

By October 1991, 21,465 women (including 17,474 IDUs) had been interviewed in the program. While women participants in the NADR program cannot be considered representative of all female drug users, data on these women do provide valuable insights into the women most at risk for HIV infection.

Most of the 21,465 women in the NADR study were young and in their prime childbearing years: 35% of IDUs and 55% of non-IDUs were under 30 years of age. The vast majority of these women were members of ethnic minorities. Among the IDUs, 48% were black and 20% Hispanic; among non-IDUs, 56% were black and 28% Hispanic.

Among these women, 36% of the IDUs and 55% of the non-IDUs had children living with them. Many of the women were homeless (10–12%); many others lived in makeshift arrangements with family and friends.

Of the IDU women, 65% were unemployed; only 14% of these women reported that a job was their major source of income. Many relied for their income primarily either on government programs (37%), a spouse or sexual partner (11%), or illegal activities (26%).

The second study from which many data for this chapter are drawn is a 5-year research and demonstration grant, funded by the NIDA, called Nontraditional Supports for Drug Using Women (NIDA grant 5R18

DA06983, V. B. Brown, principal investigator). This project is evaluating the efficacy of two intervention models for maintaining drug-free life-styles and limiting the spread of HIV infection among 1200 women reached through street outreach. Target populations include women who are: sexual partners of drug users, injection-drug users, non-injection-drug-users, former drug users, and those who exchange sex for money or drugs. The target populations reside in low-income, inner-city neighborhoods in Los Angeles County.

Data from an initial group of women are included in this chapter. The women received the NIDA Risk Behavior Assessment (RBA); the Women's Supplement to the RBA, which was developed to examine specific women's issues such as sexual and physical abuse; the Center for Epidemiological Studies Depression Scale; and a Social Support Interview developed for this study by the investigators.

Of the 887 women, 687 (77.5%) are African Americans, 180 (20.3%) are Latinas, and the remaining 20 (2.2%) are Caucasians or other ethnicities. Further, 64% are between the ages of 20 and 39 years, 73.8% live with children, and 20.6% say they are homeless or do not have a permanent home.

Addiction

In the case of IDU women, the most efficient route of infection with HIV is clear—the use of potentially contaminated needles, syringes, and other paraphernalia. Among the IDU women in the NADR study, despite good levels of knowledge about the dangers associated with shared injection equipment, the baseline level of risky injection behaviors was high. However, the frequency of these behaviors at baseline decreased over time; it appears that messages about the dangers of needle-sharing are being increasingly heard and heeded. This change has been true even in those areas of the country in which AIDS death rates among IDUs are still low. Cocaine, either alone or in combination with heroin, is the drug of choice for these injection users. Of those women who had injected drugs during the past 6 months, 55% had two or more partners with whom they shared needles, syringes, and other paraphernalia; only 20% reported no needle-sharing. Approximately a fifth of these women share only with a sex partner, but this circumstance may in fact make introducing safer needle practices more difficult, not less, since issues of power, trust, and love are usually involved in these relationships.

In terms of needle hygiene, at baseline 20% of the IDU women in the NADR study always used new needles, and another 15% always cleaned their equipment with alcohol, bleach, or boiling water; 65% of these women did not always use "safe" injection equipment at baseline.

The Sex–Drug Connection: Multiplication of Risk

In order to support their habits, many women turn to sex work, which places them at additional risk for sexual acquisition of HIV. Many others have partners who also inject drugs (almost all the IDU women in the NADR study also had IDU sexual partners) and thus are doubly at risk for HIV. Many IDU women are dependent on these partners for obtaining their drugs; for such a woman to insist that her partner wear a condom is extremely problematic.

Most of these women reported having engaged, during the 6 months prior to intervention, in sexual activities that place them at considerable potential risk for HIV. Vaginal sex was engaged in by 85% of the IDU women and 97% of the non-IDU women interviewed, but only 11% and 8%, respectively, always used condoms. Among these women, 13% of the IDUs and 15% of the non-IDUs reported engaging in anal sex, but only 2% in each group always used condoms during this activity.

Condoms were used with greater consistency among women who exchanged sex for money or drugs than among those who did not and among those with multiple partners than among those with a single partner. Among IDU women, the trend was even more dramatic. Of those with one partner, 18% sometimes or always used a condom, as opposed to 33% of those with two to four partners and 83% of those with five or more partners. These women may have heard and heeded the message about the dangers of multiple partners, but it may have been the wrong message. For some drug-using women, reducing the number of partners may not reduce risk, particularly if the remaining partner or partners inject drugs (G. Weissman & Brown, 1991).

Special Features of Crack Use

Data from the NADR program leave little doubt that, as has been reported elsewhere (G. Weissman, Sowder, Young, & the NARC, 1991; Fullilove, Fullilove, Bowser, & Gross, 1990; Sterk, 1988; Chiasson *et al.*, 1991), crack-using women have an extremely high level of risk for HIV. These data show that crack use adds significantly to risk for women already at high risk for HIV infection through their own injection-drug use or that of their male partners or both. Sexual risk factors appear to be particularly exacerbated by crack use. Among the women in the NADR study, crack users, whether or not they also injected drugs, were more likely than non-crack-users to have larger numbers of sexual partners (10 or more in the last 6 months), to engage in unprotected vaginal and oral sex, and to be involved in the trade of sex for money or drugs or both. Frequency of crack use was significantly correlated with degree of sexual risk behavior. Crack use was also significantly associated, among these women, with their reporting a diagnosed STD in the past 6 months.

While many IDU women traditionally have engaged in prostitution, it appears that there is a new group of women who are at great risk for HIV infection and other STDs because of sexual behaviors directly related to their crack use. While the proportion of women who engage in crack use may vary across ethnic groups or across geographic regions, the relationship of frequency of crack use to increased frequency of risk behaviors holds for all ethnic and regional groups.

History of Sexual/Physical Abuse

Another issue that seems to cut across all racial and ethnic groups of women is violence and abuse. Many of these women, probably most, have been victims of sexual or physical abuse, or both, by men. We need to learn a great deal more about how such abuse affects risk-taking and risk reduction. However, we already know that for such women, serious issues regarding boundaries, power, and sexuality make introducing condoms into a relationship extremely problematic.

A number of current studies are looking at these issues. For example, the Nontraditional Supports for Drug Using Women project (described above) has found that a significant percentage of the women interviewed report that they have been abused sexually or physically. Specifically, 25% of respondents report having been touched sexually during childhood and 14.5% during adolescence. In addition, 27.7% report that they were physically abused as an adult by a partner, and 20.2% report being sexually abused by a partner. These reports are probably underestimated.

Another current study, the Women Helping to Empower and Enhance Lives (WHEEL) Project, is a five-site field test of an AIDS-prevention model for women at risk developed for the NIDA (Rosenshine, Sowder, Weissman, & Young, 1990). This study has just completed all data collection. Preliminary analysis of data from 2781 female sex partners of IDUs (many of whom are non-IDUs themselves) shows that approximately 36% of the women report childhood sexual abuse, 34% report teenage sexual abuse, 45% report adult physical violence, 25% report rape/sexual abuse by a stranger or casual partner, and 31% report forced sex by a main partner.

For women currently in abusive relationships, the risks of introducing condoms are very real indeed and may, in fact, be much more immediate than the risk of contracting HIV. Telling such women that they should learn how to "negotiate" with their partners is neither sensitive nor relevant advice.

Dual Diagnosis/Depression

In a recent study (Melchoir, Brown, & Huba, 1995) of drug-using women in a residential substance-abuse treatment program in Los Angeles, 118 women completed the Basic Personality Inventory (BPI)[1] (Jackson, 1989) and the Center for Epidemiological Studies Depression Scale (CES-D)[2] (Radloff, 1977). Scores on these measures were correlated with drug-abuse history, previous treatment history, and time in program. In this study, the sample is 38.1% Caucasian, 23.7% African American, 34.7% Latina, and 3.3% Asian, Native American, and other ethnicities. Of the women, 91.5% are between the ages of 20 and 39 years. Approximately one woman in three (31.4%) is identifiable as homeless.

The most frequent drug of abuse in this sample is cocaine or crack; 49.2% of the women presented cocaine or crack as their primary drug problem, with another 23.7% reporting it as a secondary or tertiary problem. Heroin use is cited by 29.7% of the women as their primary drug problem and by 7.6% as a secondary or tertiary problem.

The initial assessment (BPI and CES-D) for each client was performed when she was judged by the clinical staff to be sufficiently detoxified and stable to provide reliable responses, i.e., approximately 45 days after intake. The BPI and CES-D were given again before the woman was discharged from the program.

Results from initial psychological testing suggest a substantial amount of psychological distress among the women. It should be noted that the testing measured both situational distress (e.g., acute depression related to removal of children) and more long-standing psychological disorder (e.g., thought disorder). Initial CES-D scores show that 59.3% of the women score above the clinical cut-point of 16 on this measure. The mean CES-D score was 19.5, with a standard deviation of 11.0. Compared to the national norms, in which approximately 20% of the general population can be expected to score above this cut-point, a significant proportion of this sample appears to suffer from acute depression. Similar rates were found

[1]The BPI is a 240-item instrument designed to measure "abnormal" forms of personality functioning. The BPI includes 11 scales with excellent psychometric properties: Hypochondriasis, Depression, Denial, Interpersonal Problems, Alienation, Persecutory Ideas, Anxiety, Thought Disorder, Impulse Expression, Social Introversion, and Self Depreciation. Drug abusers have been reported to score relatively high on the Interpersonal Problems, Alienation, Deviation, and Impulse Expression scales and relatively low on the Denial scale (Jackson, 1989).

[2]The CES-D (Radloff, 1977) is a short self-report measure of depressive symptomatology for the general population. Scores higher than 16 are generally considered to be clinically significant (M. M. Weissman, Sholomskas, Pottenger, Prusoff, & Locke, 1977).

in community samples of women reached through outreach programs; this finding is discussed below.

More than two thirds of the sample have one or more BPI T-scores elevated greater than or equal to the clinical cut-point of 70. The most frequent codes involve Alienation, by itself (6%) or in combination with other scales such as Impulse Expression (5%), Persecutory Ideas (9%), Social Introversion (4%), or Interpersonal Problems (3%).

While some of the women with identifiable levels of psychopathology can be considered to be typical of drug abusers, there appear to be distinct clusters of women with additional problems that require clinical intervention. Cluster analysis of BPI scores suggested five types of mental health issues. Two clusters (52%) had mean BPI scores at levels representative of an unselected population. Other groups were classified as Alienated (14%), Thought Disorder Problems (20%), and Withdrawn (13%). Thus, the BPI results characterize approximately half the women in the treatment program as suffering from significant patterns of psychological problems, while CES-D results suggest that as many as 63% of the women may suffer from significant psychological distress.

Current depression levels also were measured in the Los Angeles Nontraditional Supports study with the CES-D scale. In this outreach study, 70.6% of the women in the sample score at or above the clinical cut-point. The mean CES-D score in this group is 22.5%, with a standard deviation of 11.7.

It is very clear that the women in these high-HIV-risk samples tend to feel powerless, hopeless, and depressed. These samples have been formed from precisely those target groups of women who are likely to contract HIV because of their drug-use behaviors, their sexual practices, and their sex partners. These very high base rates of psychological distress suggest that these women would be ill-equipped to deal with the additional stress that might develop if they were told they were HIV-infected or if a potentially abusive sex partner were informed of HIV infection and reacted with physical or psychological violence or abandonment (V. B. Brown, Melchior, Reback, & Huba, 1994). Given their lack of ability to "defend" themselves from the many non-medical consequences potentially associated with HIV, it is not surprising that denial of HIV risk is widespread among these women. For example, when asked what they estimated the chance to be of becoming HIV-infected, despite high levels of knowledge about HIV transmission, 41.1% of those in the Nontraditional Supports study who expressed an opinion thought that it was "none," 44.9% thought that it was "somewhat," 8.9% thought that there was "half a chance," 3.4% thought that there was a "high chance," and 1.6% thought that it was "certain." This denial compounds the many difficulties facing those implementing prevention programs with this population, particularly when coupled with the sense of powerlessness many of these women also evince.

Lack of Social Supports

Given the very high levels of depression documented among this population, it is important to determine whether or not the women have reasonably intact systems of social support. As is well known from the literature relating stress, illness, and depression, social support systems can buffer the individual against additional stressors (Aneshensel & Huba, 1984).

In general, the women in the Nontraditional Supports sample lack strong social support systems. Several major findings emerge from a large dataset of more than 100 variables. For example, when asked how many good friends they have, 19.8% of the women indicated that they have no good friends, 62.2% said that they have a few good friends, and only 18.0% said that they have many good friends. Only 52.7% of the women said they have as many good friends as they want.

Of the 718 women completing the social support index, 72.0% have a spouse or significant other. Of the women in a relationship, 11.7% said that they did not get along well, 35.0% indicated that they got along fairly well with their significant other, and 33.3% indicated that they got along very well. Of the women responding, 49.6% said their partner makes a difference when they are stressed out, 58.9% said their partner makes them feel better, and 30.2% indicated that their partner makes them feel worse.

When these women were asked about different potential sources of social support if they had a problem, they ranked several of these sources much higher than they ranked their partners. Many of the sources of support are also sources of problems for the women in this sample. A significant percentage of the women cite many traditional sources of social supports, such as extended family members, as actually making their problems worse.

Counseling, Testing, and Partner-Notification Issues

Given the documented high levels of depression and other psychological problems among drug-using women and their frequently inadequate social support systems, there are special issues for counseling, testing, and partner notification in this population. For example, conventional pretest counseling protocols may not be adequate to allow these women—particularly those actively using drugs—to understand all the ramifications of the decision to be tested and to give truly informed consent. Both posttest counseling protocols and procedures for the waiting period between testing and results must incorporate the need for skilled crisis intervention and the knowledge that fear about results, a positive test result, and a negative test result can all lead to increased drug use or the possibility of relapse.

Partner notification, as alluded to earlier, poses other issues for drug-using women (V. B. Brown *et al.,* 1994; Rothenberg & North, 1991). Given the high levels of victimization among these women, it is likely that many might be subject to retaliatory violence from their partners if it becomes known that they are HIV-infected and the partners blame the women for exposing them to the infection. Some of these women may be engaging in sexual acts with partners who assert their power and control by insisting on performing especially high-risk behaviors (such as anal intercourse) without using condoms. Many of these women have significant levels of psychological distress and lack strong social support networks that might allow them to deal with potentially abusive or otherwise stressful behaviors from their sex partners and others.

Pregnant substance-abusing women who are victims of abuse are doubly at risk. In addition to direct physical harm that may be caused by battering, pregnant women who are abused by their partners are more likely to delay seeking prenatal care, potentially increasing the risk for developmental problems for the fetus (Amaro, Fried, Cabral, & Zuckerman, 1990; McKinney, 1993).

Many drug-using women also will lack the social, psychological, financial, and other resources to limit or deal with the potential violence or abandonment or both that may result from notifying their partner of their HIV status.

Although partner notification seems an appealing public health measure in such a high-risk population for sexual transmission of HIV, partner-notification and contact-tracing programs for this population must deal with these realities and take these issues into account in a systematic manner.

OUTREACH ISSUES

We have outlined a number of issues that clearly make HIV-risk reduction for drug-using women problematic: addiction itself, violence and victimization, depression, lack of social supports, and denial. Stigma, discrimination, and distrust of authority are other barriers (V. Brown & Weissman, 1993; G. Weissman & the NARC, 1991a,b; G. Weissman & Brown, 1991). While the AIDS epidemic has made reaching drug-using women more important than at any other time, it has also increased the difficulties both researchers and service providers face in reaching them. Frequently, they are women who have long been stigmatized and made to feel unwelcome—or welcome only as interesting subjects of research. Thus, it is no surprise to find them initially somewhat suspicious of all the hands now being stretched out to them. Certainly, their being labeled as "vectors" in the AIDS epidemic has not helped this situation. For pregnant women, concern that they will be urged to terminate their pregnancies if they are HIV-positive or at high risk also increases mistrust. The very real fear women have of losing their children to the authorities if they reveal drug use has become an increasingly significant barrier to outreach.

For these reasons, it seems clear that outreach efforts to this population must be very aggressive, but at the same time very sensitive. Because there is so much fear and suspicion on the part of these women about the medical and social services establishment, it is critical to assign outreach activities to those who know these women best. In order to be successful at outreach, individuals must be trusted and respected by the women being targeted and, most important, must not be judgmental.

It has in general been the policy of health care and drug treatment service providers to wait for drug-using women to come to their door. This tactic appeared to make sense for several reasons. First, programs—particularly for poor women—were already unable to meet the needs of those who did show up asking for services; long waiting lists are still a reality for drug-abuse treatment programs. Second, it was felt that treatment would work best with those who were "motivated" to seek it. The assumption was that a woman's desire to change her behaviors regarding substance abuse could be measured by her attempts to enter drug treatment and that, eventually, when she was ready, she would enter treatment, probably fail a few times, but eventually succeed.

AIDS—and the threat it posed to the public's health—jolted all of us into trying to do business in a different way. AIDS outreach programs found that it was indeed possible to reach large numbers of drug-using women—injection drug users and their partners, crack users, women in the sex industry, runaway and homeless adolescent women—many of whom were not accessing care of any kind, *and* to help them change the behaviors that put them at risk for disease.

From these successful outreach programs, it is now abundantly clear that the so-called "hard to reach" have been hard to reach only because few ever really tried to reach them. There are barriers, but they are definitely not insurmountable. In reaching drug-using women at risk for HIV, it was crucial to go beyond traditional points of access to this population and beyond accepted outreach strategies, strategies that have been oriented toward finding men. For example, while male drug users are often very accessible to street outreach in copping and drug-using areas, these areas may be too dangerous or simply "off limits" for female users.

The best strategy has been to wait neither for the woman's partner nor for the woman herself to come forward, but to go to her. When we do find them, these women make it clear that they wish to access services.

However, the barriers to access are often insurmountable—barriers such as lack of child care, of transportation, and of staff who speak their language, literally and figuratively. Staff of the NADR projects learned that when they go where these women are—where they live, where they work, where they already feel comfortable obtaining other health or social services—and when they make an effort to remove some of the barriers, by providing child care or transportation, the women are eager to participate (Gross & Brown, 1993). These projects have had considerable success contacting women through outreach in laundromats, beauty parlors, factories, and bars; through health fairs and other community events; through public health and family planning clinics; through hospital emergency rooms, OB-GYN, and well-baby clinics; through social services agencies (including WIC and AFDC); through jails and prisons; through battered women's and homeless shelters; through housing projects; and through door-to-door outreach.

Successful Models of Preventive Intervention

The experiences of the projects described briefly in this chapter, as well as many others around the country,[3] suggest a number of critical intervention principles for working with drug-using women around HIV prevention issues (V. Brown & Weissman, 1993; G. Weissman & the NARC, 1991a,b; G. Weissman & Brown, 1991). Many of these principles have been incorporated into a model prevention program developed for NIDA and field-tested in the WHEEL project (Rosenshine *et al.,* 1990). In engaging and retaining women in interventions, as in conducting outreach, staff of these projects have found that sensitivity to the women's perceived needs and understanding of the context of their lives are key. Intervention strategies should address the issues, problems, and concerns that these women identify as the most pressing in their lives, rather than those that the area's funders, researchers, program designers, and service providers may identify as most pressing. While prevention programs for women may be organized around or funded for a single, specific issue, such as substance abuse, or prenatal care, or AIDS prevention, the women with whom the programs

[3]For example, in addition to the NIDA studies mentioned, a number of preventive intervention studies have been funded by the Centers for Disease Control and Prevention (CDC). Some have been completed; others are still in progress. Study designs and findings are summarized in three recent CDC publications: *What We Have Learned from the AIDS Community Demonstration Projects* (June 15, 1992); *Behavioral and Prevention Research Branch Summary of MMWR Articles, 1992–1993; Research Summaries: Behavioral and Prevention Research Grants* (January 1994).

are trying to work cannot be categorized so neatly. As the data suggest, most of these women have multiple needs and multiple problems. In designing and delivering programs for these women, it appears crucial to be mindful of the many contexts that shape the lives of these women, including the psychological, familial, social, economic, cultural, political, medical, and spiritual. The NADR projects have found that staff cannot talk to women about AIDS prevention without also talking about health, about parenting, about sexuality, about domestic violence, about addiction and recovery, about relationships and dependency, about death and dying, and about love and loss.

These projects have seen firsthand that many women at risk for AIDS—even when they are assisted to recognize and personalize that risk—still do not view AIDS as a primary concern. In an attempt to meet some of the needs that clients identify as most pressing, staff in these projects have performed such services as rape counseling, suicide prevention, and home visits, as well as medical and legal advocacy. Several programs offer women a cup of soup or a sandwich, a safe place to drop in with their children, or used-clothing "boutiques." Educational sessions, support groups, and individual counseling on parenting issues have been extremely well received, as has pediatric care in nontraditional settings, such as mobile vans. Reaching clients "where they are" often means literally that. Programs need to take place in nonthreatening, familiar, and easily accessible community settings.

In many of these projects, peer-led interventions have been the rule. In others, indigenous outreach workers serve as the bridge between the women being reached and those delivering the intervention services. Assistance is provided by walking them through systems that may be unfamiliar or traditionally unwelcoming and acting as "translators" for both the women and the service delivery systems. In addition to being able to establish rapport and gain access, there is every indication that "natural," or "indigenous," leaders can themselves *be* an intervention, by serving as positive role models and believable message bearers. Group interventions, which focus on helping women to support and empower each other and to remedy the isolation and stigma they face, are being tried in many projects. However, some are finding that cultural and psychological issues, as well as the logistics of women's complicated lives, make group participation problematic for some women. Many projects report that group interventions are well received, but only after considerable one-on-one work is done. While the experience of the NADR projects suggests that AIDS-prevention programs must focus on empowering women individually and building those inner resources (self-esteem, sense of power, specific skills) that may help women initiate behavior changes, they have also found that they need to devote considerable attention and resources to advocacy activities focused on building the external resources (e.g., affordable housing, adequate and appropriate drug treatment programs, child care) needed to provide these women with some real power over their lives and to sustain changes.

Outcome data from the NADR projects suggest that the strategies used were effective in helping women reduce their risk for HIV, particularly in those areas in which behavior change is within their power. While reducing risk is not an easy matter, many of the women in this national study began to take important steps to protect themselves and others from infection. First, among the IDU women, overall injection-drug use decreased fairly dramatically. More than two thirds of the IDU women in the study either decreased (45%) their frequency of heroin injection or maintained a low level (23%) of use. At baseline, 48% of these women reported daily heroin injection; of these women, 29% reported no heroin injection during the 6-month follow-up period, and an additional 32% reported less frequent injection. Among cocaine injectors, almost half (48%) decreased their frequency of use. A little less than a third (31%) of the IDU women in the sample reported daily cocaine injection at baseline. One third (32%) of these women reported no cocaine injection during the follow-up period, and an additional 37% reported less frequent injection. There were also decreases in crack use. A third of the women who initially reported daily crack use indicated no use at follow-up (33% for the IDUs, 31% for the non-IDUs).

Making changes in sexual risk, for all the reasons mentioned above, is a much more difficult endeavor for women. The NADR study, like many others, shows that drug-use practices are changing faster and more dramatically than sexual practices. Nevertheless, there was a significant decrease in unprotected sex reported by the women in our study. Overall, 37% of the IDU women and 45% of the non-IDU women reduced the frequency with which they had vaginal sex without a condom.

These women may not meet the traditional standards of success for drug-abuse treatment—many continue to use drugs—but they have demonstrated that they are capable of positive change and they have taken important first steps to improve their lives. These are not insignificant accomplishments, and they are not the work of "unmotivated" women.

Role of Drug Treatment Programs in HIV Prevention

For women whose primary risk for HIV is their own drug use, entering drug-abuse treatment is clearly a desirable risk-reduction measure. However, the realities are that the United States lacks sufficient treatment slots for both men and women and that, for many women, treatment is not a viable alternative. Women encounter special barriers in entering drug treatment services. Many women have the additional responsibility of child-rearing, which is often jeopardized by their drug dependency. Most traditional therapeutic communities do not accommodate women and their children or pregnant addicted women. When and if women find a drug treatment slot, many are faced with leaving their children in the care of someone else—which they often cannot afford or understandably do not want—or declining the opportunity for treatment.

This is only one of a number of factors that continue to impede women's access to and successful engagement in drug-abuse treatment. When women are placed in treatment settings in which males dominate the client rosters or staff, special concerns for women—such as resolving issues of physical and sexual abuse, learning effective parenting, learning how to deal with a pregnancy and the threat that drug use can have to the unborn child, and how to develop independent skills that will allow them to provide for themselves and their children—are likely to be overlooked (Cohen, Hauer, & Wofsy, 1989; DiMatteo & Cesarini, 1986; Reed, 1985, 1987; Tiblier, Walker, & Rolland, 1989; V. B. Brown, 1992; Levy & Broudy, 1975; Kaubin, 1974; Maglin, 1975; Doshan & Bursch, 1982; Marsh & Miller, 1985).

One of the major goals of the NADR outreach programs was to provide referrals to and help in entering drug treatment. Here, too, outcome data were very encouraging. In these programs, 9% of the non-IDU women and an impressive 35% of the IDU women enrolled in drug treatment programs between baseline and follow-up. In addition, 20% of non-IDU women and 26% of IDU women participated in a self-help program during that period. These results appear to support the effectiveness of targeted outreach to women, particularly in facilitating entry into treatment. The use of recovering individuals as outreach workers was a crucial element. These data also support the need for close ties between AIDS-prevention programs and drug treatment programs.

Role of Needle-Exchange Programs

Needle-sharing is a main cause of the escalation of HIV infection among IDUs. Studies have shown that between 30% and 78% of drug users share needles. In many large cities, shooting galleries are places where drug users congregate to inject drugs, and syringes and needles are often shared.

Advocates of needle-exchange programs believe that legal access to sterile injection equipment would have the most immediate and far-reaching effect on reducing the spread of HIV among IDUs. Many European countries and Australia have instituted needle-exchange programs (University of California, 1993). Since 1988, over 20 needle-exchange programs have been implemented in the United States. These programs vary in size, legal status, degree of official recognition, and community support.

While opponents of needle exchange believe that these programs may condone or even encourage drug use, in fact most needle-exchange programs offer more than just trading new sterile syringes for used equipment. Drug users get education about transmission of HIV (sexual and perinatal), condoms, bleach, on-site health care such as HIV testing or TB testing, or both, and referral to drug-abuse treatment. There is growing evidence that needle exchanges reduce the spread of HIV. A mathematical model (Kaplan, 1992) created for the program in New Haven concludes that there is a 33% reduction in the annual incidence of new infections in program participants.

One of the limitations of the programs is that they often have difficulty reaching women and young users. Utilization in the United States shows only 14–25% women. Additional work would need to be done to increase utilization of these programs by women.

CONCLUSION

This chapter has addressed the major issues of risk reduction for drug-using women at high risk for HIV. The experiences of the projects described briefly in this chapter, as well as many others throughout the country, suggest a number of critical intervention principles. These include the need for: aggressive and sensitive outreach by indigenous workers; understanding the context of women's lives, including familial and cultural issues, violence and victimization, and feelings of powerlessness and psychological distress; and integration of empowerment and advocacy strategies into all interventions. In developing prevention programs, designing risk-reduction strategies, and implementing policies to meet the needs of drug-using women, these principles must be incorporated.

REFERENCES

Amaro, H., Fried, L. E., Cabral, H., & Zuckerman, B. (1990). Violence during pregnancy and substance abuse. *American Journal of Public Health, 80,* 575–579.

Andersen, M. (1977). *Medical needs of addicted women and men and the implications for treatment,* WDR Report No. 4. Ann Arbor: Women's Drug Research Project, University of Michigan.

Andersen, M. (1980). Health of heroin dependent clients: Focus on women. *Women and Health, 5*(1), 23–33.

Aneshensel, C. S., & Huba, G. J. (1984). An integrated causal model of the antecedents and consequences of depression. In J. R. Greenley (Ed.), *Research in community and mental health,* Vol. 4 (pp. 35–72). Greenwich, CT: JAI.

Brown, B. S., Garvey, S. K., Meyers, M. B., & Stark, S. D. (1971). In their own words: Addicts' reasons for initiating and withdrawing from heroin. *International Journal of Addictions, 6,* 635–645.

Brown, V. B. (1992). Drug and alcohol treatment and recovery services for pregnant addicted women. In M. Jessup (Ed.), *Drug dependency in pregnancy: Managing withdrawal* (pp. 251–267). Sacramento, CA: State of California Department of Health Services.

Brown, V. B., Melchior, L. A., Reback, C. J., & Huba, G. J. (1994). Partner notification of HIV test results: Psychosocial and social issues for women. *AIDS and Public Policy Journal, 6,* 86–92.

Brown, V. B., Ridgely, M. S., Pepper, B., Levine, I. S., & Ryglewicz, H. (1989). The dual crisis: Mental illness and substance abuse: Present and future directions. *American Psychologist, 44,* 565–569.

Brown, V., & Weissman, G. (1993). Women and men injection drug users: An updated look at gender differences and risk factors. In B. S. Brown & G. M. Beschner (Eds.), *Handbook on risk of AIDS: Injection drug users and sexual partners* (pp. 173–194). Westport, CT: Greenwood Press.

Centers for Disease Control and Prevention (1992). *What we have learned from the AIDS community demonstration projects* (June 15, 1992). Atlanta: Centers for Disease Control and Prevention.

Centers for Disease Control and Prevention (1992–1993). *Behavioral and Prevention Research Branch summary of MMWR articles, 1992–1993.* Atlanta: Centers for Disease Control and Prevention.

Centers for Disease Control and Prevention (1994). *Research summaries: Behavioral and Prevention Research grants* (January 1994). Atlanta: Centers for Disease Control and Prevention.

Chiasson, M. A., Stoneburner, R. L., Hildebrandt, D. S., Ewing, W. E., Telzak, E. E., & Jaffe, H. W. (1991). Heterosexual transmission of HIV-1 associated with the use of smokable freebase cocaine (crack). *AIDS, 5,* 1121–1126.

Clarkin, J. F., & Kendall, P. C. (1992). Comorbidity and treatment planning: Summary and future directions. *Journal of Consulting and Clinical Psychology, 60,* 904–908.

Cohen, J. B., Hauer, L. B., & Wofsy, C. B. (1989). Women and IV drugs: Parental and heterosexual transmission of human immunodeficiency virus. Special issue: Intravenous drug use and AIDS. *Journal of Drug Issues, 19,* 39–56.

Comfort, M., Shipley, T. E., White, K., & Griffith, E. M. (1990). Family treatment for homeless alcohol/drug-addicted women and their preschool children. Special issue: Treating alcoholism and drug abuse among homeless men and women: Nine community demonstration grants. *Alcoholism Treatment Quarterly, 7,* 129–147.

DiMatteo, T. E., & Cesarini, T. M. (1986). Responding to the treatment needs of chemically dependent women. *Journal of Counseling and Development, 64,* 452–453.

Doshan, T., & Bursch, C. (1982). Women and substance abuse: Critical issues in treatment design. *Journal of Drug Education, 12,* 229–239.

Faulkner, K. K., Cogan, R., Nolder, M., & Shooter, G. (1991). Characteristics of men and women completing cognitive/behavioral spouse abuse treatment. *Journal of Family Violence, 6,* 243–254.

Fiks, K. B., Johnson, H. L., & Rosen, T. S. (1985). Methadone-maintained mothers: 3-Year follow-up of parental functioning. *International Journal of the Addictions, 20,* 651–660.

Flaherty, E. W., Bencivengo, M., & Olson, K. (1978). *The causes of demand reduction: An exploratory study.* Philadelphia: Philadelphia Health Management Corp.

Fullilove, R. E., Fullilove, M. T., Bowser, B. P., & Gross, S. A. (1990). Risk of sexually transmitted disease among black adolescent crack users in Oakland and San Francisco, California. *JAMA, 263,* 851–855.

Gross, M., & Brown, V. (1993). Outreach to injection drug–using women. In B. S. Brown & G. M. Beschner (Eds.), *Handbook on risk of AIDS: Injection drug users and sexual partners* (pp. 173–194). Westport, CT: Greenwood Press.

Jackson, D. N. (1989). *Manual for the Basic Personality Inventory.* Port Huron, MI: Sigma Assessment Systems.

Hser, Y., Chou, C., & Anglin, M. D. (1990). The criminality of female narcotics addicts: A causal modeling approach. *Journal of Quantitative Criminology, 6,* 207–228.

Hurley, D. L. (1991). Women, alcohol and incest: An analytical review. *Journal of Studies on Alcohol, 52,* 253–268.

Ingram-Fogel, C. (1991). Health problems and needs of incarcerated women. *Journal of Prison and Jail Health, 10,* 43–57.

Jackson, D. N. (1989). *Basic Personality Inventory: BPI manual.* Port Huron, MI: Sigma Assessment Systems.

Kaplan, E. H. (1992). Needle exchange or needless exchange? The state of the debate. *Infectious Agents and Disease, 1,* 92–97.

Kaubin, B. J. (1974). Sexism shades the lives and treatment of female addicts. *Contemporary Drug Problems, 3,* 471–484.

Levy, S. J., & Broudy, M. (1975). Sex role differences in the therapeutic community: Moving from sexism to androgyny. *Journal of Psychedelic Drugs, 7,* 291–297.

Lex, B. W., Teoh, S. K., Lagomasino, I., Mello, N. K., & Mendelson, J. H. (1990). Characteristics of women receiving mandated treatment for alcohol or polysubstance dependence in Massachusetts. *Drug and Alcohol Dependence, 25,* 13–20.

Maglin, A. (1975). Casework with pregnant women on methadone maintenance. *Social Casework, 56,* 131–137.

Marsh, J. C., & Miller, N. A. (1985). Female clients in substance abuse treatment. *International Journal of the Addictions, 20,* 995–1019.

McKinney, L. E. (1993). The relationship between violence and female patterns of addiction. *Clearinghouse for Drug Exposed Children Newsletter, 4* (Spring).

Melchior, L. A., Brown, V. B., & Huba, G. J. (1995). A typology of mental health problems among women in residential drug treatment (submitted).

Mondanaro, J. (1981). Reproductive health concerns for the treatment of drug dependent women. In G. M. Beschner, B. G. Reed, & J. Mondanaro (Eds.), *Treatment services for drug dependent women,* Vol. I (pp. 258–292). DHHS Publication No. (ADM) 81-1177. Rockville, MD: National Institute on Drug Abuse.

Pearlman, P., West, M., & Dalton, J. (1982). Mothers and children together: Parenting in a substance abuse program. In B. G. Reed, G. M. Beschner, & J. Mondanaro (Eds.), *Treatment services for drug dependent women,* Vol. II (pp. 532–571). DHHS Publication No. (ADM) 82-1219. Rockville, MD: National Institute on Drug Abuse.

Radloff, L. S. (1977). The CES-D scale: A self-report depression scale for research in the general population. *Applied Psychological Measurement, 1,* 385–401.

Reed, B. G. (1985). Drug misuse and dependency in women: The meaning and implications of being considered a special population or minority group. Special issue: Intervening with special populations. *International Journal of the Addictions, 20,* 13–62.

Reed, B. G. (1987). Developing women sensitive drug dependence treatment services: Why so difficult? *Journal of Psychoactive Drugs, 19,* 151–164.

Rosenshine, N., Sowder B., Weissman G., & Young, P. L. (1990). *AIDS prevention model: Reaching women at risk.* Bethesda, MD: NOVA Research.

Roskies, E., Iida-Miranda, M. L., & Strobel, M. G. (1975). The application of the life events approach to the problems of immigration. *Journal of Psychosomatic Research, 19,* 235–240.

Rothenberg, K. H., & North, R. L. (1991). The duty to warn "dilemma" and women with AIDS: Redefining the "forseeable victim." *Courts, Health Science, & the Law, 2,* 90–98.

Sterk, C. (1988) Cocaine and HIV seropositivity (letter). *Lancet, 2,* 1052–1053.

Tiblier, K. B., Walker, G., & Rolland, J. S. (1989). Therapeutic issues when working with families of persons with AIDS. *Marriage and Family Review, 13,* 81–128.

Tucker, M. B. (1979). A descriptive and comparative analysis of the social support structure of heroin addicted women. In *Addicted women: Family dynamics, self perceptions, and support systems.* NIDA Services Research Monograph Series, Department of Health, Education and Welfare Publication No. ADM-80-762. Washington, DC: U.S. Government Printing Office.

Uhlenhuth, E. H., Lipman, R. S., Balter, M. B., & Stern, M. (1974). Symptom intensity and life stress in the city. *Archives of General Psychiatry, 31,* 759–763.

University of California (1993). Institute for Health Policy Studies. *The public health impact of needle exchange programs in the United States and abroad,* Vols. I and II. San Francisco: University of California.

Weissman, G., & the National AIDS Research Consortium (NARC) (1991a). AIDS prevention for women at risk: Experience from a national demonstration research program. *Journal of Primary Prevention, 12*(1), 49–63.

Weissman, G., & the National AIDS Research Consortium (NARC) (1991b). Working with pregnant women at high risk for HIV infection: Outreach and intervention, May–June 1991. *Bulletin of the New York Academy of Medicine, 67,* 291–300.

Weissman, G., & Brown, V. B. (1991). Drug use and sexual behaviors among sex partners of injecting-drug users—United States 1988–1990. *Morbidity and Mortality Weekly Report, 40,* 855–860.

Weissman, G., Sowder, B., Young, P. L., & the National AIDS Research Consortium (NARC) (1991). The relationship between crack cocaine use and other risk factors among women in a national AIDS prevention program. *Proceedings of the Sixth International AIDS Conference* (San Francisco, June 20–24, 1990), Vol. 3 (p. 126) (abstract).

Weissman, M. M., Sholomskas, D., Pottenger, M., Prusoff, B. A., & Locke, B. Z. (1977). Assessing depressive symptoms in five psychiatric populations: A validation study. *American Journal of Epidemiology, 106,* 203–214.

9

Female Sex Workers

Scapegoats in the AIDS Epidemic

JUDITH BLACKFIELD COHEN and PRISCILLA ALEXANDER

INTRODUCTION

From the volume of stories in newspapers, and studies reported in medical and health journals, one could conclude that prostitutes are a major influence in the spread of the epidemic of HIV infection. Women who earn their living by selling their sexual services have been portrayed in both media as "reservoirs" or "pools" of infection, "vectors" for the sexual transmission of HIV to unsuspecting heterosexual men and their "innocent" wives and children. Even in the absence of evidence, print media leaders such as *The New York Times* and *The Washington Post* have printed many stories supporting the thesis that heterosexual prostitution plays a major role in the HIV epidemic in the United States (King, 1990). A recent search of the Centers for Disease Control and Prevention National AIDS Clearinghouse NEWS database found 452 separate articles with references to prostitution that had been included in the CDC AIDS Daily Summary since 1988. A common subject of these articles is that a female prostitute has been charged with attempted murder, or willful endangerment of an undercover officer, because even though she tested positive for HIV at some point in the past, she continued to stand on street corners. In none of the articles was there any evidence that the woman in question had either infected anyone or engaged in any behavior likely to permit someone to be infected. It was enough that she was identified as a "prostitute."

JUDITH BLACKFIELD COHEN • Project AWARE, Oakland, CA 94612. *PRISCILLA ALEXANDER* • National Task Force on Prostitution, New York, NY 10025.

Women at Risk: Issues in the Primary Prevention of AIDS, edited by Ann O'Leary and Loretta Sweet Jemmott. Plenum Press, New York, 1995.

The purpose of this chapter is to examine the evidence on HIV infection among women who work in the sex trade in this country, and in some other countries, in terms of both their own risk of infection and the risk of their transmitting HIV infection to others. Some of the questions to answer include: What is the prevalence of infection among women who sell sex? What kinds of sex workers, and in what geographic areas, show significant rates of HIV infection? How do women in the sex trade become infected? What is the likelihood that a female sex worker with HIV infection will infect a customer? What kinds of programs are in place that can help reduce sex workers' risk of infection? And what are the public policy issues raised by prostitution in the age of AIDS?

Definitions

Before we address those questions, it may be useful to define such terms as "prostitution," "sex work," "sex trade," and "sex exchange," terms that are not entirely interchangeable in either meaning or social value.

"Sex work" is a term that has come into use in recent years, first used by a San Francisco sex worker, performance artist, and activist named Carol Leigh, also known as Scarlot Harlot (Alexander, 1987). Leigh first used the term in order to focus attention on the fact that prostitution is a form of paid sexual labor, or work, that is affected by forces similar to those that affect other kinds of paid labor. Rapidly claimed as a self-representative term by prostitutes and other sex workers—dancers, strippers, pornography models and performers, and some sex therapists—it also came into wide use in the international arena of AIDS research and prevention politics. In the context of AIDS, "sex work" is a useful term to clarify the issue of workplace and occupational risk. That is, sex workers, like health care workers, may be at risk due to occupational hazards or because of their behavior off the job. For example, health care workers may be at risk of HIV infection through needle sticks, invasive procedures, and other occupational activities, but may also be at risk because of sexual or drug-use practices in their personal lives. So too, sex workers may be at risk due to unprotected sex on the job, or through unprotected sex with their personal partners and/or needle sharing behavior unrelated to their work, as well as through blood transfusions and/or injections with unsterile equipment, especially in countries without the capacity to ensure blood safety or sterile conditions in the health care system.

At the same time, many people who engage in behaviors that outsiders clearly identify as "prostitution" do not, themselves, see it that way, or think of themselves as professional prostitutes or sex workers with the responsibility and ability to prevent disease. Nonetheless, some public health researchers have used very broad classifications—e.g., "a woman who has exchanged sex or sexual services for money or drugs at least once since 1978," used by the Centers for Disease Control and Prevention for its multicenter study of the epidemiology of HIV infection among female prostitutes (Darrow *et al.*, 1990). Such a definition includes women who have, on rare occasions, had sex with a friend who gave them money to help with the rent, or who have used sex to secure a place to sleep for the night, or to obtain a meal, as well as women who went to work on a regular basis in a stroll district, massage parlor, or other sex-work venue. The more often such a "sex exchange" or "sex trade" takes place, the more likely it is that one of the partners will be infected with HIV or some other sexually transmitted disease (STD). However, to the extent that the participants define the exchanges as the normal run of things, or possibly as a question of survival, they are unlikely to see these actions as recognized "risk behaviors" or as "prostitution" and are therefore less likely to think of protecting themselves, or their partners, from AIDS, or indeed any STD.

Some of the terms used around the world to refer to people who engage in some sort of sexual activity in exchange for some kind of economic support include: "women who go out" and "free women," both common in sub-Saharan Africa; "bar ladies," "bar workers," and "working girls" or women, common in many countries; "ladies of the evening," "nightwalkers," and "streetwalkers," and the terms related to covert businesses, such as "masseuses," "hostesses," "hospitality workers," "escorts," "guides," and "entertainers." Then there are the more familiar terms, such as "prostitutes," "sex workers," "hookers," "whores," "putains," and "putas." In any case, although many of the terms, translated into local languages, are understood by many to refer to "prostitutes," in fact many of the practitioners, who may use some of those terms to describe themselves, may not consider themselves "prostitutes." In many parts of the world, women live in communities that have grown up around the major trucking routes, communities that become, as it were, "truck stops," where they may provide a haven for a number of drivers in succession, their home away from home, receiving "help" with the rent and the cost of the food they provide. In societies where male polygamy is the norm, these women are polyandrous, but are they , or do they see themselves as, "prostitutes"? In this country, among the women who roam the streets, homeless, having sex is often a way to sleep in a warm room for the night (or a cool one, depending on the city and the season), and perhaps get a meal, and a bit of money to help them through the next day. Is that "prostitution"? And when is the line crossed between the normal barter of American life and an overtly commercial transaction, for women who have sex with the men who provide them with the nirvana of heroin or crack? The point is, every one of these situations carries the potential for HIV to move from one person to another, and every one of these people needs to know how to protect herself, or himself.

Meanwhile, most research, whether in this country or elsewhere, blurs the distinction between sex *work* and sex *exchange,* failing to recognize significant differences in behavior between the two extremes, and in fact conflating the extremes under the general term "prostitution." This practice can result and has resulted in serious misreadings of some research data.

To summarize, a wide variety of cultural and economic conditions influence sexual behavior, and only a small portion of sex with others that involves some kind of extrinsic exchange is defined as "sex work" by those involved. Moreover, the risk of transmission of any STD is independent of such labels as "prostitution" or such factors as "payment." The risk is strictly dependent on (1) the probability of infection in either of the parties involved and (2) the nature of the sex act and whether or not it is protected. Other factors that become subsumed under the mythic resonance of such terms as "prostitution," and to a lesser extent "sex work," include the types of services provided, how often the services are provided and under what conditions, and the extent of the provider's control over each transaction. That having been said, what follows is a review of some of the research regarding HIV infection among women involved in various parts of the sex trade and, to a much lesser extent, men who identify as clients.

EPIDEMIOLOGY OF HIV INFECTION IN THE CONTEXT OF PROSTITUTION

Estimates of the number of prostitutes—male as well as female—working in the United States range from about 150,000 to a million or more. More than 100,000 people are arrested on prostitution charges annually in the United States, 65–70% of them women, perhaps 20–25% male prostitutes, and 10% or so male clients. Almost all these arrests are made on the street, which the National Task Force on Prostitution (NTFP) estimates as representing between 10% and 30% of prostitution, depending on the community. However, since prostitution is an illegal occupation, outside a few small towns in Nevada, no agency has been able to collect accurate statistics about it, and few people identify themselves as "prostitutes" on IRS forms, in general population surveys, or other venues that could provide such statistics. In terms of clients, if you accept the lowest estimate of the number of prostitutes, the NTFP estimates that the actual number of individual men who engage in commercial sex transactions in 1 year could be anywhere from around 800,000 to more than 12 million, depending on, for example, the average number of clients a prostitute sees per day and the average frequency with which the client seeks the services of prostitutes. When you move outside the United States, particularly into countries with much less of an obsession for statistics, it is even less possible to estimate the overall size of either population.

In the absence of clear information about the number of people engaging in something called "prostitution," and its myriad forms, it is almost impossible to get a representative sample of either population. As a result, all the studies that have been done to be understood as snapshots of particular groups of sex workers or clients, in specific sex work contexts, at specific points in time. Most studies in this country have focused on the easiest "prostitutes" to identify—women who work on the street, many of whom were contacted in jail, in drug treatment programs, and in STD clinics, further skewing their representativeness. Studies that have used "outreach," in an effort to be more inclusive, have also tended to focus on the women working on the street in recognized stroll districts. In the United States, only a small number of studies have looked at women working in massage parlors or brothels or for escort services, although in developing countries, most research has focused on women who work in off-street venues. Even fewer studies have looked either at male sex workers or clients of workers of either gender (e.g., of 134 separate abstracts listed in the index of the 1993 International AIDS Conference, only 37 were listed under the entry for clients and 18 under the entry for male prostitutes).

The largest study of the epidemiology of HIV infection among female sex workers in the United States, conducted in eight cities, was coordinated by the Centers for Disease Control from 1986 through 1989 (Darrow *et al.*, 1990). Women were recruited from a wide range of sites, including brothels, STD clinics, drug treatment programs, escort services, and streets with a reputation for being prostitution "stroll" districts. HIV infection rates were generally low, although they ranged from zero among brothel workers in Nevada—a state with a very low population prevalence of HIV infection—few of whom had ever injected drugs, to a high of 47.5% among women recruited in a methodone maintenance program and an STD clinic in northern New Jersey, most of whom had a history of injecting drug use (Table 1). Without the data from New Jersey, however, the range was from zero to 15%, the prevalence among women in a Miami detention center. The prevalence among the entire study population was 12.3%. However, the infection rate among those who had injected drugs was 19.9%, while

Table 1. HIV Prevalence among Female Sex Workers in the United States and Europe

Location/date	Study	HIV+/all women tested (%)	Data collection source
Europe			
Amsterdam, Netherlands (1990)	van Doornum et al. (1990)	2/472 (0.4%)	STD clinic
Ghent, Belgium (1988–1989)	Mak et al. (1990)	1/123 (0.8%)	Windows, bars, clubs, saunas
Catalonia, Spain (1990)	Casabona et al. (1990)	8/71 (11.3%)	Sex work bars
Vienna, Austria (1989)	Stary et al. (1991)	0/713 (0.0%)	Registered prostitutes
United States (1986–1989)	Darrow et al. (1990)		
Southern Nevada		0/37 (0.0%)	Brothels, brothel applicants
Atlanta		1/123 (0.8%)	Street and call girl outreach; tabloid advertisements
Colorado Springs		2/98 (2.0%)	STD, methadone, and HIV screening clinics
Los Angeles		12/300 (4.0%)	Detention center
San Francisco		10/212 (4.7%)	Street outreach
Miami		66/440 (15.0%)	Detention center
South New Jersey		6/28 (21.4%)	Methadone and STD clinics; street outreach
North New Jersey		75/158 (47.5%)	Methadone and STD clinics; street outreach
TOTAL		172/1396 (12.3%)	

the rate among those who had not was 4.8%; indeed, a personal history of injecting drug use and/or an ongoing sexual relationship with a man who injected drugs, or both, were the two factors associated with a positive test result. The marked difference in infection rates among women in different geographic areas who injected drugs—1.5% in Atlanta vs. 58.3% in northern New Jersey—reflected the context of injecting drug use in the different cities and was consistent with the prevalence of diagnosed AIDS cases among other women who injected drugs or had other identifiable risk factors in each area. The factor most closely associated with higher rates of infection was the use of "shooting galleries," a milieu more common in the cities around New York and New Jersey than elsewhere. In all the cities, researchers found high rates of condom use with clients (Darrow *et al.,* 1990; Darrow, 1992; Miller, Turner, & Moses, 1990).

One of the participating centers was the San Francisco Bay Area, where the research group had been looking at HIV seroprevalence among women, including both sex workers and non-sex workers, since 1985. In 1985–1986, the infection rate among both groups of women was 4.4%, rising in 1987–1988 to 5.8% in women who had not engaged in sex work and 5.7% in those who had. Consistently, among the women who had traded sex for money, HIV infection was associated with the women's own injecting drug use, in contrast to the situation for no-sex-workers, some of whom had only sexual-contact risk factors (Cohen *et al.,* 1989).

The situation in other industrialized countries is quite similar. The prevalence of infection ranged from zero among 101 women tested in Copenhagen, Denmark, and 387 women tested in Sydney, Australia, to 77.8% among 18 women tested in Zurich, Switzerland. As in the United States, HIV infection was closely associated with both injection-drug use and the context within which the drugs are injected. For example, in Madrid, Spain, 1.5% of 165 women who did not inject drugs were infected, in contrast to 70.9% of 148 women injectors (Darrow, 1992).

The picture in developing countries appears to be quite different, however. Studies conducted in sub-Saharan Africa, Southern and Southeast Asia, and Latin America (Table 2) have found the factors associated with HIV infection to be low rates of condom use and a high prevalence of infection with other STDs, with little or no evidence of Western-style injection-drug use either by the women themselves or by their ongoing partners. As in industrial countries, the rates of infection varied widely according to the population studied, the locus of their work, and the geographic region. In sub-Saharan Africa, none of 89 women tested in Mogadishu, Somalia, 0.5% of 767 women tested in Borno, Nigeria, 16% of 50 women in Juba, southern Sudan, and rising sharply to 87.9% of 33 women in Ngoma, Rwanda, tested positive. In one city, Nairobi, Kenya, the infec-

Table 2. HIV Prevalence among Female Sex Workers in Africa, Asia, and Latin America

Location/date	Study	HIV+/all women tested (%)	Data collection source
Africa			
Yaoundé, Cameroon (1989)	Kaptue et al. (1989)	12/168 (7.1%)	Peer-recruited effort, bar workers
Mogadishu, Somalia (1990)	Burans et al. (1990)	0/89 (0.0%)	STD clinic
Mogadishu, Somalia (1990)	Ahmed et al. (1991)	1/155 (0.6%)	Four-district sample
Nairobi, Kenya (1985)	Simonsen et al. (1990)	259/418 (62%)	Pumwani district sex workers' STD clinic
Arusha and Moshi, Northern Tanzania (1991)	Nkya et al. (1991)	75/106 (73%)	Not available
Kinshasa, Zaire (1988)	Nzila et al. (1991)	432/1233 (35%)	Sex workers' STD clinic
The Gambia (1989)	Pepin et al. (1991)	6/355 (1.7%)	Not available
Asia			
Delhi, India (1988)	Singh et al. (1990)	1/701 (0.1%)	STD clinic
Philippines			
(1985)	Hayes et al. (1990)	203/25,391 (0.8%)	Registered prostitutes
(1987)		N/A (0.2%)	Registered prostitutes
Sydney, Australia (1986–1988)	Philpot et al. (1991)	0/231 (0.0%)	STD centre
Changmai, Thailand (1989)	Siraprapasiri et al. (1991)	87/238 (36.5%)	Workers at 14 brothels
Latin America			
Tijuana, Mexico (1989)	Guerena-Burgueno et al. (1991)	2/415 (0.5%)	Not available
Tegucigalpa, Honduras (1990)	Venegas et al. (1991)	8/181 (4%)	Registered prostitutes
Mexico City (1992)	Juarez et al. (1992)	0/482 (0.0%)	Not available
São Paulo, Brazil (1990–1991)	Fernandes et al. (1992)	66/600 (11%)	Not available
Buenos Aires, Argentina (1987)	Multare et al. (1989)	12/199 (6%)	Street workers

tion rate among 26 higher-class sex workers, women who work with businessmen and tourists, was 30.8%, compared with 65.6% among 64 working-class prostitutes, most of whose clients were migrant workers and others living in the same impoverished neighborhood. In the latter group, infection rose from 8% in 1980 to 59% in 1985 (Simonsen *et al.,* 1990), even though the women were participating in a long-term study of STDs.

In Asia, the rate of infection ranged from 0.1% of 701 women tested in an STD clinic in Delhi, India, to 36% of 238 female brothel workers tested in Changmai, Thailand. Although injection-drug use was closely associated with the early cases of HIV infection in Thailand, many researchers say that it is not a factor related to infection among female sex workers. It is interesting to note that the high rate in Changmai exists even though prostitutes are regularly examined for STDs by physicians. In Latin America, the infection rate ranged from zero among 482 women working in Mexico City to 11% of 600 women, most of whom worked in bars or on the street, in São Paulo, Brazil.

Although the prevalence of infection is high among some groups of prostitutes in each geographic region, the prevalence of infection is relatively low among other groups in each region. In each region, the prevalence of infection is greatest among the women who earn the least money, a factor that is also associated with higher rates of other STDs, and, in Latin America and the industrial countries, with injection-drug use.

The Nature of the Risk to the Workers

In the industrial countries, the risk of HIV infection for sex workers is most directly related to behavior, especially injection-drug use, that is not directly connected to their work. Data from the CDC multicenter study show that the rate of infection is 4 times higher among women who report a history of injection-drug use (19.9%) than among those who do not (4.8%) (Darrow *et al.,* 1990). The study of women working in Nevada's brothels (Darrow *et al.,* 1990) and other studies among call girls in Miami (Fischl, Dickinson, Flanagan, & Fletcher, 1987) and New York City (Seidlin *et al.,* 1989) found no HIV infection among women who had no injection-drug use history.

More recently, increased rates of both syphilis and HIV infection have been found among women who used crack, a smokeable form of cocaine, associated with increased numbers of both paying and nonpaying partners (Chiasson, Stoneburner, Telgak, Hildebrandt, Schultz, & Jaffe, 1989). One factor that may affect the women's vulnerability to HIV infection through fellatio is that many of them have cuts and burns on their lips, and burns on the roofs of their mouths, leaving a portal of entry for the virus (Judith Porter, personal communication; Joyce Wallace, personal communication). A 1991 review of research on crack cocaine use and STDs, including HIV infection, found that in five studies, it was increased sexual activity/number of partners, rather than selling sex, per se, that was associated with HIV infection (Marx, Aral, Rolfs, Sterk, & Kahn, 1991). However, in three of the five studies reviewed, the populations studied had other confounding markers of risk, such as injecting drug use or pelvic inflammatory disease, that made it more difficult to interpret the results.

In terms of sexual transmission, for sex workers as for any other population, the risk of HIV depends on a variety of factors including the background prevalence of infection in the population from which one or the other partners comes and the nature of the sexual encounter itself. It is generally agreed that the risk of infection from unprotected sex is greatest for anal intercourse, less high for vaginal intercourse, significantly lower for fellatio or cunnilingus, and negligible for hand genital contact, and that the use of condoms and other latex (or in some cases polyurethane) barriers substantially reduces that risk [Alexander, 1993 (draft)]. Therefore, where the predominant sexual activities are those at the lower end of the risk scale, and where the use of condoms and other barriers is high, the workplace risk to the sex worker should be low. Although the frequency with which female sex workers provide anal intercourse in their work is not well documented, most of those who have been asked this question have said they do not offer this service. Those who do generally charge more for it, which may reduce the demand. In terms of condom use, studies in the United States have found that 70–90% of sex workers report using condoms with clients (Darrow and Fischbein, personal communication).

Indeed, the greatest sexual risk prostitutes face in industrial countries appears to be from primary and casual personal relationships with men who are infected, primarily men who inject drugs but in some cases men who also have sex with men. Prostitute women, like most other women, are least likely to use condoms during sex with a primary partner, for reasons having to do with the nature of intimate relationships and issues of trust, common to all women, as well as the need for a way to distinguish between work sex and personal sex (Bailey, Fox, & Oliver, 1992; Cohen *et al.,* 1989; Day, 1988).

In terms of occupational risk, there is some evidence that the relative risk for HIV and other STD infection differs according to the work setting, the level of professionalism, the type of sexual contact involved, and the relationships between the partners (Cohen, Derish, & Sweat, 1992). In most countries, next to nothing is known about the prevalence of infection among the general population of heterosexual men from whom clients come, although a few studies have looked at specific subpopulations, such as truck drivers, military men, and migrant laborers. A limited amount of ethnographic information suggests that there are both class and cultural differences in the types of sexual services preferred by clients. The majority of transactions between sex workers and clients who contact each other on the street and in bars involve manual stimulation or fellatio (usually with a condom) and take less than 15 minutes. On the other hand, transactions involving sex workers and clients who connect through escort services or individual workers' newspaper ads involve greater privacy and a wider variety of sexual techniques and are more likely to last an hour or more. In this context, condom use has also become the norm, except in those establishments in which the management does not support, or actively discourages, routine use of condoms (Miller *et al.,* 1990; Shedlin, 1987). Thus, to the extent that sex workers define much of their sexual activity as occupational, risk of transmission of all STDs is reduced.

From Prostitutes to Clients?

Since 1978, epidemiologists and others who have written about STDs have used such terms as "core group of high-frequency transmitters" and "reservoirs of infection" to describe female prostitutes (D'Costa *et al.,* 1985; Holmes & Aral, 1991; Ronald & Aral, 1992; Yorke, Hethcote, & Nold, 1978). One particularly telling statement was this one in Piot *et al.,* (1987):

> Prostitutes are a major reservoir of STDs in Nairobi and are now probably playing an important role in the spread of AIDS virus as well. In this retrospective survey, evidence of AIDS virus infection was detected earliest in prostitutes and at a higher rate than in men with STDs, who are their customers. Prostitutes have probably contributed significantly to the introduction and dissemination of HIV in Nairobi.

The question is, if it was detected first in prostitutes, does this mean it first appeared in prostitutes? Or does it mean that prostitutes were studied first? Sometimes it seems that many epidemiologists think that prostitutes become infected from mosquitos. Nonetheless, it is important to know whether prostitutes are, in fact, playing a major role in the spread of the epidemic to others. As much as researchers have looked at the prevalence of infection among female sex workers, however, and expressed serious concern about the risk they pose to men, far fewer have conducted similar studies among clients or among groups of men likely to be clients.

One factor likely to affect client risk is the lower efficiency of female-to-male transmission than of male-to-female transmission (Padian, Shiboski, &

Jewell, 1991). It is therefore obvious that where the prevalence of infection is low among sex workers, the risk to clients from their prostitution connection will be negligible, and there is some indirect data that indicate that the risk of HIV infection is extremely low for male clients in industrial countries. For example, one study, in an STD clinic in New York City, found the same rate of infection (1.4%) among 138 men who reported no risk factors for AIDS except contact with female prostitutes as among 222 men who reported no risk factors at all (e.g., contact with either female sex workers or other men or injection-drug use)[1] (Chiasson *et al.,* 1988). In another study in New York City, 6 of 340 men (2%) who reported an average of 94 contacts with female prostitutes were HIV+. Upon further questioning, however, 3 of the 6 admitted other risk factors. The other 3 each had an average of 575 contacts with female prostitutes (Wallace, Mann, & Beatrice, 1988).

Looking at the statistics concerning diagnosed AIDS cases in the United States, as of September 1993, there were 27,783 AIDS cases initially reported with no identified risk. After attempts were made to follow up these cases, information remained incomplete for 15,184; of 12,599 who were followed up, 11,943 were reclassified as having become infected through the standard identified practices, 17 were probable health-care-setting infections, and 639 remained as unidentified risk. Of these, 342 adult males were interviewed, of whom 123 reported contact with a prostitute (sex unspecified). These 123 men represented 0.04% of 292,665 adult and adolescent males diagnosed with AIDS, which was a smaller proportion than the 0.8% reported in September 1987. Thus, the proportion of reported AIDS cases that may be attributed to sexual contact with a female prostitute is much lower than the proportion attributed to for example, homosexual contact (62%), injection-drug use (21%), documented heterosexual contact (3%), and even blood transfusion (1%). Of course it is possible that there are additional cases in which unprotected sex with a female sex worker was the mode of transmission, but other risk factors were reported that were higher on the CDC ordering of priority (Castro *et al.,* 1988; Centers for Disease Control and Prevention, 1993).

There remains, however, the question about the level of risk to uninfected clients who have sex with female sex workers among whom the prevalence of infection is relatively high. There are some indications that

[1]There is some evidence that crack may alter that picture, as a 1989 study found that HIV+ men (66.7%) were more likely to report contact with a female prostitute than men who were not infected (40.7%). However, the small sample size of men with HIV ($N = 12$), in contrast to the larger sample size of uninfected men ($N = 428$), makes it difficult to generalize from the study result (Chiasson et al., 1989).

the risk to the male clients is lower than the risk to female sex workers in developing counties, as well. For example, in Nairobi, Kenya, in 1986, 38 of 340 men (11.2%) who reported "frequent contact with prostitutes" were seropositive, at a time when 85% of the prostitutes in the same community were infected, even though condom use was rare (Simonsen *et al.,* 1988).

In the end, however, whether the risk to either prostitute or client is high or low, if we are to control the spread of HIV, it will be important to reduce that risk still further. Therefore, it is appropriate to develop prevention interventions that enable female (and male) sex workers to protect themselves from infection and, if they are infected, to protect their sex partners—paying or not—from HIV and other STDs.

PREVENTING THE PREVENTABLE: SEX-WORK-BASED INTERVENTIONS

Most of the research related to HIV and prostitution has focused on determining the prevalence of infection among female sex workers, with relatively little emphasis on determining the best approaches to take to reduce their risk. To some extent, this focus obtains because of a kind of bias in favor of "research" over the less quantifiable process of trying to change community-wide behaviors. However, to some extent, research in this area is complicated by the illegality of some or all aspects of sex work in most countries, not to mention the stigma that can affect researchers almost as much as it does sex workers.

Nonetheless, there are quite a large number of projects around the world. When one of the authors was with the World Health Organization Global Programme on AIDS, she reviewed the literature and talked with countless consultants and representatives of such projects, identifying 138 projects in 55 developing countries. Although industrialized countries were not included in the review, she was also in contact with representatives of more than 25 sex work projects in Europe and 10 in Australia and New Zealand. Before we review the characteristics of projects that have been well received by sex workers, we think it is important to look at the legal context within which such interventions have to be designed and implemented.

The Legal Context of Sex-Work Interventions

As is the case with some other populations that are highly vulnerable to HIV infection—men who have sex with men and injection-drug users (IDUs)—there is a long history of efforts to control or abolish the activity.

In terms of prostitution, one of the oldest laws was incised on clay tablets some 3244 years ago, in Sumer, requiring that good women be veiled on the street and prohibiting independent prostitutes from veiling themselves. After more than three millenia of dress codes, zoning laws, curfews, health regulations, banishments, and outright prohibitions, prostitution continues to flourish, affected more by economic up- and downturns than by police or health department activities. In no country is prostitution treated in the same way as other occupations, with the same paid vacation and sick leave, health insurance, workers' compensation, retirement pensions, and OSHA regulations found in other occupations.

Laws prohibiting prostitution are on the books in all 50 states in this country,[2] although the enforcement of the laws varies widely. Moreover, there are minor variations in the basic laws, as some states make it a crime to agree to, as well as to solicit or engage in, the exchange of sex and money or other compensation, while other states have yet to legalize such entrapment. Moreover, some states have enacted laws requiring anyone convicted on prostitution charges to be tested for HIV—a law that routinely bypasses clients, as thier charges are routinely dismissed—and, in some cases, laws making it a felony to continue to work after testing positive. California is one of those states, and in the spring of 1994, 20 people, including 12 women and 8 men, were serving time in state prison on felony prostitution charges (Teri Goodson, personal communication). Such measures have curbed neither the spread of HIV or other STDs nor the prevalence of prostitution (Alexander, in press; Institute of Medicine/National Academy of Sciences, 1988). The threat of such restrictive actions, however, may cause the persons most at risk—the homeless women, the injecting drug user working to pay for her drugs—to avoid HIV testing, and even routine health care, in order to escape identification. Moreover, where extensive police crackdowns have been implemented, prostitutes have

[2]As noted before, Nevada is the only state in which any form of prostitution is legal. The state law grants rural counties with less than 250,000 population the option to legalize brothels locally, with a mandatory health scheme requiring weekly examinations for gonorrhea and monthly examinations for syphilis and HIV, all at the workers' expense. As is the case in the Philippines, Thailand, Senegal, and other countries where mandatory health checks are in place, the examinations are often brief, perfunctory, and provided in a rude manner. Nor do most health examiners respond to other health care problems (Laurie Anderson, personal communication). The prevalence of STDs was stable, at a rather low rate, for most of the life of this system; however, when the state enacted a law requiring clients to use condoms, the low rate dropped almost to zero (Alexander, 1987), suggesting that condoms, not regular checkups, should be the primary prophylaxis against STDs.

tended to move elsewhere, to the next town or across a national boundary, until the repression lets up.

Mandatory health schemes, in which prostitutes are required to register with police or public health units, are often implemented in conjunction with prohibition, with the police, or special public health enforcement units, having the responsibility to check on sex workers' health and to arrest them if their health cards are not up to date. However, such schemes have a sorry history and have never had much success in reducing the prevalence of STDs (Brandt, 1987; Gibson, 1986; Harsin, 1985). The authors have been repeatedly impressed with the high incidence of STDs, sometimes including HIV, in groups of sex workers who are regularly examined by health care providers (e.g., in Chiangmai, Olangopo/Angeles City, and Mombasa, where such examinations are mandatory, and even in Nairobi, where they are voluntary).

Centuries of repression, and centuries-old distrust, make it difficult to establish effective HIV and AIDS prevention interventions through law enforcement agencies and detention centers, or even in STD clinics and other health programs. If the message is delivered by those who have been hounding them, the sex workers have a hard time seeing the message as something new, something for rather than against them.

Sex workers are quick to detect when the primary motivation for an intervention is to protect the clients or, worse, the "general population," from them, and they will tend to stay away. Such efforts are often accompanied both by media campaigns designed to deter men from having sex with prostitutes, thus hurting business, and periodic police "sweeps," to clear the streets of prostitutes, thus hurting prostitutes' lives. In some cases, police have waited on the sidelines while outreach workers have distributed information, condoms, and sometimes sterile injection equipment, only to swoop down when they leave, arresting everyone who has the incriminating materials on them.[3]

Other Barriers to Interventions

Sex workers and clients find each other in a wide range of places and resort to even more places to complete their transactions. In almost every country, both the contact site and the transaction site are to a greater or lesser extent underground, as sex workers and clients try to avoid being

[3]The first night Project AWARE outreach workers walked through San Francisco's Tenderloin District, police rounded up all the women to whom the outreach workers had talked, a common complaint of outreach projects everywhere in this country.

harassed, or arrested and fined or incarcerated by police. The exceptions are so few they are notable, being pretty much limited to a few cities in Europe.

Living on the margins of society affects sex workers' vulnerability to HIV infection and their openness to HIV/AIDS prevention interventions. The average work life of female prostitutes seems to be about 4 or 5 years, no matter what the country, and every country has some very young workers and quite a few in their 30s and 40s (Delacoste & Alexander, 1987; Pheterson, 1989). Because sex workers are outside the law, their ability to negotiate for safer working conditions, if they work for someone else, is often sharply restricted [Alexander, 1987, 1993 (draft); Day, 1988]. Although the primary motivation for working as a prostitute is economic, and sex work usually pays better than other available work, many prostitutes are in a precarious financial position because of the need to remain one step ahead of the law or an endless pattern of work interspaced with incarceration. For those who use drugs, the need to earn money to pay for the next fix can sometimes be overwhelming. All these factors contribute to sex workers' vulnerability to clients' offers of extra money for unprotected, or otherwise riskier, acts (Leonard, 1990).

The predominant sex work transactions can vary, considerably, from one place to another. In the United States, hand jobs and fellatio have become the most common transactions, considered to be easy to provide in cramped quarters and easy to control (Alexander, 1987; Miller *et al.*, 1990). In Australia, on the other hand, vaginal sex is the most common transaction, again considered to be easy to provide and control (Julie Bates, personal communication). In Nairobi, Kenya, only a small percentage of women who work around the tourist hotels include fellatio in their repertoire (although that may change, as a group of women working in a poor, urban workers' community were quite impressed when one of the authors demonstrated how to put a condom on a client orally). On the other hand, AIDS prevention projects have introduced the fellatio-condom tactic in such sites as Olangapo and Angeles City, and it has spread to other working communities in the Philippines (Norma Ravelo, personal communication).

Community-Based Harm-Reduction Approaches

Because of the urgency of reducing the rate of transmission, and the failure of traditional, repressive approaches, many countries have adopted a "harm reduction" model of HIV/AIDS and STD prevention. The term was first used in relation to injecting drug users, as projects to distribute sterile injection equipment were set up in such places as the Netherlands,

Scotland, and Australia, to reduce the likelihood that drug users would share needles contaminated with HIV. Gay men in many countries organized on their own behalf, sometimes with and sometimes without government funding, to begin the process of shifting the norms of sexual behavior to reduce their risk of HIV. By 1985, prostitutes and other sex workers in Western, industrialized countries had also begun to look at the need to change their practices, to insist on the use of condoms and other barriers in the workplace. The goal of all these groups was not to eliminate prostitution—as is often the goal of police, for example—but to reduce the risk, or harm, that AIDS has brought to the work.

The earliest behavior changes were made by people who openly acknowledged their behavior—self-defined sex workers, gay men, injectors. However, the growing body of research from around the world, and the growing body of experience in the field, has made it clear that the sex trade is extremely diverse, including both independent and arranged, or organized, transactions, with full-time, part-time, and casual itinerant workers. Those who are the most "professional" about their work (i.e., usually those who work on a regular schedule over an extended period of time) are the first to adopt routine safer sex practices.

The programs with the greatest success in reaching the often "hidden" populations of sex workers have involved the more self-aware sex workers in the design and the carrying out of project activities. Sometimes called "peer education," the most successful forms of this approach become more and more involved in what is really "community organizing," over time, as the sex workers on the staff, and the sex workers being reached, identify obstacles to the workers' safety and work out solutions, where possible. Prostitutes' collectives in Australia came up with the idea of "Ugly Mug Lists," flyers or newsletters containing enough information about dangerous clients—men who have raped, or tried to rape, sex workers—to enable their colleagues to avoid working with them. Within only a few years, this strategy has spread to projects in other countries, in every region of the world, laying the groundwork for a collective, community response to violence against prostitutes. A project in Calcutta, and another in Kathmandu, are supporting prostitutes' efforts to form unions, to negotiate with the managers of brothels with bad working conditions. In Yaoundé, Cameroon, Accra, Ghana, and Davao City, The Philippines, sex workers formed credit unions to enable women faced with family crises to borrow money. In Nairobi, a similar credit union enabled women to take turns having a day off, a day to take care of themselves.

Some projects—in Australia, in the United States—have opened drop-in centers where street workers, often homeless women, can take a shower, wash their clothes, even find some almost-new clothes in a clothing exchange, have a cup of coffee or something to eat, even take a much-needed nap. Many projects have used mobile vans—in San Francisco, New York, and Amsterdam, for example—to take services to the streets where the women are working, instead of waiting for the women to come to their offices. Vans are especially suited to providing health care, including STD diagnosis and treatment, anonymous HIV testing, methadone and other drug services, and emergency services to help women deal with the sometimes violent nature of their lives on the street. Sometimes, the van becomes a place of refuge, a way to get out of a neighborhood where police action is heavy or where there are drive-by shootings. And they are a good place to store large quantities of condoms, lubricant packets, bottles of bleach, and sterile needles to be distributed as you go.

Many projects have established good working relationships with drug treatment programs and have pressured the government to open additional programs, especially programs sensitive to women's needs, to reduce the time lag between applying and being admitted to them. It can also be useful to establish good relationships with other service providers, especially those that respond to violence against women (e.g., rape crisis centers and battered women's shelters), the staffs of which sometimes require sensitization before they can effectively meet the needs of sex workers without judging them.

When projects respond to a range of immediate needs, then the messages about AIDS prevention are easier to hear. However, it is important not to expect too much change too rapidly. One of the authors has been struck by the fact that many women, in many countries, have told her that it took them about a year before they completely shifted to safer sex practices, including condom use and lower-risk services. As with other populations, there is a lag between understanding the risk, understanding the need to use a barrier to prevent transmission, and changing the way they have sex. The changes are likely to happen first in the work situation, where it is relatively easy to tell a client, especially a new one, to use a condom, or even just assume the client's agreement to use one and put it on. It is not so easy to use condoms with regular clients, who are accustomed to not using condoms, or with lovers. With the latter, the decision to use a condom is complicated by the same issues of trust that other women face, as, despite the prostitution, the primary relationship is often emotionally monogamous. Moreover, after a day of exerting control over one client after another, most sex workers want to take off that mask and be themselves, spontaneous and intimate at the end of the day. For the behavior at home to change, their partners will also need to be involved (Alexander, 1987, in press; Day, 1988). It would also help to have a wider variety of barrier methods available, including nonirritating intravaginal microbicides. The female condom, already available in some European countries and beginning to be available in the United States, may also make a difference.

CONCLUSION

In summary, sex-work-related interventions to prevent HIV/AIDS and other STDs need to be designed with the interests of the sex worker as the main agenda. They need to consider the legal context and the effect of years of repression on sex workers' ability to care about, and take care of, themselves. Education is only one part of AIDS prevention, which also has to involve community organizing to change the context of the way they work and live. Handing condoms out, for example, is not very effective if the police confiscate them or use their possession as evidence of intent to commit a crime, as they do in San Francisco, London, and Bombay. If police hound women to keep a health card up to date, the women are not likely to trust the clinic to which the police send them. Laws that force them to get tested and jail them if they have no option but to continue to work will further interfere with the development of effective interventions. These practices and policies have to change.

If interventions are to effectively reduce the spread of AIDS, the messages and the message sources must be trustworthy, meeting and reflecting the interests and needs of the target groups (i.e., sex workers, managers, and clients). Prevention messages that warn men not to have sex with prostitutes have never reduced either prostitution or STDs. The intervention must start with the recognition that selling sex is a transaction that involves buyers as well as sellers and has flourished throughout human history. By involving the sex workers in the design and implementation of a project, it is possible to overcome some barriers and to help the women begin to change the context of their lives. In terms of the clients, who are significantly male, they need to be told to use condoms—with prostitutes, with casual partners, with girlfriends, with their wives—and perhaps reminded that prostitutes are, after all, experts in the art of having pleasure safely.

The picture is not terribly encouraging, however. The Centers for Disease Control and Prevention is preparing for a new prevention initiative, to begin in the summer of 1995. States are currently working with community-based organizations to decide how to allocate those resources, and while many are discussing supporting projects to work with female sex workers, few are thinking about how to get heterosexual men—whether clients or not—to be willing, or even eager, to use condoms. Although safe sex prevention messages are widely visible in some cities, such as San Francisco, they are all but invisible in others, such as New York. One of the authors has been dismayed that in more than a year, she has seen two subway ads promoting condoms and three television public service announcements in New York City, the epicenter of the epidemic in industrialized countries. One thing that has become clear, especially with the increase in reports that some gay men are negotiating away from the gold standard of 100% condom use—denying their risk in some relationships, daring the odds in others—is that HIV/AIDS and STD prevention campaigns and interventions have to be ongoing, for the long term. Virtually every study that has looked at the question has found that there is a major discrepancy between knowledge and behavior, something that should not surprise us, given that so many smokers continue to smoke. Changing community norms, which everyone agrees is necessary, requires more than ideologies and messages; it requires active, positive reinforcement in the communities and sites where people are most at risk.

In terms of sex work, policy makers need to address the impact of the law, and law enforcement practices, on the ability of sex workers to retain any control over their lives and, more specifically, their ability to insist on condom use with clients and to negotiate from a position of strength with lovers. A number of researchers are beginning to look at the impact of frequent incarceration on, for example, drug users' behavior when out of prison. Similar research needs to be done for prostitutes, especially those on the street, who also suffer from inordinate amounts of violence. One question that sex workers' rights groups are asking all over the world is, if prostitution were not a crime, and prostitutes were free to carefully negotiate with clients before they get in their cars, enter their hotel rooms, or let them into their homes/work spaces, would they be better able to recognize trouble before it starts and feel sure enough of themselves to get out of danger when it occurs?

In San Francisco, the Board of Supervisors formed a Task Force on Prostitution to examine the situation as it currently stands and to recommend some alternatives. If every city would do that, it might be possible to begin changing the laws or, barring that, to change local policies and procedures, such as confiscation or evidentiary use of condoms.

In the meantime, existing projects that work with sex workers need to be funded on a long-term basis, and funders need to consider a broader range of services than merely distributing condoms, information, and even needles. The stronger the community of sex workers is, the more will they be able to control the way they work, reducing both their own and their sex partners' risk of HIV infection and AIDS.

REFERENCES

Ahmed, H. J., Omar, K., Adan, S. Y., Guled, A. M., Grillner, L., & Bygdemem, S. (1991). Syphilis and human immunodeficiency virus seroconverstion during a 6-month follow-up of female prostitutes in Mogadishu, Somalia. *International Journal of STD and AIDS, 2,* 119–123.

Alexander, P. (1987). Prostitution: A difficult issue for feminists. In F. Delacoste & P. Alexander (Eds.), *Sex work: Writings by women in the sex industry* (pp. 184–214). San Francisco: Cleis Press.

Alexander, P. (draft, 1993). *Making sex work safer: A guide to HIV/AIDS prevention interventions.* Geneva: Global Programme on AIDS, World Health Organization.

Anonymous (1988). AIDS and sex (editorial, Jan. 29). *Lancet, 1,* 8573–8576.

Bailey, P., Fox, L., & Oliver, R. (1992). Heterogeneity among commercial sex workers and commonalities of condom use (abstract Po.D. 5600). Eighth International Conference on AIDS, Amsterdam.

Brandt, A. M. (1985). *No magic bullet: A social history of venereal disease in the United States since 1880.* New York: Oxford University Press.

Burans, J. P., Fox, E., Omar, M. A., Farah, A. H., Abbass, S., Yusef, S., Guled, A., Mansour, M., Abu-Elyazeed, R., & Woody, J. N. (1990). HIV infection surveillance in Mogadishu, Somalia. *East African Medical Journal, 67,* 466–472.

Casabona, J., Sanchez, E., Salinas, R., Lacase, C., & Verani, P. (1990). Seroprevalence and risk factors for HIV transmission among female prostitutes: A community survey. *European Journal of Epidemiology, 6,* 248–252.

Castro, K. G., Lifson, A. R., White, C. R., Bush, F. J., Chamberland, M. E., Lekatsas, A. M., & Jaffe, H. W. (1988). Investigations of AIDS patients with no previously identified risk factors. *JAMA, 259,* 1338–1342.

Centers for Disease Control and Prevention (1993). *HIV/AIDS surveillance report, 5*(3), 7, 17.

Chiasson, M. A., Stoneburner, R. L., Lifson, A. R., Hildebrandt, D., & Jaffe, H. W. (1988). No association between HIV-1 seropositivity and prostitute contact in New York City (Abstract 4053). Fourth International Conference on AIDS, Stockholm.

Chiasson, M. A., Stoneburner, R. L., Telzak, E., Hildebrandt, D., Schultz, S., & Jaffe, H. (1989). Risk factors for HIV-1 infection in STD clinic patients: Evidence for crack-related heterosexual transmission (abstract T.A.P. 112). Fifth International Conference on AIDS, Montreal.

Cohen, J., Derish, P., & Sweat, M. (1992). Different types of prostitution show wide variation in HIV and other STD disease risk (abstract Po.D. 5609) Eighth International Conference on AIDS, Amsterdam.

Cohen, J. B., Lyons, C. A., Lockett, G. J., McConnell, P. A., Sanchez, L. R., & Wofsy, C. B. (1989). Emerging patterns of drug use, sexual behavior, HIV infection and STDs in high-risk San Francisco areas from 1986–1989 (abstract W.D.P. 52). Fifth International Conference on AIDS, Montreal.

Darrow, W. W. (1992). Assessing targeted AIDS prevention in male and female prostitutes and their clients. In F. Paccaud, J. P. Vader, & F. Gutzwiler (Eds.), *Assessing AIDS prevention* (pp. 215–231). Basel: Birkhäuser Verlag.

Darrow, W. W., Deppe, D. A., Schnable, C. A., Hadler, S. C., Larsen, S. A., Khabbaz, R. F., Jaffe, H. W., Cohen, J. B., Wofsy, C. B., French, J. F., Gill, P. S., Potterat, J. J., Ravenholtd, O., Sikes, R. E., & Witte, J. J. (1990). Prostitution, IV drug use, and HIV infection in the United States. In M. A. Plant (Ed.), *AIDS, drugs, and prostitution* (pp. 18–40). London: Routledge.

Day, S. (1988). Prostitute women and AIDS: Anthropology. *AIDS, 2,* 413–319.

Delacoste, F., & Alexander, P. Eds. (1987). *Sex work: Writings by women in the sex industry.* San Francisco: Cleis Press.

D'Costa, L. J., Plummer, F. A., Bowmer, I., Fransen, L., Piot, P., Ronald, A. R., & Nsanze, H. (1985). Prostitutes are a major reservoir of sexually transmitted diseases in Nairobi, Kenya, *Sexually Transmitted Diseases, 12:*64–67.

Fernandes, M. E., Reingold, A., Hearst, N., Inglesi, E. A., Huges, V., Lima, V. C. P., Padian, N., & Frini, I. G. (1992). HIV in commercial sex workers in São Paulo, Brasil (abstract Po.C. 4190). Eighth International Conference on AIDS, Amsterdam.

Fischl, M. A., Dickinson, G. M., Flanagan, S., & Fletcher, M. A. (1987). Human immunodeficiency virus (HIV) among female prostitutes in South Florida (abstract). Third International Conference on AIDS, Washington, DC.

Gibson, M. (1986). *Prostitution and the state in Italy, 1860–1915.* New Brunswick, NJ: Rutgers University Press.

Guerena-Burgueno, F., Benenson, A. S., & Sepulveda-Amor, J. (1991). HIV-1 prevalence in selected Tijuana sub-populations. *American Journal of Public Health, 81,* 623–625.

Harsin, J. (1985). *Policing prostitution in nineteenth century Paris.* Princeton, NJ: Princeton University Press.

Hayes, C. G., Manaloto, C. R., Basaca-Sevilla, V., Padre, L. P., Laughlin, L. W., O'Rourke, T. F., Espinosa, G. E., Adrada, A. B., Mejia, P., & Cano, D. (1990). Epidemiology of HIV infection among prostitutes in the Philippines. *Journal of AIDS, 3,* 913–920.

Holmes, K. K., & Aral, S. O. (1991). Behavioral interventions in developing countries. In J. N. Wasserheit, S. O. Aral, & K. K. Holmes (Eds.), *Research issues in human behavior and sexually transmitted diseases in the AIDS era* (pp. 318–344). Washington, DC: American Society for Microbiology.

Institute of Medicine/National Academy of Sciences (1988). *Confronting AIDS: Update 1988.* Committee for the Oversight of AIDS Activities. Washington, DC: National Academy Press.

Juarez, L., Uribe, F., Hernandez, P., Urbide, P., Hernandez, G., Conde, C., & Calderon, E. (1992). Prevalence and determinants of HIV and other STDs in a population of commercial sex workers in Mexico City (abstract Po.C. 4191). Eighth International Conference on AIDS, Amsterdam.

Kaptue, L., Zekeng, L., Djoumessi, S., Monny-Lobé, M., Nichols, D., & Debuysscher, R. (1989). HIV and chlamydia infections among prostitutes in Yaoundé, Cameroon. *Genitourinary Medicine, 67,* 143–145.

King, D. (1990). Prostitutes as pariah in the age of AIDS: A content analysis of coverage of women prostitutes in *The New York Times* and *The Washington Post,* September 1985–April 1988. *Women and Health, 16,* 156–176.

Leonard, T. L. (1990). Male clients of female street prostitutes: Unseen partners in sexual disease transmission. *Medical Anthropology Quarterly, 4,* 41–55.

Mak, R., Plum, J., & Van Renterghem, L. (1990). Human immunodeficiency virus (HIV) infection, sexually transmitted diseases and HIV-antibody testing practices in Belgian prostitutes. *Genitourinary Medicine, 66,* 337–341.

Marx, R., Aral, S. O., Rolfs, R. T., Sterk, C. E., & Kahn J. G. (1991). Crack, sex and STD. *Sexually Transmitted Diseases, 18,* 92–101.

Miller, H. G., Turner, C. F., & Moses, L. E., (Eds.) (1990). Interventions for female prostitutes. In *AIDS: The second decade* (pp. 253–287). Washington, DC: National Academy Press.

Multare, S., Zarate, M., Boxaca, M., Martinez Paeralta, L., & Weissenbacher, M. (1989). Anti-

HIV antibodies in male and female streetwalkers in Buenos Aires City (abstract W.G.P. 21). Fifth International Conference on AIDS, Montreal.

Nyka, W. M., Gillespie, S. H., Howlett, W., Elford, J., Hyamuryekunge, C., Assenga, C., & Nyombi, B. (1991). Sexually transmitted diseases in prostitutes in Moshi and Arusha, Northern Tanzania. *International Journal of STDs and AIDS, 2,* 432–435.

Nzila, N., Laga, M., Thiam, M. A., Mayimona, K., Edidi, B., Van Dyck, E., Behts, F., Hassig, S., Nelson, A., & Mokwak (1991). HIV and other sexually transmitted diseases among female prostitutes in Kinshasa. *AIDS, 5,* 715–721.

Padian, N. S., Shiboski, S. C., & Jewell, N. P. (1991). Female-to-male transmission of human immunodeficiency virus. *JAMA, 266,* 1664–1667.

Pepin, J., Dunn, D., Gaye, I., Alonso, P., Egboga, A., Tedder, R., Piot, R., Berry, N., Schellenberg, D., & Whittle, H. (1991). HIV-2 infection among prostitutes working in The Gambia: Association with serological evidence of genital ulcer diseases and with generalized lymphadenopathy. *AIDS, 5,* 69–75.

Pheterson, G., (Ed.) (1989). *A vindication of the rights of whores.* Seattle: Seal Press.

Philpot, C. R., Harcourt, C. L., & Edwards, J. M. (1991). A survey of female prostitutes at risk of HIV infection and other sexually transmissible diseases. *Genitourinary Medicine, 67,* 384–388.

Piot, P., Plummer, F. A., Rey, M. A., Ngugi, E. N., Rouzioux, C., Ndinya-Achola, J. O., Veracauteren, G., D'Costa, L. J., Laga, M., Nsanze, H., Fransen, L., Haase, D., van der Groen, G., Brunham, R. C., Ronald, A. R., & Brun-Vézinet, F. (1987). Retrospective seroepidemiology of AIDS virus infection in Nairobi populations. *Journal of Infectious Diseases, 155,* 1108–1112.

Ronald, A., & Aral, S. O. (1992). Assessment and prioritization of actions to prevent and control reproductive tract infections in the third world. In A. Germain, K. K. Holmes, P. Piot, & J. N. Wasserheit (Eds.) *Reproductive tract infections: Global impact and priorities for women's reproductive health* (pp. 199–225). New York: Plenum Press.

Seidlin, M., Krasinski, K., Bebenroth, D., Itri, V., Paolino, A. M., & Valentine, F. (1989). Prevalence of HIV infection in New York call girls. *Journal of AIDS, 1,* 150–154.

Shedlin, M. G. (1987). If you wanna kiss, go home to your wife: Sexual meanings for the prostitute and implications for AIDS prevention activities. Annual Meeting of the American Anthropological Association, Chicago, November 18–22.

Simonsen, J. N., Cameron, W., Gakinya, M. N., Ndinya-Achola, J. O., D'Costa, L. J., Karasira, P., Cheang, M., Ronald, A. R., Piot, P., & Plummer, F. A. (1988). Human Immunodeficiency Virus infection among men with sexually transmitted diseases. *New England Journal of Medicine, 319,* 274–278.

Simonsen, J. N., Plummer, F. A., Ngugi, E. N., Black, C., Kreiss, J. K., Gakinya, M. N., Waiyaki, P., D'Costa, L. J., Ndinya-Achola, J. O., Piot, P., & Ronald, A. (1990). HIV infection among lower socioeconomic strata prostitutes in Nairobi. *AIDS, 4,* 139–144.

Singh, Y. N., Malaviya, A. N., Tripathy, S. P., Chaudhuri, K., Ghargava, N. C., & Khare, S. D. (1990). HIV serosurveillance among prostitutes and patients from a sexually transmitted diseases clinic in Delhi, India. *Journal of AIDS, 3,* 287–289.

Siraprapasiri, T., Thanprasertsuk, S., Rodklay, A., Srivanichakorn, S., Sawanpanyalert, P., & Temtanarak, J. (1991). Risk factors for HIV among prostitutes in Chiangmai, Thailand. *AIDS, 5,* 579–582.

Stary, A., Kopp, W., & Soltz-Szots, J. (1991). Medical health care for Viennese prostitutes. *Sexually Transmitted Diseases, 18,* 159–165.

van Doornum, G. J., Hooykaas, C., Huisman, J. G., van der Linden, N. M., & Coutinho, R. A. (1990). Prevalence of human T-cell leukemia virus antibody among heterosexuals living in Amsterdam, The Netherlands. *Journal of Medical Virology, 32,* 183–188.

Venegas, V. S., Madris, J. P., Lorenzana, I., Grillner, L., Cosenza, H., & Bygdeman, S. (1991). Human immunodeficiency virus infection and syphilis in Honduran female prostitutes. *International Journal of STD and AIDS, 2,* 110–113.

Wallace, J. I., Mann, J., & Beatrice, S. (1988). HIV-1 exposure among clients of prostitutes (abstract 4055). Fourth International Conference on AIDS, Stockholm.

Yorke, J. A., Hethcote, H. W., & Nold, A. (1978). Dynamics and control of the transmission of gonorrhea, *Sexually Transmitted Diseases, 5,* 51–56.

Women and AIDS in Developing Countries

MARCELA RAFFAELLI and JENNIFER PRANKE

Increasing numbers of women worldwide are being infected with HIV, the virus that causes AIDS. In the last year alone, 1 1/2 million women around the world were infected, and the number of HIV-positive women is expected to increase in coming years [World Health Organization (WHO), 1994a]. The WHO projects that by the year 2000, 13 million women will have been infected with HIV, and 4 million will have died of AIDS, since the pandemic began (WHO, 1993a). Until recently, women were "missing persons in the AIDS epidemic" (Rosser, 1991, p. 231), partly because of the initial definition of AIDS as a gay male disease and partly because of a tendency to focus on women as "vectors" of transmission, with emphasis on their roles as mothers or commercial sex workers (de Bruyn, 1992; Carovano, 1991; Hankins & Handley, 1992; Nichols, 1990; Preble, 1990). As the incidence of HIV has increased among women from all segments of the population in all parts of the world, attention has finally turned to understanding the factors that put women at risk and working to decrease the number being infected.

Over three quarters of the world's population is in developing countries,[1] which include all of Africa, Latin America, Asia (excepting Japan), and Oceania (excepting Australia and New Zealand) (United Nations, 1986). HIV/AIDS will have its greatest impact on women in the developing

[1]While we recognize that some readers may find the term "developing country" objectionable, we use it in this chapter for lack of a widely accepted alternative.

MARCELA RAFFAELLI • Department of Psychology, University of Nebraska, Lincoln, NE 68588-0308. *JENNIFER PRANKE* • Department of Psychology, Rutgers University, New Brunswick, NJ 08903.

Women at Risk: Issues in the Primary Prevention of AIDS, edited by Ann O'Leary and Loretta Sweet Jemmott. Plenum Press, New York, 1995.

world, where unprotected heterosexual intercourse has been and will continue to be the predominant mode of HIV transmission (WHO, 1993b). In this chapter, we describe factors that contribute to women's risk of HIV infection, summarize the HIV/AIDS situation in developing countries, and discuss ways of preventing the further spread of HIV/AIDS among women. Due to space constraints, we do not discuss issues of treatment, disease progression, and reproductive rights among HIV-positive women; although these issues are of critical importance, their complexity puts them beyond the scope of this chapter.

FACTORS THAT CONTRIBUTE TO WOMEN'S RISK OF HIV INFECTION

Three main sets of factors contribute to the increasing number of HIV infections among women (WHO, 1993a). First, women are more biologically vulnerable to HIV infection during heterosexual intercourse, which is now the predominant mode of HIV transmission in many parts of the world; male-to-female transmission of HIV during intercourse is more efficient than female-to-male transmission (Brunham & Ronald, 1991; Padian, Shibowski, & Jewell, 1991). One reason for women's increased vulnerability is that during vaginal or anal intercourse, women have a large mucosal surface exposed, increasing the likelihood of transmission if their partner is infected. In addition, semen contains a higher concentration of HIV than does vaginal fluid. The presence of other sexually transmitted diseases (STDs) also increases the risk of transmission (Merson, 1993; Wasserheit, 1992) (also see Chapter 2), and many women have asymptomatic or undiagnosed STDs. For example, STD rates among women seeking care at antenatal, family planning, or gynecological clinics in developing countries range up to 18% for gonorrhea, 17% for syphilis, and 30% for trichomoniasis (Lande, 1993).

A second factor that contributes to women's risk of HIV infection is epidemiological vulnerability. Women's partners tend to be older men who are likely to have had previous sexual partners and are thus more likely to be infected with HIV (de Bruyn, 1992; Carovano, 1991). This being the case, women are infected at younger ages than men; for example, in sub-Saharan Africa, HIV rates peak for women in the 20–24 age group and for men in the 25–29 age group (Decosas & Pedneault, 1992). In addition, large numbers of women in developing countries receive blood transfusions to treat anemia during pregnancy or childbirth (de Bruyn, 1992) or hemorrhage after childbirth or illegal abortions (Kimball, Gonzalez, & Zacarias, 1991). Because many countries lack reliable blood-testing programs, blood transfusions continue to be a risk factor for HIV infection among women of reproductive age.

Sociocultural factors that constrain life options and sexual behavior represent a third set of influences on women's vulnerability to HIV infection. Women are more likely to be poor and uneducated than men (Holmes & Aral, 1991) and are thus likely to be dependent on men for their survival and for the survival of their children. In the context of unequal relationships, and in settings where their wage-earning abilities are limited, women may be afraid to risk angering or losing their partners by bringing up monogamy or condom use, and leaving an uncooperative partner is not seen as a realistic option (Weiss & Gupta, 1993). Furthermore, women who do have to support themselves may find that they have to exchange sex for money, goods, favors (including career advancement), and other services (Carballo, Tawil, & Holmes, 1991), placing themselves at risk of exposure to HIV.

Other sociocultural factors that enhance women's vulnerability are beliefs about sexual behavior and gender roles. Many societies value female virginity at marriage but grant sexual freedom to unmarried men; in addition, women are expected to be less knowledgeable about sex than men and may be stigmatized or punished for seeking information about sex (Carovano, 1991; Weiss & Gupta, 1993). Additionally, sex is often nonconsensual (Heise, 1992), limiting women's ability to control their sexual behavior and protect themselves from HIV infection (Weiss & Gupta, 1993). Finally, the most effective ways of preventing HIV infection—abstinence and condom use—also prevent pregnancy, which is problematic in cultures in which a woman's primary role is that of mother. Many women in developing countries do not use any method of family planning; contraceptive prevalence ranges from under 10% in sub-Saharan Africa to around 60% in Latin America, and condoms are rarely the method of choice (Robey, Rutstein, Morris, & Blackburn, 1992).

For a variety of reasons, then, women are at ever-increasing risk of HIV infection. Women in different countries are affected to varying degrees by these risk factors. In the next section, we present regional reports on the HIV/AIDS situation and describe the special challenges faced by women in different parts of the developing world.

REGIONAL DIMENSIONS OF THE HIV/AIDS PANDEMIC

Africa

Epidemiology of HIV/AIDS

As of June 1994, 329,538 cumulative adult and pediatric AIDS cases had been reported by African countries. However, these statistics seriously underrepresent the scope of the epidemic, due to underdiagnosis, underreporting, and delays in reporting. The WHO estimates that in fact over 2.5 million African adults have developed AIDS since the pandemic began (WHO, 1994b). The impact of HIV/AIDS has not been uniform across the African continent; the epidemic is highly variable from country to country and even within countries (de Zalduondo, Msamanga, & Chen, 1989). Sub-Saharan Africa (particularly east and central Africa) has been most affected, with an estimated 10 million adult HIV infections, and 2 million AIDS deaths, as of June 1994 (WHO, 1994b). North Africa and the Middle East have been less affected, with an estimated 100,000 HIV infections to date (WHO, 1994b).

HIV/AIDS is having a devastating impact on the female populations of many African nations. Indeed, it is estimated that 80% of all HIV-positive women in the world are currently found in sub-Saharan Africa (Orubuloye, Caldwell, & Caldwell, 1993). Heterosexual transmission has been the main route of spread of HIV in most African countries since the beginning of the epidemic, and cases among women outnumber those among men by a ratio of 6:5. Thus far, over 5 million African women of childbearing age have been infected (WHO, 1994a), and HIV infections among women are expected to increase. As the number of HIV-positive women rises, millions of infants will also be infected, and millions more will be healthy but orphaned before the age of 10 (Preble, 1990).

Although women who engage in commercial sex continue to be at the highest risk of HIV infection, the pandemic moved into the general population several years ago. Extremely high seroprevalence rates (ranging from 31% to 88%) were reported for small samples of commercial sex workers during the 1980s (e.g., Kreiss *et al.,* 1986; Van de Perre *et al.,* 1985). More unexpectedly, recent sentinel studies of women from the general population show that growing numbers are HIV-positive. Seroprevalence rates among large samples of women attending prenatal or antenatal clinics in urban settings were 4.9% in Kenya (Hunter, Maggwa, Mati, Tukei, & Mbugua, 1994), 5.9% in Zaire (Batter, Nsuami, Baangi, & Ryder, 1993), 15% in Tanzania (Kigadye *et al.,* 1993), 18.7% in Burundi (Buzingo *et al.,* 1993), and 32% in Rwanda (Allen *et al.,* 1991). In addition, surveys of women in rural areas, considered to be at the lowest risk, reveal lower but ominous infection rates: 1.3% in Kenya (Valadez & King, 1993), 2.1% in Burundi (Buzingo *et al.,* 1993), 2.7% in Rwanda (Dushimimana *et al.,* 1993), 3.8% in Zaire (Green *et al.,* 1994), and 8.8% in Uganda (Wagner, Kamali, Nunn, Kengeya-Kayondo, & Muldur, 1993).

It is clear from these statistics that African women, particularly those from east and central African countries, are at tremendous risk of HIV infection. Perhaps most alarmingly, many women at low behavioral risk are being infected. In one large-scale study, 25% of urban Rwandan women with one lifetime sex partner, and 40% of those with two lifetime sex partners, tested positive for HIV (Allen *et al.,* 1991). Another study demonstrated that Kenyan women with two lifetime sexual partners were 2.5 times as likely to be HIV-positive as women with only one lifetime partner (Hunter *et al.,* 1994). Researchers conclude that for many African women, the main risk of HIV infection is not their own sexual behavior but that of their male partners, posing a challenge to intervention development.

Regional Considerations

Much has been written about the cultural, social, historical, economic, and political factors that shaped the AIDS epidemic in Africa (e.g., Barnett & Blaikie, 1992; Hickson & Mokhobo, 1992; Hrdy, 1987; Jochelson, Mothibeli, & Leger, 1991; Kane *et al.,* 1993; McGrath *et al.,* 1993; Sanders & Sambo, 1991; Schoepf, 1993; Scott & Mercer, 1994; Ulin, 1992; Van de Walle, 1990). Contributing factors include not only cultural definitions of gender roles, which influence sexual behavior most directly, but also poverty; overpopulation; civil unrest; inadequate medical systems and general ill-health (including high rates of STDs); the migrant labor system; the trucking industry; rural-to-urban migration and displacement of populations due to war, drought, and famine; and limited economic opportunities for women. These factors facilitated the rapid spread of HIV in Africa and represent major barriers to women's ability to decrease their risk of infection.

One topic that has been the focus of much attention is prostitution [although the use of the term "prostitution" to characterize the varied forms taken by survival sex in Africa has been questioned (e.g., Seidel, 1993; de Zalduondo, 1991) (see also Chapter 9)]. Because of economic constraints and the disruption of traditional family and social systems, many women must exchange sex to survive; strategies range from the straightforward exchange of sex for money to relationships involving friendship, gifts, and other forms of support. Women who migrate to cities, unable to pursue traditional women's work of growing food crops and trading but unprepared for the urban job market, are particularly likely to engage in sex as a means of survival (Ulin, 1992).

Another issue that has received a great deal of attention is vertical transmission of HIV in sub-Saharan Africa, where over 80% of the world's HIV-infected children are found (WHO, 1994a). A major barrier to preventing vertical transmission is that in most African cultures, childbearing is strongly valued (e.g., Hickson & Mokhobo, 1992; Scott & Mercer, 1994). Women who do not have children may be subject to divorce, physical harm, and public censure; because of this attitude, HIV-positive women are unwilling to tell their partners of their serostatus (Heyward *et al.,* 1993; Ryder *et al.,* 1991). Given the value placed on childbearing, programs aimed at limiting the fertility of HIV-positive women have been largely unsuccessful (e.g., Allen *et al.,* 1993; Heyward et al., 1993).

Asia

Epidemiology of HIV/AIDS

As of June 1994, 8739 AIDS cases had been reported to the WHO by the countries of south and southeast Asia (WHO, 1994b). The AIDS pandemic is a recent arrival in this part of the world, with extensive spread of HIV beginning only in the mid to late 1980s, and the epidemiological picture is changing rapidly. Official numbers greatly underrepresent the scope of the epidemic; the WHO estimates that in the past year there has been an 8-fold increase in AIDS cases, which are thought to number 250,000. Asia now accounts for 6% of the world's estimated AIDS cases, up from 1% a year ago (WHO, 1994a). Because over half the world's population is found in Asia, many analysts fear that the impact of the HIV/AIDS pandemic in this region will ultimately surpass that in Africa (e.g., Merson, 1993). The WHO estimates that over 2.5 million Asian adults are already infected with HIV and projects that over 10 million will be infected by the year 2000 (WHO, 1994a).

The majority of AIDS cases in Asia have been reported in Thailand, India, and Myanmar (WHO, 1994b). Initial AIDS cases occurred among injection-drug users (IDUs), and HIV seroprevalence rates of over 50% were found by the late 1980s among IDUs in Bangkok (WHO, 1992), Myanmar (WHO, 1993b), and northeast India (Sarkar *et al.,* 1993). The HIV/AIDS situation in Asia is dynamic and is evolving rapidly in other countries and among specific populations within countries; during the last few years, transmission has spread rapidly to other groups, including women. Currently, HIV prevalence ratios among adult men and women in south and southeast Asia are around 1.5:1 (WHO, 1993a), but women are now being infected at much higher rates than men (Moodie & Aboagye-Kwarteng, 1993).

Women who engage in commercial sex constitute the group at greatest risk for HIV infection in Asia. Recent dramatic increases in seroprevalence rates have been observed among sex workers in Thailand (from 3.5% in 1989 to 23.8% in 1992) and Bombay (from 1.1% in 1986 to 18.1% in 1990 and 34.4% in 1992) (Berkley, 1993). Although few studies have been conducted with women in the general population, there is evidence that they are at heightened risk. One indicator of women's risk is that their partners are increasingly likely to be infected. HIV seroprevalence rates among men seeking care for conventional STDs increased from zero in 1989 to 6% in 1992 in Thailand and from 2% in 1990 to 9% in 1991 in

Myanmar (Merson, 1993). High infection rates are also found in males from the general population; e.g., in 1992, 3.5% of 21-year-old Thai military recruits tested positive for HIV (WHO, 1994a). These growing infection rates among men are having repercussions in their partners: Seroprevalence rates among new mothers in Thailand went from zero in 1989 to 1% in June of 1992 (Berkley, 1993); in several provinces, prevalence rates were over 4% (WHO, 1993b). Asian women will be increasingly affected by HIV/AIDS in the next few years, and the potential for devastation is tremendous, given the rapidity with which HIV is spreading.

Regional Considerations

The HIV/AIDS epidemic in south and southeast Asia has been firmly linked in the popular, medical, and academic press to the sex industry (Lyttleton, 1994). More so than in any part of the world, female commercial sex workers are held responsible for the heterosexual spread of HIV. While it is true that engaging in commercial sex has been shown to put men at significant risk for HIV infection (e.g., Celentano *et al.,* 1993; Nopkesorn *et al.,* 1993), the emphasis on sex workers as a "reservoir" of infection obscures the magnitude of the threat to the women themselves. In fact, for Asian women, sex work is becoming an increasingly dangerous profession; one longitudinal study found seroconversion rates of 10% per month among women working in 14 brothels in one province (Siraprapasiri *et al.,* 1991).

The sex industry has a long history in Asian countries, and large segments of the population are thought to be involved as either purchasers or providers of commercial sex services. Although the international press has focused on sex tourism, it appears that local demand plays the most significant role in the spread of HIV; between 43% and 97% of Thai men surveyed have patronized a brothel at some point in their lives (Celentano *et al.,* 1993; Lyttleton, 1994; Nopkesorn et al., 1993; Weniger *et al.,* 1991). On the supply side, the figures are equally overwhelming; estimates of the number of female prostitutes in Thailand range from government figures of under 100,000 to the more generally accepted figure of 500,000 (Berkley, 1993; Lyttleton, 1994), and *Time* magazine reports a figure of 2 million (Hornblower, 1993).

Efforts to halt heterosexual transmission of HIV in Asia have focused on the commercial sex industry, and innovative programs targeting brothel owners, sex workers, and clients have achieved some measure of success (Berkley, 1993; Celentano *et al.,* 1993). However, given the rapidity with which HIV is spreading and its movement into the general population, further efforts are desperately needed. The success of prevention efforts is also threatened by a disturbing trend for ever-younger girls to become involved in the sex industry. The AIDS epidemic has resulted in an increased demand for child prostitutes, who are thought to be "clean." The number of girls involved in the sex industry is unknown, but appears to be large. One survey in northern Thailand found only 5 girls ages 13 and 14 in nine villages studied; the others had gone south to work in brothels (Simons, 1994). Many of these children are kidnapped or purchased by brothel owners and live a life of virtual slavery (Simons, 1994). Further, because children's tissues often tear during sex with adults, young prostitutes quickly become infected with HIV. The coerced involvement of young women and girls in the commercial sex industry is unlikely to be reversed without government (and international) intervention and represents a great source of risk for HIV infection as well as a human rights violation.

Latin America and the Caribbean

Epidemiology of HIV/AIDS

As of June 1994, approximately 102,000 AIDS cases had been reported in Latin America and the Caribbean. As in other regions, these figures underestimate the actual extent of the epidemic; the WHO estimates that to date, over 450,000 adults have developed AIDS, and over 2 million have been infected with HIV (WHO, 1994b). Brazil and Mexico account for the majority of cases in this region.

Transmission patterns differed by subregion in the early years of the epidemic. In Latin America, initial HIV infections occurred among homosexual or bisexual men, with heterosexual transmission becoming a significant mode of spread only in the late 1980s. Dramatic changes in the male-to-female ratio of AIDS cases have been seen in recent years; e.g., in Brazil, the ratio dropped from 9.7:1 in 1987 to 4.6:1 in 1992, and a similar trend was observed in Mexico (Pan American Health Organization, 1993). In contrast, heterosexual transmission has predominated in most of the Caribbean for at least a decade, and the male-to-female ratio has remained at about 2:1 for the past 6 years.

Most AIDS cases (80%) in the Latin American and Caribbean region have occurred in men, but in recent years the epidemiological pattern has shifted, and increasing numbers of women are becoming infected. Seroprevalence studies of different subgroups reveal that although women who exchange sex for money are at the greatest risk, HIV is also increasingly found among so-called "low-risk" women, including women seeking prenatal care. For example, surveys conducted in Salvador, Brazil, during 1989 found seroprevalence rates of 13.3% among female prostitutes and 0.9% among new mothers (Ivo-dos-Santos *et al.,* 1991). A similar study in Costa Rica revealed that 2% of sex workers presenting at an STD clinic, and 0.4% of pregnant women surveyed, tested positive for HIV (Elizondo,

Shultz, Baum, & Herrera, 1993). In large-scale surveys, 0.82% of women randomly sampled from 14 postpartum wards in Rio de Janeiro hospitals (May, Perez, Pinto, Schechter, & Ramos-Filho, 1993) and 0.97% of pregnant women tested in São Paulo (Santos *et al.,* 1993) were HIV-positive. Although the seroprevalence rates currently found in Latin countries are low compared to those found in other developing countries, it is apparent that HIV has moved into the general population of women and that cases among women (and their children) will continue to increase in the near future.

Regional Considerations

In addition to barriers that are common to poor women around the world, Latin women must deal with additional ones that are typical of the countries in which they live. One feature of Latin culture that contributes directly to women's risk of HIV infection is that a high proportion of men engage in sexual activity with both same-sex and opposite-sex partners (Carrier, 1976, 1985; Parker, 1987; Parker & Carballo, 1990). For example, a six-city study of Mexican men recruited at "gay" locations (e.g., gay discos and bars, gay organizations, parks frequented by gay men) revealed that 27% of the sample had engaged in sex with women as well as men in the previous year (Izazola-Licea *et al.,* 1991). In contrast to North America and Europe, where the majority of early AIDS victims were homosexual men, in most Latin American countries, a sizable proportion of early AIDS cases occurred in bisexual men (Parker, 1987; Quinn, Zacarias, & St. John, 1989). The rapid spread of HIV into the general population of women can be attributed in part to high seroprevalence rates among bisexual men (e.g., Cortes *et al.,* 1989), particularly since heterosexual anal intercourse (a practice that facilitates HIV transmission) is common in Latin countries (Carrier, 1976, 1985; Parker, 1987).

An additional feature of many Latin countries is the culture of machismo, or male superiority and female subordination (Carrier, 1976; Pick de Weiss, Atkins, Gribble, & Andrade-Palos, 1991). Although machismo has positive connotations (e.g., the belief that a "real man" is one who protects and supports his wife and children), it also has negative connotations (e.g., a "real man" needs to have many partners; a "real man" controls his woman's behavior). There is reason to believe that machismo may be a risk factor for HIV infection. For example, research in the United States has shown that less acculturated (i.e., more traditional) Hispanic men are more likely to have multiple partners (Marin, Gomez, & Hearst, 1993). Another potential source of HIV risk is the acceptance of violence as a means to control, which has been linked to high levels of assault in some Latin countries (e.g., Robinson & Epstein, 1994) and may result in female powerlessness and inability to negotiate safer sex.

COMBATING AIDS IN DEVELOPING COUNTRIES

All over the world, many women are at risk of HIV infection not primarily because they engage in "high-risk" behavior but because they are constrained by social, economic, and cultural factors beyond their control. In the continued absence of a vaccine, the long-term solution to preventing AIDS among women is to bring about major structural changes that result in reduced poverty, improved availability of and access to health services, creation of affordable housing for women and their families, education and job training, and the removal of legal barriers to women's financial independence. Obviously, such changes will not be achieved in the near future, but they will ultimately be necessary to ensure the well-being of women. In the short term, immediate action is needed to fight the spread of HIV among women. During the last decade, much has been learned about helping individuals protect themselves from HIV infection. In this section, we make specific recommendations for reducing women's risk of HIV infection in developing countries.

Empower Women and Girls

One feature common to women all over the world is that they have little power relative to men, and so are often unable to insist on preventive measures such as condom use or monogamy. Programs are needed not only to give women information about HIV and their options for protecting themselves, but also (and more importantly) to teach them skills for negotiating with their partners and to foster community norms that support prevention (Weiss & Gupta, 1993). It appears that small-group interventions involving skill-building for negotiation can be successful in helping some women change their sexual behavior (for a review, see O'Leary & Raffaelli, in press). Programs that are responsive to women's situations and needs, and that reflect the reality of their lives, hold the most promise of success (Carovano, 1991; Levine *et al.,* 1993), although interventions that focus primarily on the individual ignore the fact that many women will not be able to change their sexual behavior because their partners are uncooperative.

Target Men in Prevention Programs

It has been said that "[a]s a locus for change in the AIDS epidemic, women have the most limited options" (Sanders & Sambo, 1991, p. 160). This being so, prevention programs should also target men, emphasizing their role in protecting their partners and children (Merson, 1993). One successful intervention with long-distance truck drivers and their assistants in Tanzania led to an increase in condom use during sex with commercial sex workers; another program for Rwandan military recruits resulted in a drop in the incidence of STDs (*Public Health Reports,* 1992). Another intervention (Allen *et al.,* 1992) involved HIV-discordant couples in a longitudinal study. Couples watched an educational video, participated in a discussion group, and were given free condoms. After 1 year, 57% of the discordant couples enrolled in the study were using condoms (compared to 16% of couples in which only the woman was tested for HIV); however, it appears that men are more motivated to protect themselves than to protect their partners. Condoms were used more frequently when the man was the HIV-negative partner; only 2 of 23 men (8.7%) in discordant couples seroconverted, compared to 6 of 30 women (20%) whose partners were HIV-positive. These studies suggest that men can be induced to reduce unsafe sex, at least in the context of sex with nonprimary partners or when they are aware of their own risk. Motivating men to use condoms to protect their primary sex partners will be more challenging, but will be necessary as rates of HIV infection in men increase.

Promote Alternatives to Condoms

Condoms are a highly effective barrier to HIV transmission and can reduce the spread of HIV (e.g., Centers for Disease Control and Prevention, 1993; Liskin, Wharton, Blackburn, & Kestelman, 1990; Ngugi et al., 1988). However, experts recognize that it is probably unrealistic to expect consistent condom use in low-seroprevalence situations, particularly in long-term partnerships (e.g., Holmes & Aral, 1991). There are many reasons for this difficulty, including low perceptions of risk; cost and availability issues; association in many cultures of condoms with infidelity, mistrust, and prostitution; misconceptions about condoms (e.g., belief that they cause infertility or illness); and perceptions of diminished sexual enjoyment.

Because of these and other barriers to condom use in long-term relationships, alternative prevention strategies are urgently needed. One innovative approach developed to promote monogamy in India uses illustrations of poses from the *Kama Sutra* (an ancient Sanskrit treatise on the art of physical love) to deliver the following message: "Many postures with one, better than one with many" (WHO, 1993c). Another strategy for long-term couples involves being tested for HIV together, using condoms for 6 months, and being tested again. If both partners are HIV-negative at both time points and neither is engaging in other risk behaviors, condom use can be discontinued within the partnership. One drawback to this strategy is that it demands a high level of trust and commitment on the part of both partners and may involve a degree of equality not granted to women in many cultures. The ideal solution for women would involve technological advances to develop a female-controlled method that is unobtrusive and permits conception while inhibiting HIV transmission (Weiss & Gupta, 1993).

Expand STD Treatment Services to Other Health Care Delivery Settings

Many analysts have pointed out that one way to reduce the spread of HIV is to increase efforts to diagnose and treat conventional STDs (e.g., Holmes & Aral, 1991; Wasserheit, 1992). There are several reasons this approach would work. First, the presence of other STDs facilitates HIV transmission in both women and men (Wasserheit, 1992), and thus a decrease in STDs would lessen HIV infection rates. Second, in many countries, STDs are more salient to the general population than is HIV, so incorporating HIV/AIDS into broader STD prevention programs could increase responsiveness to interventions. Third, if existing STD delivery services can be expanded to include HIV prevention, scarce resources will not be expended in creating new systems to deliver HIV/AIDS preventive services.

Because women often avoid STD clinics (where they may be stigmatized) or do not know they are infected, STD detection, treatment, and preventive services should be delivered in those health care settings where women seek care for themselves or their children. These settings could include primary care clinics, maternal and child health (MCH) clinics, or even pharmacies (Holmes & Aral, 1991). In addition, because childbearing is tremendously important to most women, integrating HIV/AIDS prevention into MCH programs would make HIV prevention more salient. In recent decades, significant progress has been made in MCH promotion, and valuable lessons have been learned about creating community-based programs and training indigenous health care providers (Lettenmaier, Liskin, Church, & Harris, 1988). Much of what has been learned about MCH promotion could be readily adapted to HIV prevention programs.

Educate Children and Adolescents about Sex

Because it is difficult to change a behavior once it becomes established, the best time to teach individuals how to avoid HIV infection is before they become sexually active. Although adults in many societies oppose early sex education because they fear that it promotes sexual activity, a growing body of research suggests that the reverse is true. Well-designed sex education programs have been linked to the postponement of sexual initiation as well as to effective contraceptive use once sexual activity is initiated (Grunseit & Kippax, 1993). In addition, industrialized countries that have the most open attitudes toward sex and make information and contraceptive services readily accessible to teenagers have the lowest rates of pregnancy, abortion, and childbearing (Jones *et al.*, 1985). The WHO has urged all countries to implement school-based sex education as a means of curtailing the AIDS pandemic (WHO, 1993d); because many youth in developing countries (particularly girls) leave school at early ages, sex education should begin in primary school and be supplemented by community-based programs. Broad-based education efforts are the best way of implementing long-term changes in norms and attitudes and should be considered a key strategy in the fight to prevent the further spread of HIV.

CONCLUSION

The AIDS epidemic highlights the lack of control women in most parts of the world have over their own bodies and destinies (Carovano, 1991). Since its appearance nearly 15 years ago, AIDS has gone from being a disease of rich men from developed nations to being a disease of the poor and disenfranchised (Kapila, 1990), and women's subordinate status contributes directly to their risk of HIV infection (Holmes & Aral, 1991; Merson, 1993). Many promising prevention efforts have been developed and encouraging results obtained in different parts of the world. However, in the continued absence of a vaccine to prevent HIV transmission, the bleak reality is that unless significant improvements are made in women's social status, millions will become infected with HIV during the coming decades. Until women have the power to decide for themselves such fundamental questions as when, with whom, and under what circumstances they want to have sex, they will be unable to control their risk of HIV infection.

REFERENCES

Allen, S., Lindan, C., Serufilira, A., Van de Perre, P., Rundle, A. C., Nsengumuremyi, F., Carael, M., Schwalbe, J., & Hulley, S. (1991). Human immunodeficiency virus infection in urban Rwanda. *JAMA, 266,* 1657–1663.

Allen, S., Serufilira, A., Gruber, V., Kegeles, S., Van de Perre, P., Carael, M., & Coates, T. J. (1993). Pregnancy and contraception use among urban Rwandan women after HIV testing and counseling. *American Journal of Public Health, 83,* 705–710.

Allen, S., Tice, J., Van de Perre, P., Serufilira, A., Hudes, E., Nsengumuremyi, F., Bogaerts, J., Lindan, C., & Hulley, S. (1992). Effect of serotesting with counselling on condom use and seroconversion among HIV discordant couples in Africa. *British Medical Journal, 304,* 1605–1609.

Barnett, T., & Blaikie, P. (1992). *AIDS in Africa: Its present and future impact.* New York: Guilford Press.

Batter, V., Nsuami, M., Baangi, M., & Ryder, R. (1993). Stable HIV-1 seroprevalence in child-bearing women (CBW) in Kinshasa, Zaire, masks a stable epidemic (abstract WS-C18-1). Ninth International Conferenceon AIDS, Berlin.

Berkley, S. (1993). AIDS in the developing world: An epidemiologic overview. *Clinical Infectious Diseases, 17,*(Supplement 2), S329–S336.

Brunham, R. C., & Ronald, A. R. (1991). Epidemiology of sexually transmitted diseases in developing countries. In J. N. Wasserheit, S. O. Aral, & K. K. Holmes (Eds.), *Research issues in human behavior and sexually transmitted diseases in the AIDS era* (pp. 61–80). Washington, DC: American Society for Microbiology.

Buzingo, T., Alexandre, Y., Kamuragiye, A., Nkurikiya, S., Shepard-Perry, M., & Herah, B. (1993). The epidemiology of HIV and AIDS in Burundi (abstract PO-CO7-2750). Ninth International Conference on AIDS, Berlin.

Carballo, M. C., Tawil, O., & Holmes, K. (1991). Sexual behaviors: Temporal and cross-cultural trends. In J. N. Wasserheit, S. O. Aral, & K. K. Holmes (Eds.), *Research issues in human behavior and sexually transmitted diseases in the AIDS era* (pp. 122–139). Washington, DC: American Society for Microbiology.

Carovano, K. (1991). More than mothers and whores: Redefining the AIDS prevention needs of women. *International Journal of Health Services, 21,* 131–142.

Carrier, J. M. (1976). Cultural factors affecting urban Mexican male homosexual behavior. *Archives of Sexual Behavior, 5,* 103–124.

Carrier, J. M. (1985). Mexican male bisexuality. *Journal of Homosexuality, 11,* 75–85.

Celentano, D. D., Nelson, K. E., Suprasert, S., Wright, N., Matanasarawoot, A., Eiumtrakul, S., Romyen, S., Tulvatana, S., Kuntolbutra, S., Sirisopana, N., Akarasewi, P., & Theetranont, C. (1993). Behavioral and sociodemographic risks for frequent visits to commercial sex workers among northern Thai men. *AIDS, 7,* 1647–1652.

Centers for Disease Control and Prevention (1993). Update: Barrier protection against HIV infection and other sexually transmitted diseases. *Morbidity and Mortality Weekly Report, 42,* 589–591.

Cortes, E., Detels, R., Aboulafia, D., Li, X. L., Moudgil, T., Alam, M., Bonecker, C., Gonzaga, A., Oyafuso, L., Tondo, M., Boite, C., Hammershlak, N., Capitani, C., Slamon, D. J., & Ho, D. D. (1989). HIV-1, HIV-2 and HTLV-I infection in high-risk groups in Brazil. *New England Journal of Medicine, 320,* 953–958.

de Bruyn, M. (1992). Women and AIDS in developing countries. *Social Science and Medicine, 34,* 249–262.

Decosas, J., & Pedneault, V. (1992). Women and AIDS in Africa: Demographic implications for health promotion. *Health Policy and Planning, 7,* 227–233.

de Zalduondo, B. O. (1991). Prostitution viewed cross-culturally: Toward recontextualizing sex work in AIDS intervention research. *Journal of Sex Research, 28,* 223–248.

de Zalduondo, B. O., Msamanga, G. I., & Chen, L. C. (1989). AIDS in Africa: Diversity in the global pandemic. *Daedalus, 118,* 165–204.

Dushimimana, A., Chao, A., Bulterys, M., Munyampeta, I., Habimana, P., & Saan, A. (1993). Socioeconomic status and preventing the spread of HIV-1 infection into rural Rwanda (abstract WS-CO6-3). Ninth International Conference on AIDS, Berlin.

Elizondo, J. A., Shultz, J. M., Baum, M. K., & Herrera, G. M. (1993). The epidemiology of AIDS and HIV infection in Costa Rica. *Bulletin of the Pan American Health Organization, 27,* 145–150.

Green, S. D. R., Cutting, W. A. M., Mokili, J. L. K., Nganzi, M., Hargreaves, F. D., Davies, A. G., Bopopi, J. M., Elton, R. E., Hardy, I. R. B., Jackson, D. J., & Klee, E. B. (1994). Stable seroprevalence of HIV-1 in antenatal women in rural Bas-Zaire, 1988–1993 (letter). *AIDS, 8,* 397.

Grunseit, A., & Kippax, S. (1993). *Effects of sex education on young people's sexual behavior.* Commissioned by the Youth and General Public Unit, Global Programme on AIDS. Geneva: World Health Organization.

Hankins, C. A., & Handley, M. A. (1992). HIV disease and AIDS in women: Current knowledge and a research agenda. *Journal of Acquired Immune Deficiency Syndromes, 5,* 957–971.

Heise, L. (1992). Violence against women: The missing agenda. In M. Koblinsky, J. Timyan, & J. Gay (Eds.), *The health of women: A global perspective* (pp. 175–195). Boulder, CO: Westview Press.

Heyward, W. L., Batter, V. L., Malulu, M., Mbuyi, N., Mbu, L., St. Louis, M. E., Kamenga, M., & Ryder, R. W. (1993). Impact of HIV counseling and testing among child-bearing women in Kinshasa, Zaire. *AIDS, 7,* 1633–1637.

Hickson, J., & Mokhobo, D. (1992). Combatting AIDS in Africa: Cultural barriers to effective prevention and treatment. *Journal of Multicultural Counseling and Development, 20,* 11–22.

Holmes, K. K., & Aral, S. O. (1991). Behavioral interventions in developing countries. In J. N. Wasserheit, S. O. Aral, & K. K. Holmes (Eds.), *Research issues in human behavior and sexually transmitted diseases in the AIDS era* (pp. 318–344). Washington, DC: American Society for Microbiology.

Hornblower, M. (1993). The skin trade. *Time,* June 21, 45–51.

Hrdy, D. B. (1987). Cultural practices contributing to the transmission of human immunodeficiency virus in Africa. *Review of Infectious Diseases, 9,* 1109–1119.

Hunter, D. J., Maggwa, B. N., Mati, J. K. G., Tukei, P. M., & Mbugua S. (1994). Sexual behavior, sexually transmitted diseases, male circumcision and risk of HIV infection among women in Nairobi, Kenya. *AIDS, 8,* 93–99.

Ivo-dos-Santos, J., Couto-Fernandez, J. C., Santana, A. J., Luna, T. M. S., Cunha, G. C. M., Moreira, L., Lemos, A. C., Dutra, M., Miranda, C., & Galvao-Castro, B. (1991). Prevalence of HIV-1 antibodies in selected groups of a Brazilian city with African sociodemographic characteristics (letter to the editor). *Journal of Acquired Immune Deficiency Syndromes, 4,* 448–449.

Izazola-Licea, J. A., Valdespino-Gomez, J. L., Gortmaker, S. L., Townsend, J., Becker, J., Palacios-Martinez, M., Mueller, N. E., & Sepulveda-Amor, J. (1991). HIV-1 seropositivity and behavioral and sociological risks among homosexual and bisexual men in six Mexican cities. *Journal of Acquired Immune Deficiency Syndromes, 4,* 614–622.

Jochelson, K., Mothibeli, M., & Leger, J. P. (1991). Human immunodeficiency virus and migrant labor in South Africa. *International Journal of Health Services, 21,* 157–173.

Jones, E. F., Forrest, J. D., Goldman, N., Henshaw, S. K., Lincoln, R., Rosoff, J. I., Westoff, C. F., & Wulf, D. (1985). Teenage pregnancy in developed countries: Determinants and policy implications, *Family Planning Perspectives, 17*(2), 53–63.

Kane, F., Alary, M., Ndoye, I., Coll, A. M., M'boup, S., Gueye, A., Kanki, P. J., & Joly, J. R. (1993). Temporary expatriation is related to HIV-1 infection in rural Senegal. *AIDS, 7,* 1261–1265.

Kapila, M. (1990). An international perspective on the impact of AIDS and national AIDS education policies and programmes. *Hygiene, 9,* 8–12.

Kigadye, R. M., Klokke, A., Nicoll, A., Nyamuryekung'e, K. M., Borgdorff, M., Barongo, L., Laukamm-Josten, U., Lisekie, F., Grosskurth, H., & Kigadye, F. (1993). Sentinel surveillance for HIV-1 among pregnant women in a developing country: 3 Years' experience and comparison with a population serosurvey. *AIDS, 7,* 849–855.

Kimball, A. M., Gonzalez, R., & Zacarias, F. (1991). AIDS among women in Latin America and the Caribbean. *Bulletin of the Pan American Health Organization, 25,* 367–373.

Kreiss, J. K., Koech, D., Plummer, F. A., Holmes, K. K., Lightfoot, M., Piot, P., Ronald, A. R., Ndinya-Achola, J. O., O'Costa, L. J., Roberts, P., Ngugi, N., & Quinn, T. J. (1986). AIDS virus infection in Nairobi prostitutes. *New England Journal of Medicine, 314,* 414–418.

Lande, R. (1993). Controlling sexually transmitted diseases. *Population Reports,* Series L, No. 9. Baltimore, MD: Population Information Program, Johns Hopkins School of Public Health.

Lettenmaier, C., Liskin, L., Church, C. A., & Harris, J. A. (1988). Mothers' lives matter: Maternal health in the community. *Population Reports,* Series L, No. 7. Baltimore, MD: Population Information Program, Johns Hopkins School of Public Health.

Levine, O. H., Britton, P. J., James, T. C., Jackson, A. P., Hobfoll, S. E., & Lavin, J. P. (1993). The empowerment of women: A key to HIV prevention. *Journal of Community Psychology, 21,* 320–334.

Liskin, L., Wharton, C., Blackburn, R., & Kestelman, P. (1990). Condoms—now more than ever. *Population Reports,* Series H, No. 8. Baltimore, MD: Population Information Program, Johns Hopkins University.

Lyttleton, C. (1994). Knowledge and meaning: The AIDS education campaign in rural northeast Thailand. *Social Science and Medicine, 38,* 135–146.

Marin, B. V. O., Gomez, C. A., & Hearst, N. (1993). Multiple heterosexual partners and condom use among Hispanics and non-Hispanic whites. *Family Planning Perspectives, 25,* 170–174.

May, S. B., Perez, M. A., Pinto, M. E., Schechter, M., & Ramos-Filho, C. G. (1993). High prevalence of HIV-1 infection in a representative sample of childbearing women in Rio de Janeiro, Brazil (abstract PO-C11-2856). Ninth International Conference on AIDS, Berlin.

McGrath, J. W., Rwabukwali, C. B., Schumann, D. A., Pearson-Marks, J., Nakayiwa, S., Namande, B., Nakyobe, & Mukasa, R. (1993). Anthropology and AIDS: The cultural context of sexual risk behavior among urban Baganda women in Kampala, Uganda. *Social Science and Medicine, 36,* 429–439.

Merson, M. H. (1993). Slowing the spread of HIV: Agenda for the 1990s. *Science, 260,* 1266–1268.

Moodie, R., & Aboagye-Kwarteng, T. (1993). Confronting the HIV epidemic in Asia and the Pacific: Developing successful strategies to minimize the spread of HIV infection. *AIDS, 7,* 1543–1551.

Ngugi, E. N., Plummer, F. A., Simonsen, J. N., Cameron, D. W., Bosire, M., Paiyaki, P., Ronald, A. R., & Ndinya-Achola, J. O. (1988). Prevention of transmission of human immunodeficiency virus in Africa: Effectiveness of condom promotion and health education among prostitutes. *Lancet, 2,* 887–890.

Nichols, M. (1990). Women and acquired immune deficiency syndrome: Issues for prevention. In B. R. Voeller, J. M. Reinisch, & M. S. Gottleib (Eds.), *AIDS and sex: An integrated biomedical and biobehavioral approach* (pp. 375–392). New York: Oxford University Press.

Nopkesorn, T., Mastro, T. D., Sangkharomya, S., Sweat, M., Singharaj, P., Limpakarnjanarat, K., Gayle, H. D., & Weniger, B. G. (1993). HIV-1 infection in young men in northern Thailand. *AIDS, 7,* 1233–1239.

O'Leary, A., & Raffaelli, M. (1995). Preventing the sexual transmission of AIDS: Current status and future directions. *Psychology and Health* (in press).

Orubuloye, I. O., Caldwell, J. C., & Caldwell, P. (1993). African women's control over their sexuality in an era of AIDS. *Social Science and Medicine, 37,* 859–872.

Padian, N. S., Shibowski, S. C., & Jewell, N. P. (1991). Female-to-male transmission of human immunodeficiency virus. *JAMA, 266,* 1664–1667.

Pan American Health Organization (1993). *AIDS surveillance in the Americas: Quarterly report, 10 June 1993.* Washington, DC: Pan American Health Organization.

Parker, R. (1987). Acquired immunodeficiency syndrome in urban Brazil. *Medical Anthropology Quarterly, 1,* 155–175.

Parker, R., & Carballo, M. (1990). Qualitative research on homosexual and bisexual behavior relevant to HIV/AIDS. *Journal of Sex Research, 27,* 497–525.

Pick de Weiss, S., Atkins, L. C., Gribble, J. N., & Andrade-Palos, P. (1991). Sex, contraception, and pregnancy among adolescents in Mexico City. *Studies in Family Planning, 22,* 74–82.

Preble, E. A. (1990). Impact of HIV/AIDS on African children. *Social Science and Medicine, 31,* 671–680.

Public Health Reports (1992). Prevention efforts slow worldwide spread of HIV. *Public Health Reports, 107,* 602–603.

Quinn, T. C., Zacarias, F. R. K., & St. John, R. K. (1989). HIV and HTLV-I infections in the Americas: A regional perspective. *Medicine, 68,* 189–209.

Robey, B., Rutstein, S. O., Morris, L., & Blackburn, R. (1992). The reproductive revolution: New survey findings. *Population Reports,* Series M, No. 11. Baltimore, MD: Population Information Program, Johns Hopkins University.

Robinson, L., & Epstein, J. (1994). Battered by the myth of machismo: Violence against women is endemic in Brazil. *U.S. News and World Report,* April 4, 40–41.

Rosser, S. (1991). AIDS and women. *AIDS Education and Prevention, 3,* 230–240.

Ryder, R. W., Batter, V. L., Nsuami, M., Badi, N., Mundele, L., Matela, B., Utshudi, M., & Heyward, W. L. (1991). Fertility rates in 238 HIV-1 seropositive women in Zaire followed for 3 years post-partum. *AIDS, 5,* 1521–1527.

Sanders, D., & Sambo, A. (1991). AIDS in Africa: The implications of economic recession and structural adjustment. *Health Policy and Planning, 6,* 157–165.

Santos, V. A., Salto, R., Fiszman, M., Carraro, A., Andriolo, A., *et al.* (1993). Seropositivity for HIV-1 in pregnant women attended from January 1991 to April 1992. (abstract PO-C21-3133). Ninth International Conference on AIDS, Berlin.

Sarkar, S., Das, N., Panda, S., Nail, T. N., Sarkar, K., Singh, B. C., Ralte, J. M., Aier, S. M., & Tripathy, S. P. (1993). Rapid spread of HIV among injecting drug users in north-eastern states of India. *Bulletin on Narcotics, 15,* 91–105.

Schoepf, B. G. (1993). AIDS action-research with women in Kinshasa, Zaire. *Social Science and Medicine, 37,* 1401–1413.

Scott, S. J., & Mercer, M. A. (1994). Understanding cultural obstacles to HIV/AIDS prevention in Africa. *AIDS Education and Prevention, 6,* 81–89.

Seidel, G. (1993). The competing discourses of HIV/AIDS in sub-Saharan Africa: Discourses of rights and empowerment vs. discourses of control and exclusion. *Social Science and Medicine, 36,* 175–194.

Simons, M. (1994). The littlest prostitutes. *New York Times Magazine,* January 16, 30–35.

Siraprapasiri, T., Thanprasertsuk, S., Rodklay, A., Srivanichakorn, S., Sawanpanyalert, P., & Temtanarak, J. (1991). Risk factors for HIV among prostitutes in Chiangmai, Thailand. *AIDS, 5,* 579–582.

Ulin, P. R. (1992). African women and AIDS: Negotiating behavioral change. *Social Science and Medicine, 34,* 63–73.

United Nations (1986). *Demographic yearbook, Issue 38.* New York: published by the author.

Valadez, J. J., & King, B. (June 1993). HIV prevalence among rural Maasai attending antenatal mobile clinics (abstract PO-C11-2865). Ninth International Conference on AIDS, Berlin.

Van de Perre, P., Clumeck, N., Carael, M., Nzabihimana, E., Robert-Guroff, M., de Mol, P., Freyens, P., Butzler, J. P., Gallo, R. C., & Kanyamupira, J. B. (1985). Female prostitutes: A risk group for infection with human T-cell lymphotropic virus type III. *Lancet, 2,* 524–527.

Van de Walle, E. (1990). The social impact of AIDS in sub-Saharan Africa. *Milbank Quarterly, 68,*(Supplement 1), 10–32.

Wagner, H. U., Kamali, A., Nunn, A. J., Kengeya-Kayondo, J. F., & Muldur, D. W. (1993). General and HIV-1 associated morbidity in a rural Ugandan community. *AIDS, 7,* 1461–1467.

Wasserheit, J. N. (1992). Epidemiological synergy: Interrelationships between human immunodeficiency virus infection and other sexually transmitted diseases. In L. C. Chen, J. Sepulveda, & S. J. Segal (Eds.). *AIDS and women's reproductive health* (pp. 61–77). New York: Plenum Press.

Weiss, E., & Gupta, G. R. (1993). Women facing the challenge of AIDS: Prevention and policy concerns. In G. Young, V. Samarasinghe, & K. Kusterer (Eds.), *Women at the center: Development issues and practices for the 1990's* (pp. 168–181). West Hartford, CT: Kumarian Press.

Weniger, B. G., Limpakarnjanarat, K., Ungchusak, K., Thanprasertsuk, S., Choopanya, K., Vanichseni, S., Uneklabb, T., Thongcharoen, P., & Wasi, C. (1991). The epidemiology of HIV infection and AIDS in Thailand. *AIDS, 5,*(Supplement 2), S71–S85.

World Health Organization (1992). Current and future dimensions of the HIV/AIDS pandemic: A capsule summary, January 1992. Geneva: World Health Organization.

World Health Organization (1993a). 13 Million HIV positive women by 2000 (press release WHO/69, September 7, 1993). Geneva: World Health Organization.

World Health Organization (1993b). *The HIV/AIDS pandemic: 1993 overview.* Geneva: World Health Organization.

World Health Organization (1993c). Indian NGO features *Kama Sutra* in safe sex campaign. *Global AIDSNEWS, 4,* 7–8.

World Health Organization (1993d). Sex education leads to safer behavior. *Global AIDS-NEWS, 4,* 1–2.

World Health Organization (1994a). 60% Increase in estimated AIDS cases worldwide mounting concern for epidemic in Asia (press release WHO/53, July 1, 1994). Geneva: World Health Organization.

World Health Organization (1994b). *The current global situation of the HIV/AIDS pandemic, July 1, 1994.* Geneva: World Health Organization.

11

Lesbian Women and HIV/AIDS

An Appeal for Inclusion

KATHLEEN M. MORROW

> . . . to believe that lesbians are not at risk for AIDS . . . I would have to know and agree with the standards by which we are judged to be safe . . . [and] believe that lesbians, unlike straight women, can get seven years' worth of honest answers from their lovers about forgotten past lives.
>
> ——Lee Chiaramonte (1988, p. 5)

GENERAL BACKGROUND

This chapter will focus on the unique needs of women who have sex with women. The virtual absence of women from the history of HIV prevention education efforts, with a particular focus on lesbian women and their unique needs as a subculture, will be discussed. Recommendations will be made addressing both research and prevention education needs as they pertain to this underserved population.

Initially deemed, in the United States, to be a disease of homosexual men [i.e., gay-related immune deficiency (GRID) and intravenous-drug users (IDUs)], the disease that we now call AIDS is beginning to be accepted by the scientific community and the general public alike as infecting and affecting all people, regardless of race, gender, religion, age, sexual orientation, or ability. There has been one exception to this global recognition, however, one hole in the fabric of understanding. Where do lesbians (i.e., women who self-identify as women-loving women) come into the picture?

KATHLEEN M. MORROW • Department of Psychology, Western Michigan University, Kalamazoo, MI 49008.

Women at Risk: Issues in the Primary Prevention of AIDS, edited by Ann O'Leary and Loretta Sweet Jemmott. Plenum Press, New York, 1995.

Many continue to doubt the possibility of female-to-female transmission of HIV. Even fewer seem to rally behind the need for women who have sex with women to be systematically and explicitly included in HIV prevention programming, treatment, and research. But one fact remains: Lesbian women have not only been *affected* by AIDS, they have been *infected.*

Treatment issues, as well as HIV education and prevention programs and research, historically have focused on gay males and IDUs. It seemed, if one were to rely exclusively on the early HIV/AIDS prevention literature in this country, that women did not get AIDS. And those who did appeared to have contracted the disease via injection-drug use or heterosexual contact with a male IDU or gay/bisexual male. At least that is what the surveillance statistics showed. Penetration by needle or penis has been given the most attention in prevention programming, while other routes of transmission, including oral–vaginal and oral–anal sex, have been virtually ignored. Little prevention information, whether targeted for gay men, heterosexuals, or lesbians, includes information on these modes of transmission. And even if these routes are included, the discussion is merely cursory.

Only recently has the notion of widespread infection in women become accepted as worthy of research. As political activists are aware, visibility for women who are HIV-infected has been long in coming, and even now the struggle continues. Often, it seems that what has been true for one population with this disease is not necessarily true for another. Gay men have different needs than bisexual or heterosexual men. Euro-Americans have different needs than Native Americans, African Americans, Asian Americans, and other ethnic and racial minorities. Most predominantly, it seems that women have finally been recognized as having needs unique to gender, which are further compounded by the complexities of racial and ethnic backgrounds, sexual orientation, and living situations.

After over a decade of an AIDS surveillance definition that was characterized by diseases and conditions associated almost exclusively with HIV-antibody-positive (HIV+) males, the definition was finally altered, in 1993, to include some HIV-related illnesses that are specific to women suffering from this disease (e.g., recurrent cervical dysplasia). However, as a result of years of surveillance according to the old definition, a significant number of HIV+ women, despite severe progression of the disease, often died categorized and diagnosed as HIV+, not diagnosed as having "AIDS" because they did not fit the narrowly defined list of opportunistic infections that made up the syndrome at that time. This deficiency points out that inherent in currently available surveillance statistics on AIDS in women is a gross underestimation and lack of validation of the suffering of women within this epidemic. Among these women, presumably, are lesbians.

Little attention has been given to this subset of the population within this epidemic. Heterosexual women have recently come into the forefront of the AIDS epidemic because of their rapidly increasing numbers of reported AIDS cases. Historically, they were present as partners and mothers, giving care to their partners and children dying of this disease. Similarly, throughout the history of the AIDS pandemic, the role of lesbians has been defined narrowly and almost exclusively as one of caregiver or activist or both (Corea, 1992; Reider & Ruppelt, 1988). Lesbian women stepped into the tide of the epidemic and offered emotional, physical, and financial support to their gay male counterparts hardest hit by the virus. Lesbian women began and supported many of the grass-roots political and community-based organizations that energized the AIDS movement, fighting politically to make services and treatments more easily and readily available through improved systems for drug treatment trials and more sensitive government disability services.

In the area of HIV prevention, numerous studies have been conducted with gay males, IDUs, and, most recently, heterosexual populations. If one were to scrutinize the history of the epidemic, one would find that rates of AIDS diagnoses reported today lag considerably behind the corresponding HIV infections transmitted years before. HIV prevention efforts, therefore, need to focus, not solely on the groups of people whose members are currently progressing into the final stages of AIDS, but also on those groups who currently have low, but not insignificant, prevalence figures. This would include women who engage in sexual activity with other women.

Empirically derived interventions, or components of interventions, that produce consistent and durable behavior change have been difficult to identify and generalize to all those at risk. Affecting the basic HIV/AIDS knowledge (i.e., definitions of HIV/AIDS, transmission routes) of the general population has proved a relatively easy task. Affecting consistent and *maintained* safer sexual and drug self-administration patterns has not. Possibilities for effective interventions include, but are not limited to, education to increase safer sex skills and decrease communication barriers between partners, access to HIV antibody testing, social norm changes, and efforts to use the personal impact of multiple AIDS-related losses in an individual's lifetime to affect risk perceptions of personal vulnerability to the disease (Kelly & Murphy, 1992). Lesbian women and their unique needs have not been included in HIV prevention programs. Some lesbians report experiences in which physicians and community-based HIV testing sites refuse to test them because of their status as lesbians, thus limiting their access to adequate and culturally sensitive HIV antibody testing (Morrow, Meinhold, & Fuqua, 1994b). Lesbians themselves rarely engage their own communities in dialogue about risk behaviors, let alone actively encourage and promote safer sex practices.

Lesbians have been informed from the onset of the epidemic that, due to their status as lesbians, they are not at risk for HIV infection, except through nonsexual means (e.g., injection-drug use, health-care-related accidents). One of the few seemingly effective components of HIV prevention programming (Kelly & Murphy, 1992) experienced by lesbians to date involves the tragic loss of many of their gay male counterparts. The assumption is that multiple AIDS-related losses increase a person's exposure to the mortality of AIDS and cause them to look more closely at their own risk. However, these losses (i.e., gay male friends) are still given an "other" status by lesbians (Croteau & Morgan, 1989). Armed with the rationalization from scientific and medical sources that lesbians are not at risk for HIV infection through sexual routes of transmission, lesbians view themselves as effectively separate from their male counterparts in the gay community, allowing them to distance themselves emotionally and cognitively from their own potential risk through unprotected sex. They do not equate their life-styles with those of gay or bisexual men and hence do not see the risk they subject themselves to with each episode of unsafe behavior. Because lesbian sexuality does not fit neatly into currently utilized categories of risk behavior, they are not considered at significant risk by medical, research, or prevention strategists. Few prevention programs currently address issues unique to these women: acceptable safer sex activities, accessible and usable safer sex materials, communication skills necessary to practice safer sex within the context of a lesbian relationship, and personal risk perceptions accurately appraising one's own risk as it pertains to the sexual relationship between women.

Intervention strategies in general continue to encounter difficulties in their widespread acceptance, efficacy, and use. Results are often correlational. Conclusions and recommendations drawn from the results are often broad and speculative. Within the drug-using populations, for instance, research to date has resulted in few empirically derived solutions to education and prevention questions. Generalities, however, include notions that the success of safer injection practices among IDUs is greatest with those who have injection patterns that are less frequent and less established. There is also a greater success among opiate users, as opposed to cocaine users, and among those users who are older (Kelly & Murphy, 1992). Consistent and regular use of condoms among IDUs remains infrequent. Within the gay male community, there was, initially, a vast amount of behavior change. Large-scale community outreach and social norm change programs resulted in more gay men consistently practicing safer sex, or at least using condoms for penile–anal and oral–penile sexual activities.

However, behavior maintenance remains inconsistent, and there is new evidence that suggests that younger gay males are not consistently engaging in safer sex [Centers for Disease Control and Prevention (CDC), 1993b]. Much of the behavior change initially noted within the gay male community was evident in white, well-educated, high-socioeconomic-status males and cannot necessarily be generalized to persons of other racial, economic, or education status (Kelly & Murphy, 1992). The CDC has long recommended the consistent and correct use of latex condoms during sexual intercourse to prevent the transmission of HIV and other sexually transmitted diseases (STDs). The use of the female condom is recommended secondary to male condom use, and nonoxynol-9 is recommended as well (CDC, 1993c). Interestingly, there has been no known study to date that includes issues related to protected oral–vaginal or oral–anal sex for the purpose of HIV prevention through the use of latex barriers for *any* community or population.

The majority of our knowledge base regarding HIV/AIDS, whether it be from the perspective of prevention, treatment, or psychosocial effects, is based on research with males. Gay men, in particular, and IDUs, have been most often studied. Many of these studies are descriptive or epidemiological or both in nature and have been reviewed elsewhere (Becker & Joseph, 1988; Kelly & Murphy, 1992; Kelly, Murphy, Sikkema, & Kalichman, 1993). Much of the difficulty surrounding definitive answers to the question of behavior change and maintenance is compounded by the virtual nonexistence of experimentally controlled HIV prevention outcome research. This is not to say that the vast numbers of descriptive and group intervention studies are unimportant or useless. On the contrary, epidemiological and descriptive studies often provide the theory from which controlled outcome studies can expand. However, behavior maintenance continues to be a significant problem in AIDS prevention, and attention needs to be given to discovering workable and effective individualized program components in this arena as well. This emphasis may yield sound data that can then be generalized back to larger community efforts. According to Kelly *et al.* (1993), there are only seven published controlled intervention outcome studies to date, only two of which include females in their subject pool. Neither included lesbians nor focused on barrier protection other than latex condoms.

Despite the lack of sound experimentally controlled outcome strategies (i.e., in which one independent variable is manipulated at a time and dependent variables are measured for indications of changes in behavior due to the effect of the treatment), there continue to be some common threads throughout the literature that offer hope to future prevention efforts. We know that substance use, especially that immediately preceding sexual activity, is associated with increased risk-taking. We also know that such factors as an individual's underestimation of his or her personal risk, his or her perception that safer sex is not the norm within the community, and the high reinforcement value of unprotected sexual activity are all associated with risk behaviors. Prevention strategists are also becoming increasingly aware of the impediments to maintaining behavioral change: competing survival responses, socioeconomic disadvantage, lack of access to health care, and cultural differences, to name a few (Kelly & Murphy, 1992). All these issues need to be addressed within lesbian communities, framed in a culture-specific context.

HIV/AIDS knowledge is quite well established: Most people can identify the most common forms of HIV transmission. Still to be determined, however, is the role that subcultural traditions, values, and belief systems play in providing the rationale for engagement in both precautionary and risk behaviors. There is particular difficulty when the behaviors to be targeted are socially stigmatized (Hahn, 1991). AIDS prevention programs continue to be impeded by our inability to effectively address these arenas. Again, lesbians and lesbian cultures need to be addressed in these arenas, as well.

Kelly *et al.* (1993) present three basic models for HIV prevention and education work that seem to offer the greatest promise of effectiveness: cognitive–behavioral skills training models, social norm change models, and multifaceted community mobilization efforts. It remains imperative that epidemiological and survey research continue. However, given the continued rapid escalation of HIV infection and the cost-effectiveness of primary prevention, it is also imperative that increased efforts be placed on experimentally controlled outcome studies (Kelly *et al.,* 1993).

THE ABSENCE OF WOMEN

Women are almost completely absent from HIV/AIDS-related research. It is this absence, and in particular the absence of focus on lesbian women, that this chapter attempts to address. There are, admittedly, a number of descriptive studies and reviews that include women as either primary IDUs or partners of IDUs; however, few even mention lesbians. Mondanaro (1987) neglected to mention lesbians at all in his article, which suggested avenues of approach in motivating health behaviors in drug-dependent women, one subgroup of women among whom it seems lesbians would at least be given some credence. Cohen, Hauer, and Wofsy (1989) are credited by this author for mentioning lesbians in the context of HIV as early as 1989. Their statements were inclusive only of lesbian IDUs; however, they did mention that lesbian sex should be included in discussions of sex in drug treatment programs. Feucht, Stephens, and Roman (1990) cite evidence of HIV transmission from female to male and state clearly that partners of IDUs, whether male or female, are at risk. Further, they report that more than 10% of black female IDUs in their sample reported having engaged in sexual activities with women. If female-to-male transmission of HIV is possible, it should be clear that female-to-female transmission of the virus is possible as well. Obviously, what literature exists remains inconsistent, as well as inconclusive, with regard to the necessity of including lesbians in HIV prevention programming.

Several studies specifically address women of color, appropriately so given their disproportionate representation among female AIDS cases in this country. However, only a few even remotely address *lesbian* women of color. DiClemente, Boyer, and Morales (1988), in their study regarding knowledge and attitudes among minority adolescents, included one true/false statement concerning lesbians: "All gay women have AIDS" (p. 56). It is not clear, however, whether any of the participants were lesbians themselves. Kalichman, Hunter, and Kelly (1992) surveyed both minority and non-minority women, 22% of whom reported high-risk behavior. Data on the sexual orientation of respondents were not collected, however, and questions regarding sexual behaviors engaged in did not seem to include female-to-female sexual activities. Kalichman, Kelly, Hunter, Murphy, and Tyler (1993) address the unique cultural needs of urban African American heterosexual women and speak to the need for cultural specificity in *all* HIV prevention education. All these authors, despite various degrees of inclusion of lesbians in their presentations, emphasize the necessity for culture-specific prevention strategies. Mays and Cochran (1988) recommended that AIDS prevention education be disseminated by people with whom the target individuals can identify. Prevention specialists must be influenced by, and influence, group norms. And programs must include skill-building that effectively meets the needs of specific cultural identities and living situations, including lesbian women.

Within the last few years, surveillance statistics kept by the CDC show a disproportionate increase in AIDS cases diagnosed among women. Recent reports from the CDC (1993a) state that women now comprise approximately half of all new AIDS cases in the United States. Historically, it has been assumed by the scientific and medical communities that HIV is transmitted primarily to women via sexual intercourse with males (i.e., penile–vaginal penetration) and the sharing of HIV-contaminated injection equipment. Admittedly, a majority of female AIDS cases currently being reported by the CDC can be categorized as cases of male-to-female transmission or injection-related transmissions. However, the basis of transmission of nearly 10% of AIDS cases in women is still classified as "risk not identified." This rate is over twice that of male cases in the same category (CDC, 1993a). In addition, among AIDS cases in persons age 25 years or younger, 11% of female cases are classified as "risk not identified," while only 4% of males are so classified (CDC, 1993a). The CDC readily admits that female-to-male transmission of HIV occurs, but mentions only theoretically the possibility of female-to-female transmission (CDC, 1993d). It is possible that the discrepancy between rates of male and female AIDS cases classified as "risk not identified" is due, at least in part, to a lack of data collection protocol relevant to female-to-female transmission.

It is important to note that, historically, women, as stated earlier, have enjoyed only cursory inclusion in prevention and treatment efforts within the AIDS epidemic. They have been denied access to clinical drug treatments trials, resulting in their being prescribed drugs that are still untested on women. Until 1993, many women died without an AIDS diagnosis because the opportunistic infections and diseases often contracted by HIV+ women were not included in the surveillance definition of "AIDS." As a result, many died without validation of their suffering or without having had medical and social benefits routinely given to their male counterparts (e.g., disability status and its federally mandated benefits)(Stevens, 1993). Additionally, this data collection practice omitted thousands of HIV+ women from our current AIDS statistics. It is impossible to calculate what AIDS case totals would be now if the current definition had been in use since the early stages of the AIDS epidemic (Corea, 1992; Young, Weissman, & Cohen, 1992)!

THE CASE FOR INCLUSION OF WOMEN WHO HAVE SEX WITH WOMEN

The rate of AIDS cases among women in the "risk not identified" category is currently twice as high as the rate among men. Additionally, there is a long latency between infection and onset of symptomatology of HIV disease. AIDS case diagnoses, as a result, lag considerably behind transmission and therefore presumably underestimate the growing rates of HIV seroprevalence in, as yet, undetected populations. It is thus imperative that any population that appears to be in initial stages of dissemination of HIV be strongly considered for HIV prevention education. One such population is the lesbian population, in which HIV seroprevalence is low, but not insignificant. Not to include this population is to be negligent.

Within the context of subcultural values and traditions, lesbians may be at risk of HIV infection through seemingly "nontraditional" modes of transmission. It is important to note that lesbian women are not the only people engaging in the sexual activities highlighted here. Males who engage in these behaviors with women or men or both, as well as bisexual women who do so, subject themselves to similar risk.

What are these routes of transmission? It is a long-accepted fact that four basic body fluids act as vehicles of HIV infection: semen, blood, vaginal secretions, and breast milk. This view remains undisputed. It is also undisputed that any person who engages in any single activity that allows for contact between any of these fluids of an infected partner and that person's own uninfected blood or mucous membranes is at potential risk of contagion. The bottom line is this: Behaviors that allow for this type of contact are risk behaviors, and lesbians engage in these behaviors (Morrow *et al.,* 1994b).

Lesbians can be IDUs and may share contaminated injection equipment. Lesbians have unprotected sex with men, risking exposure to HIV-infected semen. Lesbians use semen in alternative insemination procedures, again risking exposure. Lesbians are health care workers and, unfortunately, are sometimes involved in health-care-related injuries (e.g., needle sticks). Not insignificantly, lesbians engage in unprotected sex with other women and put themselves at risk of exposure to HIV-contaminated fluids by doing so. Vaginal secretions, blood, and menstrual fluids are all part of the sexual lives of most sexually active lesbian women. Any sexual activities that involve potential trauma to sexual organs and body parts (e.g., sadomasochistic activities, fisting, using sex toys that are too large for particular orifices) increase the risk of lesions or tearing of membranes, thus increasing the risk of HIV exposure. Regardless of how theorists believe HIV initially entered the lesbian community, unprotected sex between women is risky.

AIDS surveillance data currently neglect the possibility of female-to-female exposure. In addition, whenever multiple risk behaviors are present in a person's sexual or drug history or both, infection is always attributed to the behavior considered most risky. The categorization system is hierarchical and identity-based and contains only mutually exclusive categories. Only recently have multiple transmission routes been reported, but individual cases are still assigned to categories on the basis of epidemiological distribution of AIDS cases in the United States and the category of transmission that is highest on the hierarchy for a particular individual. Bisexual women who are HIV+ are often similarly classified as having been infected through heterosexual contact or through injection-drug use. Lesbian women who are HIV+ are commonly classified as IDUs or "risk not identified."

The picture is further complicated by the fact that an unknown proportion of lesbians who report that their sexual partners are IDUs may be included in the "partner of IDU" category, with the implication that *male* IDUs transmitted HIV to them through heterosexual contact. It has *not* historically been the case, nor is it common practice now, for women to be asked to identify the gender of their IDU partners. Additionally, if a woman identifies herself as a lesbian, and reports sexual activity only with other women, except for one and only one episode of sex with, for instance, an IDU male, all other factors being equal, that woman could be categorized as "partner of IDU." Admittedly, this categorization may indeed be accurate. If the male partner's HIV status were unknown and remained unknown, however, it is also possible, and may be equally likely, that the woman contracted HIV via her female partner(s).

The relative risk of female-to-female sexual transmission remains essentially unknown and unaccounted for. There are few empirical data that document the frequency of risky sexual behaviors (e.g., those involving vaginal fluids, blood, or menstrual products) or rates of HIV seropositivity in women who engage in sexual activity with other women. Likewise, we know little about patterns of personal risk perception or attitudes toward safer sex practices in this population, nor have recommendations for safer sex practices specific to lesbian women been developed and tested empirically. As a result, women who have sex with other women have been underdocumented and underserved in this epidemic (Stevens, 1993; Young *et al.,* 1992).

Woman-to-woman HIV transmission has been reported in the medical literature since 1984 (Sabatini, Patel, & Hirschman, 1984). The first was a 37-year-old, non-Haitian, non-drug-using black woman who reported a lifelong sexual contact history involving only women partners. The second documented female-to-female case involved the female sexual partner of a female IDU (Marmor *et al.,* 1986). A third case involved a woman who reported having exclusively female-to-female sexual contact, denying all heterosexual contact and injection-drug use (Monzon & Capellan, 1987). Most recently, two HIV+ women were recently reported to have no other risk behaviors than unprotected female-to-female sexual activity (CDC, 1993b). It is of interest to question why *these* cases were reported when others were not. Perhaps *these* providers considered the possibility of female-to-female HIV transmission while many others have not.

The CDC conducted a retrospective epidemiological study to determine whether there is indeed a risk of lesbian transmission of HIV. In the study (Chu, Buehler, Flemming, & Berkelman, 1990), the CDC's surveillance definition of "lesbian" was used. That definition states that only women who have engaged in exclusively female-to-female sexual contact since 1977 are considered "lesbian." Despite this extremely limited view of lesbian reality, the researchers nonetheless concluded that women who engage in sexual activity with other women can be exposed to HIV. They validated their assertions by pointing to the case reports of female-to-female sexual transmission of HIV, as well as the fact that female-to-male transmission is well documented.

In addition to these reports, a number of less-known reports and presentations can conceivably add some new information to that already available. Chu *et al.* (1990) reported that between June 1980 and September 1989, 79 women with AIDS had voluntarily reported sexual behavior solely with another woman. A survey conducted in 1989 among lesbian residents of Michigan (Bybee, 1990) reported that lesbian women were, at that time, only beginning to be concerned with HIV infection. In this survey, 19% reported having been tested for HIV antibodies, and 28% reported having made behavioral changes since the beginning of the AIDS epidemic. Over half the respondents, however, reported having engaged in potentially risky sexual behaviors in the 3 years prior to the survey: 14% had had sexual contact with men, and 25% reported having had more than one sexual partner in the past year. These same women were also more likely to have a history of injection-drug use. Of the overall respondents, 11% had a history of STD, a cofactor for HIV risk. Over half reported "possible risk due to sexual practices," including oral sex during menstruation, sharing sex toys, and oral–anal sex. In another study, Martin and Battles (1989) reported that "at least 101 cases of AIDS among lesbians have been reported" (p. 1), at least 15% of which were the result of "heterosexual contact, transfusions, and *other unknown factors*" (p. 3) [emphasis added]. In addition, 23% of their respondents reported HIV transmission risk due to injection drug use, and 41% reported unprotected sex with men. It seems that injection-drug use and heterosexual contact may be efficient and sufficient modes of transmission into the lesbian community, but the virus may then spread within the community through sexual contact between females. In analyzing all the available data, one needs to take into account the definitions employed by various researchers. The CDC's criteria for "lesbian" may be convenient for data collection, but it is not necessarily realistic in terms of its accuracy in depiction of lesbian sexual behavior and, hence, its ability to adequately inform the lesbian community regarding the real possibilities of risk.

Hunter, Rosario, and Rotheram-Borus (1993) reported on adolescent lesbians attending gay and lesbian community-based agencies in New York City, stating that 20% reported exchanging sex for drugs or money, 28% reported a history of cocaine or crack use, and 75% reported being sexually active with males. Many reported higher numbers of sexual partners in their lifetimes, on average, than national adolescent norms. In a self-administered structured questionnaire, 141 mostly Caucasian, college-educated lesbian women reported their HIV risk history (Hunter, Rotheram-Borus, Reid, & Rosario, 1992). Lifetime sexual behaviors among these women included 81% penile–vaginal penetration, 18% receptive anal–penile sex, 31% active anilingus, and 69% active oral–penile sex. Additionally, 96% engaged in active oral–vaginal sex with other women, and 31% engaged in active anilingus with women partners. This sample's lifetime prevalence of STDs ranged from 0% (syphilis) to 7% (urethritis). Only 2% of these women reported using a dental dam in the past year, and 41% reported having refused active oral sex with a lover who requested the use of a dental dam. In a discussion of AIDS public policy, Young *et al.* (1992) cite a sample of 711 women, of whom twice as many self-identified lesbian and bisexual women as heterosexual women reported that they had engaged in anal intercourse with a male in the previous 3 years.

Finally, in a survey conducted by Morrow, *et al.* (1994b), significant numbers of lesbian and bisexual women reported engaging in risk behaviors relative to HIV. Questionnaires were distributed at two nationally attended women's music festivals and through outreach workers in several cities across the country. Approximately 1800 questionnaires were distributed. A total of 504 lesbian and bisexual women across the United States completed the questionnaire (a return rate of over 25%). Over 26% reported being sexually active with two or more female partners in the last year; 7% reported being sexually active with two or more male partners. Approximately 27% reported a history of having been diagnosed with at least one STD. Over 90% reported engaging in active oral–vaginal sex; 19% engaged in active oral–anal sex; 20% engaged in sexual activities involving possible exposure to blood; and 2–4% reported engaging in sexual activities at anonymous sex clubs or group sex parties or both with women or men or both. Only 42% of respondents reported *ever having tried* protective barriers during sex.

On a more positive note, 54% (266) of the respondents (Morrow *et al.*, 1994b) reported having been tested for HIV antibodies at least once, indicating some level of perceived risk. Of those women, 2 (0.7%) reported testing HIV+. Of those respondents who reported *not* having been tested, 9% reported that their reason for not being tested was that they were afraid they "were HIV positive and did not want to know." Anecdotally, 3 women voluntarily included the information that although they themselves were not HIV+, their primary female sexual partners were. HIV risk perception was also noted to be quite low within this sample, with 76% reporting a 0.0 estimated probability of exposure to HIV in the next year, and with 74% reporting that same estimate (ie., 0.0) of their probability of having been exposed to HIV in the previous year. The majority of the sample, 98%, reported a perceived risk between 0.0 and 0.25 estimated probability of HIV transmission via sexual activity in the next year. It was interesting to note that 21% (108) of the original 504 respondents reported suggesting the use of safer sex to their partner(s) at least once in a typical month. Of these 108, 86% (93) reported that as a result of their suggestion, subsequent sexual activity would occur either safely or not at all (i.e., suggestions yielded some form of safe behavior). This finding suggests that communication regarding the use of safer sex practices may be a key component for skills training within this population, especially given that the other 14% (15 women) reported that their partner(s) objected, *and* they continued to engage in sex *unprotected.* Of these 15, 8 respondents (7% of the sample) reported that *every* suggestion to practice safer sex was followed by refusal on the part of their partner(s) and subsequent acquiescence into unsafe sexual practices (Morrow, Fuqua, & Meinhold, 1994a).

Although injection-drug use may be the most likely mode of transmission of HIV into the lesbian population, sexual partners of IDU lesbians are at increased risk of exposure to the virus and would be able to transmit the virus to other sexual partners (Dicker, 1989). Women who have sex with women are at risk for HIV infection sexually via open lesions on body parts involved in sexual activity, oral sex, the sharing of sex toys, drug use, and alternative insemination. Their risk is particularly high when menstrual blood is present in the vaginal fluid (Clavreul, 1992). In addition, communication skills play a key role in whether or not safer sex techniques are employed, particularly during the time in women's lives when they are exploring their sexuality and oftentimes doing so with other women and men who are exploring as well. This time is often not one of comfort with regard to frank discussions about sex and negotiations for safer sex (Martin & Battles, 1989). Thus, unsafe sexual liaisons are more likely (e.g., adolescent lesbians may frequently have unprotected sex with men who have had sex with other men).

Lesbians do not consider themselves at risk for HIV infection. Thirteen years of myths from governmental and community organizations have given them reason to feel confident. As a result, lesbians continue to engage in potentially risky sexual behaviors (and verifiably risky injection-drug-use behaviors) (Stevens, 1993). Even in more AIDS-aware lesbian and gay communities, the advent of safer sex for women who have sex with women has not been well received. Women initially accused the gay male establishments—which at that time were doing the most to educate and prevent HIV transmission—of making them (i.e., lesbians) engage in safer sex when they did not really need to. Other women believed, and still feel, that those women who advocate for lesbians engaging in safer sex are overreacting

(O'Sullivan, 1990). However, it seems quite obvious from the data presented above that women who engage in sexual activity with women *are* at risk for being exposed to HIV. The necessary "ingredients" for transmission (i.e., vaginal secretions, blood products/by-products, and semen) are present in many of the sexual activities of lesbian women.

Despite a currently low incidence of AIDS cases among women who voluntarily report their sexual orientation as lesbian, now *is* the time to focus prevention efforts on this population, so that the seroprevalence rates of other groups do not have to be duplicated in this one. To focus only on those who are currently diagnosed with AIDS in the determination of target groups for prevention is counterproductive. Given the long incubation period from infection to symptomatic disease, such a focus would be approximately 10 years behind current infection rates and therefore negligent. The longer lesbian women are excluded from prevention education, the more likely it is that their infection rates will continue to rise (Cole & Cooper, 1990–1991).

CHANGES IN FOCUS NECESSARY TO INCLUDE LESBIAN WOMEN

The issue, then, comes down to the methodology and content of prevention research and education for this unique population. A key issue involves accurate data collection. To begin with, current surveillance systems define a lesbian as a woman who has had sexual contact exclusively with women partners since 1977 (Chu *et al.,* 1990; Stevens, 1993). As stated earlier, this may be a convenient, albeit arbitrary, definition, but it does *not* adequately represent the lesbian experience.

There is currently no category for female-to-female transmission or even for "women who have sex with women." The CDC surveillance definitions systematically exclude these women: Only recently have any data been taken on sexual orientation of HIV+ women, as there are, and have been for some time, for men. In a recent survey of 960,000 female blood donors, the CDC found no evidence for female-to-female HIV transmission (Peterson, Doll, White, Chu, & the HIV Blood Donor Study Group, 1992). However, the definition cited above was used in that study and does not allow for a realistic representation of the lesbian population. It assumes that any woman having sex with a male partner (given that he is HIV+) or using injection drugs *must* be at risk through those means rather than through female-to-female sexual contact. In addition, the study assumes that women did not select themselves out of blood donor activities due to their own personal assessment of HIV status or risk. As a result of current surveillance definitions and methods, lesbian women with HIV disease remain officially uncounted and yet are still told that evidence for HIV transmission between women is nonexistent (Clavreul, 1992; Stevens, 1993; Warren, 1993; Young *et al.,* 1992). This assessment perpetuates the notion among the general public and many service providers that lesbians remain sexually "risk-free" from HIV infection.

Beyond biases in surveillance definitions, there remains bias in research protocol. Sexual activity that is deemed responsible for HIV transmission is almost exclusively defined by the presence of a penis, with the exception of some cases of female-to-male transmission. In many studies, the term "lesbian" still excludes any woman who has had even one sexual encounter with a male since 1977. In addition, frequency of condom use is often erroneously used as an indicator of frequency of dental dam use (Young *et al.,* 1992) when there is *no* evidence to suggest a direct relationship here. If anything, the lack of discussion of dental dams in HIV prevention efforts, even among gay males and heterosexuals, is indicative of the lack of acceptability of the use of dental dams as a result of the lack of access to knowledge with regard to oral HIV transmission.

Within the lesbian community itself, there is a continued lack of risk perception. This lack is probably a function, at least in part, of a lack of emphasis on inclusion of woman-to-woman sexual practices in well over a decade of discussion about safer sex. It is also a function, presumably, of lesbians not knowing other lesbians who are HIV+, and especially not HIV+ lesbians whose only risk factor was female-to-female transmission (O'Sullivan, 1990; Young *et al.,* 1992). This low perceived risk of infection, coupled with high rates of potentially risky sexual and drug-using behaviors, necessitates a conclusion that lesbian and bisexual women are potentially at risk for HIV infection (Case, Downing, Fergusson, Lorvick, & Sanchez, 1988; Cole & Cooper, 1990–1991).

CONCLUSIONS AND RECOMMENDATIONS

A series of focus groups conducted in the winter of 1994 (Morrow *et al.,* 1994a) concluded that HIV prevention programming must include culture-specific information, rationale, and strategies unique to lesbian communities. Each lesbian community, whether urban or rural, woman of color or white, and so forth, must be individually assessed to determine its own unique needs and attitudes. This individualized needs assessment will offer more precise information necessary in the development of a culture-specific prevention program.

According to women who participated in the focus groups (Morrow *et al.,* 1994a), myths surrounding lesbian life-styles and sexual activities need to be dispelled. Risk behaviors and the body fluids involved need to be aggressively targeted and presented as risks: Risk groups per se, they recommend, should be less of an issue, especially for lesbians, given the historical myth of lesbian invulnerability to HIV infection. In terms of safer sex, safer sex barriers (e.g., dental dams, surgical gloves) need to be as readily accessible as condoms. In addition, social norms must change to accommodate healthy sexual life-styles and encourage the use of safer sex techniques. Communication skills training unique to woman-to-woman relationships need to be incorporated into prevention programming.

Prevention programs must incorporate a rationale for the adoption of safer-sex life-styles that appeal to the uniqueness of lesbian community pride. Focus group participants stressed the importance of political awareness as another aspect for the rationale as it relates to women's health care in general and to lesbian health care in particular. In addition, focus group participants expressed a desire for flexible programming (e.g., neutral, non-AIDS-related settings in which to conduct prevention programs; flexible data collection systems that accommodate those women who do and do not wish to have "penile sex" included in their information packets and on their data sheets). Despite the stereotype of a unique homogeneity within lesbian communities, there is actually a great amount of diversity. This diversity needs to be acknowledged and accommodated. As particular and insignificant as some of these recommendations may seem, adherence to them may increase the likelihood that women will participate in and respond to prevention programming and research efforts.

For the Educator/Counselor

As articulated in the quotation that began this chapter, there are many myths that contribute to the continued lack of HIV education and prevention services for lesbians. Many scientists and public health professionals continue to believe that lesbians do not have very much sex, that what sexual acts lesbians *do* engage in are not risky, that lesbians do not engage in penile–vaginal intercourse with men, that lesbians cannot or do not become pregnant, that lesbians do not use drugs, and that lesbians do not exchange sex for drugs or money (Cole & Cooper, 1990–1991). This misinformation perpetuates the confusion and lack of information that currently pervade HIV education programs, drug treatment programs, and the lesbian community itself. The data, however, do not support the myths and misinformation. Hence, HIV/AIDS education professionals and counselors need to update their knowledge base and programs to include the needs of lesbian women. In order to facilitate accurate communication between prevention workers, researchers, policy makers, and communities, a common language needs to be incorporated into all published materials, or, at a minimum, terms need to be defined clearly. The target populations themselves, in this case women who have sex with women, need to be actively involved in program development, implementation, and evaluation. The unique psychosocial context of risk behaviors among lesbians needs to be defined and addressed. And the attitudes, beliefs, and sexual practices of lesbian women need to be well understood and incorporated into education programs (Hahn, 1991).

There are potential difficulties in HIV education efforts directed at women who have sex with women. First, there is an historical impediment in this community, as in many others, to open discussion of sexual practices. Gaining access to lesbian women's language with regard to sex and promoting open communication about it will be a challenging process, but is essential (O'Sullivan, 1990). Participation by lesbians in the development and evaluation of prevention programs is imperative. It will be of the utmost importance to acknowledge the specific needs, values, and traditions of this community in that process (Cole & Cooper, 1990–1991).

For the Researcher

Additional research is needed that will document the HIV-related behavioral risks in which lesbian women currently engage. Culturally relevant and accurate prevention programs need to be developed on the basis of the needs of this population (Stevens, 1993). It will be particularly important to be aware of the differences between sexual self-identification and sexual behavior as they relate to surveillance data collection. Additionally, it will be equally important to be aware of the necessary interplay that exists between sexual identity and sexual behavior, despite the seeming behavioral differences between them. That is, it will be imperative to articulate a balance between the roles that lesbian sexual behaviors and lesbian self-identification play in the ultimate practice of safer sex between women. Lesbian communities need to be targeted for culture-specific and relevant HIV prevention programs, not necessarily because their risk behaviors are unique, but because of their potential resistance to traditionally available programs that have historically excluded them and invalidated their existence.

Given the promise of cognitive–behavioral skills training, and social norm change strategies, as well as community mobilization efforts (Kelly et al., 1993), these types of programs should be developed specifically for lesbian women. Making risk-reduction behaviors the norm within the lesbian community and producing these norm changes before the prevalence of HIV infection rises to high levels will allow for the greatest efficacy of prevention within this population. Skills specific to the lesbian woman will be of greatest value and should include the proper use of dental dams (including how to cut condoms and surgical gloves to use as dams), communications skills specific to negotiating safer sex within woman-to-woman relationships, assertiveness and unsafe-sex-refusal skills within woman–woman relationships, and proper procedures for cleaning sexual and drug paraphernalia. It is imperative that research efforts be designed as experimentally sound outcome studies, with a focus on behavior change and maintenance.

Additional issues within the lesbian culture will also need to be addressed by both researchers and educators/counselors. These issues include those of internal and external homophobia, biphobia, and erotophobia, as well as the necessity for building community support and encouragement for safer sex practices (i.e., social norm changes). In addition, future research and education programs should begin to address the unique needs of lesbian women of color, as well as those who are physically challenged, homeless, incarcerated, or make their living as sex workers.

REFERENCES

Becker, M. H., & Joseph, J. G. (1988). AIDS and behavioral change to reduce risk: A review. *American Journal of Public Health, 78,* 394–410.

Bybee, D. (1990). *The Michigan lesbian health survey: Results relevant to AIDS.* Research report: Michigan Organization for Human Rights and the Michigan Department of Public Health. Lansing: Michigan Department of Public Health.

Case, P., Downing, M., Fergusson, B., Lorvick, J., & Sanchez, L. (1988). The social context of AIDS risk behavior among intravenous drug using lesbians in San Francisco. *Fourth International Conference on AIDS: Stockholm International Fairs, Stockholm,* p. 454.

Centers for Disease Control and Prevention (1993a). *HIV/AIDS surveillance report, 5.*

Centers for Disease Control and Prevention (1993b). *AIDS daily summaries.* National AIDS Clearinghouse. Atlanta: CDC.

Centers for Disease Control and Prevention (1993c). Update: Barrier protection against HIV infection and other sexually transmitted diseases. *Morbidity and Mortality Weekly Report, 42,* 30, 589–591, 597.

Centers for Disease Control and Prevention (1993d). *HIV infection and AIDS: Are you at risk?*

Chiaramonte, L. (1988). Lesbian safety and AIDS: The very last fairy tale. *Visibilities, January/February,* 4–7.

Chu, S. Y., Buehler, J. W., Fleming, P. L., & Berkelman, R. L. (1990). Epidemiology of reported cases of AIDS in lesbians, United States 1980–89. *American Journal of Public Health, 80,* 1380–1381.

Clavreul, G. (1992). Lesbians and AIDS: The overlooked statistics: How and why lesbians should protect themselves. *Gay and Lesbian Times,* August 13, 32.

Cohen, J. B., Hauer, L. B., & Wofsy, C. B. (1989). Women and IV drugs: Parenteral and heterosexual transmission of human immunodeficiency virus. *Journal of Drug Issues, 19,* 39–56.

Cole, R., & Cooper, S. (1990–1991). Lesbian exclusion from HIV/AIDS education: Ten years of low-risk identity and high-risk behavior. *SIECUS Report, 19,* 18–23.
Corea, G. (1992). *The invisible epidemic: The story of women and AIDS.* New York: HarperCollins.
Croteau, J. M. & Morgan, S. (1989). Combatting homophobia in AIDS education. *Journal of Counseling and Development, 68,* 86–91.
Dicker, B. (1989). Risk of AIDS among lesbians (letter). *American Journal of Public Health, 79,* 1569.
DiClemente, R., Boyer, C., & Morales, E. (1988). Minorities and AIDS: Knowledge, attitudes, and misconceptions among black and Latino adolescents. *American Journal of Public Health, 78,* 55–57.
Feucht, T. E., Stephens, R. C., & Roman, S. W. (1990). The sexual behavior of intravenous drug users: Assessing the risk of sexual transmission of HIV. *Journal of Drug Issues, 20,* 195–213.
Hahn, R. (1991). What should behavioral scientists be doing about AIDS? *Social Science and Medicine, 33,* 1–3.
Hunter, J., Rosario, M., & Rotheram-Borus, M. J. (1993). Sexual and substance abuse acts that place adolescent lesbians at risk for HIV. Poster presented at the Ninth International Conference on AIDS/IV STD World Congress, Berlin.
Hunter, J., Rotheram-Borus, M. J., Reid, H., & Rosario, M. (1992). Sexual and substance abuse acts that place lesbians at risk for HIV. Poster presented at the Eighth International Conference on AIDS/III STD Congress, Amsterdam.
Kalichman, S. C., Hunter, T. L., & Kelly, J. A. (1992). Perceptions of AIDS susceptibility among minority and nonminority women at risk for HIV infection. *Journal of Consulting and Clinical Psychology, 60,* 725–732.
Kalichman, S. C., Kelly, J. A., Hunter, T. L., Murphy, D. A., & Tyler, R. (1993). Culturally tailored HIV/AIDS-risk reduction messages targeted to African-American urban women: Impact on risk sensitization and risk reduction. *Journal of Consulting and Clinical Psychology, 61,* 291–295.
Kelly, J. A., & Murphy, D. A. (1992). Psychological interventions with AIDS and HIV: Prevention and treatment. *Journal of Consulting and Clinical Psychology, 60,* 576–585.
Kelly, J. A., Murphy, D. A., Sikkema, K. J., & Kalichman, S. C. (1993). Psychological interventions to prevent HIV infection are urgently needed: New priorities for behavioral research in the second decade of AIDS. *American Psychologist, 48,* 1023–1034.
Marmor, M., Weiss, L. R., Lyden, M., Weiss, S. H., Saxinger, W. C., Spira, T. J., & Feorino, P. M. (1986). Possible female-to-female transmission of human immunodeficiency virus. *Annals of Internal Medicine, 105,* 969.
Martin, S. M., & Battles, L. L. (1989, October). Screening for HIV in the lesbian community: Is it necessary? Paper presented to the American Public Health Association Conference, Chicago.
Mays, V. M., & Cochran, S. D. (1988). Issues in the perception of AIDS risk and risk reduction activities by black and Hispanic/Latin a women. *American Psychologist, 43,* 949–957.
Mondanaro, J. (1987). Strategies for AIDS prevention: Motivating health behavior in drug dependent women. *Journal of Psychoactive Drugs, 19,* 143–149.
Monzon, O. T., & Capellan, J. M. B. (1987). Female-to-female transmission of HIV. *Lancet, 2,* 40–41.
Morrow, K. M., Fuqua, R. W., & Meinhold, P. M. (1994a). Self-reported HIV risk behaviors and serostatus in lesbian and bisexual women. Presented at the Convention of the American Psychological Association: Psychosocial and Behavioral Factors in Women's Health: Creating an Agenda for the 21st Century.

Morrow, K. M., Meinhold, P. M., & Fuqua, R. W. (1994b). Incidence of HIV-related risk behaviors and seropositivity in the lesbian/bisexual women's communities. Presented at the 15th Anniversary Convention of the Society of Behavioral Medicine.

O'Sullivan, S. (1990). MAPPING: Lesbians, AIDS, and sexuality. *Feminist Review, 34,* 120–133.

Peterson, L. R., Doll, L., White, C., Chu, S., & the HIV Blood Donor Study Group (1992). No evidence for female-to-female HIV transmission among 960,000 female blood donors. *Journal of Acquired Immune Deficiency Syndromes, 5,* 853–855.

Rieder, I., & Ruppelt, P. (Eds.). (1988). *AIDS: The women.* San Francisco: Cleis Press.

Sabatini, M. T., Patel, K., & Hirschman, R. (1984). Kaposi's sarcoma and T-cell lymphoma in an immunodeficient woman: A case report. *AIDS Research, 1,* 135–137.

Stevens, P. E. (1993). Lesbians and HIV: Clinical, research, and policy issues. *American Journal of Orthopsychiatry, 63,* 289–294.

Warren, N. (1993). Out of the question: Obstacles to research on HIV and women who engage in sexual behaviors with women. *SIECUS Report, 22,* 13–16.

Young, R. M., Weissman, G., & Cohen, J. B. (1992). Assessing risk in the absence of information: HIV risk among women injection-drug users who have sex with women. *AIDS and Public Policy Journal, 7,* 175–183.

12

Future Directions

ANN O'LEARY and LORETTA SWEET JEMMOTT

INTRODUCTION

Research on the prevention of AIDS among women is clearly just beginning. Remaining questions far outnumber lessons learned, even though women are becoming infected at a rate that is already much too high and accelerating rapidly. We conclude by presenting a brief listing of conclusions as well as some issues in need of further attention as the epidemic progresses.

LESSONS LEARNED

1. *Skill-building interventions can help many women to reduce their risk of HIV infection.* As we discussed in Chapter 1, a small number of AIDS risk reduction programs targeting women have shown some promise. Clearly, many women have the potential to be helped by fairly intensive, small-group interventions that provide opportunities for practicing condom use and sexual negotiation skills. It is of utmost urgency that such interventions be made available to community-based organizations, providers in health care settings, and other agencies serving at-risk women.

2. *Many other at-risk women have not achieved behavioral risk reduction, due not only to unavailability of such programs, but also to numerous barriers to change.* Even in the successful intervention trials, more women appear to be at risk at the trials' completion than have eliminated their

---

ANN O'LEARY • Department of Psychology, Rutgers University, New Brunswick, NJ 08903. *LORETTA SWEET JEMMOTT* • University of Pennsylvania School of Nursing, Philadelphia, PA 19104.

Women at Risk: Issues in the Primary Prevention of AIDS, edited by Ann O'Leary and Loretta Sweet Jemmott. Plenum Press, New York, 1995.

risk. Likely barriers include poverty, substance use, gender role expectations and other cultural factors, and disempowerment in sexual relationships. Further, participant samples in these trials may not accurately represent those women most at risk, e.g., homeless women or those not attached to community agencies.

UNANSWERED QUESTIONS AND UNMET NEEDS

1. Of greatest urgency is the need for controlled intervention trials. Such trials should compare different theory-based intervention strategies whenever possible, rather than simply employ a single control group. Interventions targeting women of different ethnic groups and highly at-risk women must be rigorously evaluated, and those that are shown to be successful in reducing AIDS risk behavior must be disseminated rapidly. In addition, settings and contexts providing the most support for these programs must be identified. Behavior changes not involving condom use must be studied for effectiveness in this work as well.

2. Substance use prevention and treatment must be a strong priority, both for injection-drug users to reduce their risk of HIV transmission through needle sharing and for those using other drugs that increase their sexual risk. It is clear that the use of other drugs, such as crack cocaine, leads to risk through sex–drug trades, sexual coercion and violence, and homelessness (e.g., leading to exchange of sex for a place to stay). Such programs must be delivered in humane and respectful ways (see Chapter 8).

3. Violence against women by their sex partners, as well as violence against children, must be better studied. Further, adequate services to end these situations must be provided to those affected. In the short term, woman-controlled technologies must be developed and employed to enable such women to protect themselves from HIV. In the longer term, women must become empowered in their relationships and in their gender-related beliefs and expectations. Education beginning early will be helpful in this effort. Ultimately, the "feminization of poverty" (see Pearce, 1993) must be reversed if women are to become truly empowered.

4. The control of other sexually transmitted diseases must be prioritized and adequate funding made available for this effort. Other epidemic STDs, beyond having their own severe sequelae (e.g., cervical cancer and infertility), also increase the risk of HIV transmission (see Chapter 2). In other parts of the world, it is recognized that STD control *by itself* has the capability to reduce HIV incidence substantially.

5. Societal efforts must be made to improve sex education and drug-use prevention and to improve norms for AIDS protection. The recent dismissal of Surgeon General Joycelyn Elders causes pessimism in this regard. However, early education regarding sex, drugs, and AIDS, provided in our public schools, remains a dire need in this country. The information media also carry responsibility for keeping these issues within public awareness.

CONCLUSION

It is unlikely that any of us will be untouched by AIDS or that the magnitude of the epidemic will be reduced during our lifetime. We must confront this disease with courage and persistence. While it brings immeasurable suffering, AIDS and our response to it have the capacity also to bring growth and benefit—to the women's health movement, to health care reform efforts, to awareness of poverty and its effects, to discourse concerning sexuality, and to our development as a humane society.

REFERENCE

Pearce, D. (1993). Something old, something new: Women's poverty in the 1990's. In S. Matteo (Ed.), *American women in the 1990's: Today's critical issues* (pp. 79–97). Boston: Northeastern University Press.

About the Authors

Priscilla Alexander is coordinator of the National Task Force on Prostitution, a network of sex workers' rights organizations and allies based in New York City. She was an active member of COYOTE, the San Francisco-based sex workers' rights organization, from 1979 to 1990, and cofounded the California Prostitutes Education Project (CAL-PEP), an HIV/AIDS prevention project. With Frederique Delacoste, she coedited the book *Sex Work: Writings by Women in the Sex Industry.* In 1990, she joined the Global Programme on AIDS, where she reviewed the experiences of sex-work-related HIV/AIDS and STD prevention projects in developing countries and wrote a guide to the design and implementation of such projects. In 1994, she enrolled in the M.P.H. program at Columbia University School of Public Health, where she plans to go on for a doctorate, after which she hopes to teach and start an institute of sex work studies to encourage sex workers to go to graduate school and do research on the sex industry from the inside.

Sevgi O. Aral, Ph.D., is the Associate Director for Science for the Division of STD/HIV Prevention (DSTD/HIVP), National Center for Prevention Services, Centers for Disease Control and Prevention. In this capacity, she is responsible for all aspects of the research program in the DSTD/HIVP. Dr. Aral's background is quite eclectic; she holds degrees in psychology, sociology, and demography. Dr. Aral's research for the past 17 years has focused primarily on behavioral aspects of STD and their prevention. Dr. Aral is the author or coauthor of more than 90 scientific publications.

Vivian B. Brown, Ph.D., is President and Chief Executive Officer of PROTOTYPES, a Center for Innovation in Health, Mental Health, and Social Services that she founded in 1986. Dr. Brown also holds the position of Associate Professor in the Department of Psychiatry at the University of California, Los Angeles. She has authored more than 50 works; has served as a consultant in the areas of health, substance abuse, and mental health to many organizations; and has been appointed to federal, state, and county funding review committees. Recently she was presented with the McNeill Award, a national honor given jointly by the American Psychological Association and the American Psychological Foundation, in recognition of her pioneering efforts and innovative work in the field of community mental health. In 1985, Dr. Brown was presented with the Boots Jones Humanitarian Award for Lifetime Services by the Los Angeles Commission on Assaults against Women.

Judith B. Cohen, Ph.D., directs AWARE, the Association for Womens' AIDS Risk Education in Oakland, California. She received her Ph.D. in epidemiology from the University of California, Berkeley. Her pioneering research on HIV risk among sex workers and other women has been funded by the National Institute of Allergy and Infectious Diseases, the National Institute on Drug Abuse, and the American Foundation for AIDS Research. She has published extensively in the areas of women and STD/HIV.

Maria Isabel (Isa) Fernandez, Ph.D., received her doctorate in community psychology from Michigan State University under George W. Fairweather, Ph.D., one of the founding fathers in the field. Her early research concerned dissemination of community mental health programs. She subsequently worked for the Centers for Disease Control in the National AIDS Information and Education Programs and for the National Institute of Mental Health as staff collaborator for the NIMH Multisite HIV Prevention Trial. While at NIMH, Dr. Fernandez convened a national working meeting of researchers and community-based providers entitled "Putting Knowledge to Work for Prevention." The meeting was cited in the National Commission on AIDS report as an important first step. Recently, recognizing that the private sector offered a unique opportunity to focus on dissemination issues, Dr. Fernandez joined Professional and Scientific Associates.

Mindy Thompson Fullilove, M.D., is a graduate of Bryn Mawr College and Columbia University College of Physicians and Surgeons. She did psychiatric residency at New York Hospital–Westchester Division and Montefiore Hospital. She is currently Associate Professor of Clinical Psychiatry and Public Health at Columbia University. Her current research interests include the epidemiology of HIV infection in minority communities and trauma as a cofactor in drug abuse. Previously, she served as director of Multicultural Inquiry and Research on AIDS (MIRA), a component of the UCSF Center for AIDS Prevention Studies located at the Bayview-Hunter's Point Foundation. Her recent publications are on traumatic experiences in the lives of women crack users and methods of research in minority communities.

Erica L. Gollub, Dr.P.H., received her B.S. at Stamford University and her M.P.H. (population and family health) and Dr.P.H. (epidemiology) from Columbia University. Her research interests include the risks and benefits of birth control methods, regulatory policies related to women, and new protective methods and intervention techniques for the prevention of STD/HIV in women. She has recently undertaken a series of intervention studies in clinic- and hospital-based settings, the outcomes of which include the effectiveness and acceptability of the female condom, spermicides, and other female barriers for STD risk reduction.

John B. Jemmott III, Ph.D., received his Ph.D. in psychology from the Department of Psychology and Social Relations, Harvard University. He is currently Professor of Psychology at Princeton University, where he has taught Health Psychology and Quantitative Methods since 1981. Dr. Jemmott was a National Science Foundation Graduate Fellow and is currently a Fellow of the Division of Health Psychology of the American Psychological Association. Dr. Jemmott has served on the Committee on Psychology and AIDS of the American Psychological Association and is currently on the AIDS and Immunology Research Review Committee of the National Institute of Mental Health. He has been the recipient of several grants from the American Foundation for AIDS Research, the National Institute of Child Health and Human Development, and the National Institute of Mental Health to conduct research designed to develop and test HIV-risk-reduction interventions. His current research revolves around the prevention of pregnancy, sexually transmitted diseases (including HIV), and violence-related injury among adolescents.

Loretta Sweet Jemmott, Ph.D., R.N., F.A.A.N., is an Associate Professor of Nursing at the University of Pennsylvania School of Nursing. She received her B.S.N. from Hampton Institute and her master's degree in nursing (specializing in psychiatric mental health nursing) and her Ph.D. in education (specializing in human sexuality education) from the University of Pennsylvania in 1987. She has been involved in several federally funded research projects aiming to reduce the risk of HIV infection among African American adolescents and women. She has published numerous articles on HIV risk-reduction. She was recently funded by the National Institute of Health and the National Institute for Nursing Research to conduct a research project entitled "AIDS and Black Women Testing Risk

Behavior Interventions." She is a member of Sigma Theta Tau International Nursing Honor Society, a Fellow in the American Academy of Nursing, and a member of the Advisory Council for the National Institute for Nursing Research. She has served on the New Jersey Governor's AIDS Advisory Board, where she cochaired the Education and Prevention Committee, and currently serves on the Public Policy Committee for the American Foundation for AIDS Research. Recently the Center for Disease Control's Division of Adolescent and School Health (DASH) selected her HIV risk-reduction research-based curriculum entitled "Be Proud! Be Responsible! Strategies to Empower Youth to Reduce Their Risk for HIV Infection" as a model curriculum for national dissemination in conjunction with their project entitled "Research to Classrooms: Programs That Work."

Gail E. Kennedy, M.P.H., has received a Master's of Public Health from Columbia University School of Public Health, Division of Health Promotion and Disease Prevention. Currently she coordinates services for HIV positive women and children at Metropolitan Hospital in New York City. She has participated with Dr. Mindy Thompson Fullilove in research on issues of prevention and care of HIV/AIDS in women. She is interested in the psychosocial and medical aspects of HIV/AIDS prevention and treatment.

Kate Morrow is a clinical psychology doctoral student at Western Michigan University. She has been involved in the psychological treatment of people with HIV disease and various HIV/STD prevention research projects since the late 1980s. She has presented research at conventions of the Society of Behavioral Medicine, the American Psychological Association, and the Association for Behavior Analysis.

Adeline Marie Nyamathi, Ph.D., R.N., F.A.A.N., is an Associate Professor of Nursing at the University of California, Los Angeles. Originally from New York, Dr. Nyamathi received her Bachelor of Science in Nursing from Hunter College, Bellevue School of Nursing, in New York, a Master's in Nursing and Adult Nurse Practitioner from SUNY at Stonybrook, and a Ph.D. in nursing from Case Western Reserve University.

Dr. Nyamathi has been active in research related to coping and health outcome of spouses of myocardial infarction patients and in research on homeless and drug-addicted women of color in Los Angeles. She is currently principal investigator of two studies funded by the National Institute on Drug Abuse (NIDA) and one study funded by the National Institute of Mental Health that assesses the effectiveness of culturally competent AIDS education programs delivered by nurses and outreach workers to impoverished women who are vulnerable to AIDS. She is also coprincipal investigator with researchers from the UCLA Schools of Nursing, Public Health, and Medicine and the Rand Corporation, investigating the impact of health programs in the community.

Dr. Nyamathi serves on the editorial board of several journals, is faculty chair of the UCLA Latino Advisory Board, and is chair of the Acute Care Section at UCLA School of Nursing. Dr. Nyamathi is also a Fellow of the American Academy of Nursing. She has published and lectured extensively in the area of women and AIDS, homelessness, and coping and health outcome. Her research findings have played a prominent role in scientific reports to Congress, NIH officials, NIDA advisory bodies, and a broad community of scientists and HIV prevention workers.

Ann O'Leary, Ph.D., is an Associate Professor of Psychology at Rutgers University. She received her B.A. from the University of Pennsylvania and completed her doctorate in psychology at Stanford University in 1986. She has published numerous articles on health and behavior, psychoneuroimmunology, and AIDS prevention. She has served in an advisory capacity to the National Institutes of Health, the Centers for Disease Control and Prevention, the American Cancer Society, the New Jersey Department of Health, the International Center for Research on Women, Family Health International, and the Academy for Educational Development.

Beatriz E. Perez, M.P.H., is a 1993 graduate of Columbia University School of Public Health with a concentration in health promotion and disease prevention. Much of her course work focused on violence as a public health issue. She has worked extensively with Mindy Fullilove to develop, implement, and evaluate a curriculum to address trauma in women in recovery from substance abuse as a more comprehensive approach to decreasing HIV risk-taking behavior. She also has experience working with and conducting research in other adult populations, adolescents, and pregnant women.

Jennifer L. Pranke graduated in 1994 from Rutgers University in New Jersey with a bachelor's degree in psychology. She has been working on a National HIV/AIDS Intervention Study at Rutgers for the past two years.

Marcela Raffaelli, Ph.D., is an Associate Researcher in the School of Family Resources and Consumer Sciences, University of Wisconsin–Madison. She has worked on HIV/AIDS prevention programs for street youth in Brazil and impoverished minorities in the United States. She is currently conducting research on parent–child communication about sexual issues and adolescent risk reduction.

Mary Jane Rotheram-Borus, Ph.D., is a Professor of Clinical Psychology and Director, Clinical Research Center, in the Division of Social Psychiatry, Neuropsychiatric Institute, at the University of California, Los Angeles. Dr. Rotheram-Borus received her Ph.D. in clinical psychology from the University of Southern California. Her research interests include HIV/AIDS prevention with adolescents, suicide among adolescents, homeless youth, assessment and modification of children's social skills, ethnic identity, group processes, and cross-ethnic interactions. Dr. Rotheram-Borus has received grants from the National Institute of Mental Health to study HIV prevention with adolescents, the chronically mental ill, and persons with sexually transmitted diseases; to study interventions for children whose parents have AIDS and for the HIV-positive adolescents; and to examine the effectiveness of children's mental health service programs in four cities. In 1986, her work on suicide prevention was selected as the Outstanding Child and Adolescent Mental Health Program by the New York State Department of Mental Health, and her assertiveness training with children was chosen as an exemplary model by the American Psychological Association. Her research also has been funded by the National Science Foundation, National Institute on Drug Abuse, Society for Research in Child Development, and the W.T. Grant Foundation.

Judith N. Wasserheit As director of the Division of STD/HIV Prevention, National Center for Prevention Services, Centers for Disease Control and Prevention (CDC), Judith N. Wasserheit is responsible for developing and directing CDC's national STD and HIV prevention programs and related research in behavioral science, epidemiology and surveillance, health services, and program evaluation.

Gloria Weissman, Ph.D., is Deputy Director, Office of Science and Epidemiology in the Bureau of Health Resources Development at the Health Resources and Services Administration (HRSA). She is involved in evaluations of HRSA programs, particularly Titles I and II of the Ryan White CARE Act programs in the administration of the Special Projects of National Significance and in the development of Federal initiatives to improve access to care for underserved populations—particularly women, adolescents, and drug users—with HIV disease. Prior to that, Ms. Weissman spent 11 years at the National Institute on Drug Abuse (NIDA). There she was instrumental in the design and implementation of the National AIDS Demonstration Research Program, which developed and evaluated innovative, community-based outreach and prevention projects in 63 sites focused on populations at high risk for HIV: injection drug users and their sex partners, runaway and homeless adolescents, individuals in the sex industry, and crack users. She was also responsible for the development and testing of a comprehensive model prevention program for women at risk for HIV and for coordinating NIDA's efforts in the area of women and AIDS. Ms. Weissman has published and presented extensively on women, HIV, substance abuse, and access to care for underserved populations.

Index